Kristen Wheldon

Fire Service Psychology

A Comprehensive Approach to Enhancing Firefighter Health, Safety, and Longevity

Springer

Kristen Wheldon
Fire Service Psychology Association
South Pasadena, CA, USA

ISBN 978-3-032-02125-0 ISBN 978-3-032-02126-7 (eBook)
https://doi.org/10.1007/978-3-032-02126-7

This Springer imprint is published by the registered company Springer Nature Switzerland AG
The registered company address is: Gewerbestrasse 11, 6330 Cham, Switzerland

Foreword

The first psychology textbook, The Principles of Psychology, was authored by William James and published in 1890. James Braidwood wrote the first English textbook on fire service, *On the Construction of Fire Engines and Apparatus: The Training of Firemen, and the Method of Proceeding in Cases of Fire*, in 1860. These leaders and authors understood a basic premise of professionalism…we all build on the work that came before us. James and Braidwood made significant contributions to their disciplines. Wheldon has now made a significant contribution to both fire and psychology.

Dr. Wheldon and I met 10 years ago; she had just started working for the Los Angeles City Fire Department as a psychologist and I had just retired from the National Fire Academy as the Management Science Chair. I knew the National Fire Academy had no adjunct faculty who were psychologists. I also knew there should be, so I encouraged Dr. Wheldon to join the NFA faculty. Thankfully, she did.

The Fire Service typically does not let outsiders in. If a person has not crawled down a hall full of smoke, heat, and pitch blackness, we question their ability to understand or help us. The small number of students and faculty at the National Fire Academy are not like that; they embrace outside knowledge, skill, and ability.

From this humble beginning, Kristen instantly recognized the need to bridge the gap between psychology and the fire service. She was the only licensed psychologist in the Los Angeles City Fire Department, whereas there were dozens of licensed psychologists in the surrounding police departments. There was National Fire Academy content related to psychology that had not been vetted through the psychology discipline. There were NFPA standards related to psychology that had not been vetted through the psychology discipline. Even the American Psychology Association only tacitly included the fire service by using the phrase …military, police, and other first responders. In 2024, there were only 72 psychology dissertations with the word firefighter in the title compared to 442 with the word police officer (ProQuest).

I've been in a fire service for 55 years; it became my calling. From the beginning, I have been an outlier. I now understand why because in my youth, I was a lifeguard and swimming instructor. A basic premise of water safety is that the lifeguard does not exchange their life for the person they are trying to save. When a lifeguard dies trying to rescue someone it is not considered heroic. Something went wrong. This is the exact opposite of a firefighter dying. With a firefighter it's called a line of duty death, a heroic sacrifice, part of the job. This is a deeply held construct in the fire service and in society. I see this as philosophically, psychologically, and culturally dysfunctional. And so, I am still an outlier.

"You are not wrong." This is how Dr. Wheldon repeatedly councils me and gives me courage to keep sharing my beliefs.

This book is the first of its kind, but it will not be the last. More psychologists will study, research, and share their thoughts about the fire service discipline. This can only help "…increase the professionalism of the fire service and others, engaged in fire prevention and control activity." (purpose of the NFA PL 93498). Dr. Kristen Wheldon will be the first to celebrate a 50-year career as a fire service psychologist. There will be many more. Their work will increase the quality of life for firefighters and the communities they serve and protect.

It is an honor to be part of this beginning, I am grateful.

Mount Airy, MD, USA Burton A. Clark

Prologue

Throughout society, images of firefighters and fire trucks have been woven into the fabric of our lives. From infant clothing, blankets, plush toys, television shows, and preschool lessons about "community helpers," the fire service surrounds us. Society often ignores the risk of fire, as we rely on firefighters to intervene in situations where we are faced with fire.

What do firefighters do?

> They do fire extinguishers. They do water hoses. They do it because they don't want to get anyone dead. means safely. — Archer (Age Five)

> They spray water when there is fire. — Shelby (Age Three)

Most communities are not adequately prepared for or educated about basic fire safety. Although fire can have devastating consequences, it often remains an invisible risk. In the United States alone, fire-related incidents result in approximately 3000 deaths each year, making it the ninth most common cause of unintentional injury fatalities, followed by cases of overdoses, motor vehicle accidents, and firearm-related injuries (Centers for Disease Control and Prevention [CDC], 2023). Similarly, on a global scale, the World Health Organization (WHO, 2018) estimates that burns account for 180,000 deaths annually, with the majority occurring in low- and middle-income countries where access to safe cooking and heating methods is limited. In the USA, specific populations, such as children, older adults, individuals with disabilities, and those living in poverty or substandard housing, experience a higher incidence of fire-related mortality (CDC, 2023). There is also elevated fire-related risk among those residing in wildfire-prone regions. Consequently, firefighters are faced with occupational exposure to physical and psychological trauma as well as various types of cancer. While fire-related fatalities occur less frequently than other leading causes of injury-related death, they remain a consistent and preventable component of national and global public health data. Every reasonable person should be aware of and prepared for the risks associated with fire to protect themselves and others and reduce property damage.

Firefighting begins well before the first unit arrives at the scene. It starts with public education on fire safety, ensuring that homes and businesses are equipped with functional smoke alarms, and advocacy for the widespread adoption of residential fire sprinkler systems. Proactively, communities could engage in prudent city and county planning initiatives, zoning efforts, and investments in establishing defensible space in wildfire-prone areas. Equally important are building codes and fire-safe construction practices, the enforcement of fire prevention ordinances, and accessible community risk reduction programs. Engaging at-risk populations, such as older adults, children, and individuals with limited mobility, through targeted outreach enhances overall community preparedness. Firefighters play a critical role in fire prevention by serving as educators, risk assessors, and advocates for safety in various settings long before any emergency occurs. By understanding the true nature of risk mitigation and fire danger, proactive measures become the starting point of heroism, allowing society to decide which firefighter behaviors deserve specific and thoughtful recognition.

While there has long been an awareness of the nation's high fire death rates, insufficient prevention measures, and a lack of coordinated research (National Commission on Fire Prevention and Control, 1973), fire and emergency services are now beginning to adopt a multidisciplinary strategy to increase safety and prevention. To address these challenges, some nations have started building stronger partnerships between fire and emergency services and academic institutions to support evidence-based approaches. A recent United Kingdom study introduced a framework that connects academic research with real-world incident data, showing how cross-disciplinary collaboration can help forecast risks, improve firefighter safety, and shape national policy (Hill et al., 2023). By tapping into fields such as public health, psychology, engineering, and emergency management, these partnerships offer a more organized way to understand fire risk and better protect the health and safety of firefighters. As US fire and emergency services face new and growing challenges, embracing this kind of academic and strategic collaboration could help build a stronger, more resilient, and data-driven future for public safety.

Fire Service Psychology and the Nexus Between Systems, Stakeholders, and Firefighter Health, Safety, and Wellness

Although awareness of firefighter behavioral health is increasing, psychology remains underrepresented, mainly within the institutional and operational frameworks of US fire and emergency services. Despite the presence of influential advocacy groups, such as the "Nine Sisters," psychologists are seldom included in national discussions on fire service policy. This omission limits the system's ability to address behavioral health, trauma resilience, and performance optimization through a scientific lens. The discipline of psychology is a highly regulated profession that is uniquely qualified to contribute expertise in assessment, intervention, operations, human factors, and consultation. Integrating fire service psychology as a formal stakeholder is both an ethical and strategic necessity that aligns fire service practices with the professional standards expected in other high-risk sectors.

Structural Oversight and Governance in the US Fire Service

Fire and emergency medical services (EMS) operate within overlapping local, regional, and national infrastructures. However, unlike sectors such as defense or justice, the US Fire Service lacks a single, centralized regulatory authority. The Secretary of Defense, for example, advises the President and oversees the Department of Defense under the Presidential Directive. Similarly, the Department of Justice enforces federal law and protects civil liberties. In contrast, the US Fire Administration (USFA) is a principal federal agency for fire data collection, public education, research, and training. Nevertheless, it does not possess regulatory power (U.S. Fire Administration, 2022). In this regulatory vacuum, local authorities with jurisdiction (AHJs) determine which standards, often drawn from consensus-based documents, are adopted into departmental policies and procedures.

Federal Advocacy and Representation Gaps in Fire Service Mental Health

In Washington, D.C., a constellation of fire-service advocacy groups, frequently dubbed the "Nine Sisters," lobby Congress on behalf of the needs of the fire and emergency service community, many through the Congressional Fire Services Institute's National Advisory Committee (CFSI, 2023). Notably, absent from these stakeholder dialogs is representation from the field of professional psychology. The lack of a recognized cohort of fire-service psychologists at the federal level deprives policymakers of empirical guidance on mental health best practices. This situation leaves psychological care under-emphasized in national fire-service legislation and funding decisions.

Professional Regulation and Ethical Boundaries in Fire Service Psychology

Professional psychology in the United States is governed by state licensure statutes and the APA's Ethical Principles of Psychologists and Code of Conduct (APA, 2017). Each jurisdiction establishes scope-of-practice laws akin to those for medicine, law, and accounting, designed to protect the public from incompetent or unethical practices. Integrating this rigorously regulated discipline into fire-service agencies presents unique challenges: many existing providers originate from military or law-enforcement backgrounds, and agency priorities sometimes conflict with professional ethical standards. Psychologists working in fire departments must navigate these tensions, often in professional isolation, while adhering to legal and ethical mandates.

Legal Admissibility and Scientific Standards in Fire Service Psychology

The National Fire Protection Association (NFPA), an ANSI-accredited nonprofit, publishes consensus-based codes covering nearly 300 aspects of fire and life-safety, including responder health (NFPA, 2023). Although NFPA standards undergo regular public review and revision, the Association lacks the statutory authority to mandate psychological qualifications or interventions. Establishing defensible psychological standards, such as those governing pre-employment screening or PTSD risk assessment, would require broad acceptance within the scientific community of fire-service psychology and alignment with legal criteria for evidence admissibility (e.g., the Frye standard; Frye v. United States, 293 F. 1013 [D.C. Cir. 1923]).

Fire Service Psychology as a Stakeholder

Fire-service psychologists deliver assessment, operational support, clinical intervention, and management consultation to departments across the USA and internationally (e.g., Singapore, Canada, Lithuania, New Zealand, Netherlands). Relying on professional standards from unrelated disciplines can be ineffective or unethical; instead, psychologists must collaborate with fire-service leaders to adapt evidence-based practices, such as trauma risk management and psychological autopsies, to the unique demands of firefighting (O'Brien et al., 2021).

Integrating fire-service psychology as a recognized stakeholder offers multiple benefits:

- **Enhanced Mental Health Support**: Specialized interventions can address PTSD, anxiety, depression, and suicidality at rates commensurate with firefighting's elevated risk.
- **Improved Performance and Resilience**: Psychologically informed training bolsters decision-making under pressure and fosters team cohesion.
- **Reduced Occupational Stress and Burnout**: Proactive stress-management programs can decrease absenteeism and turnover.
- **Risk Mitigation and Safety**: Human-factor analyses and psychological screening support pre-incident risk reduction (Taylor, 2019).
- **Legal Compliance and Professional Standards**: Aligning with APA ethics and legal precedents ensures that assessments and interventions withstand judicial and regulatory scrutiny (APA, 2017; Frye v. United States, 293 F. 1013).

International Model for Knowledge Exchange

Recent work in the United Kingdom underscores the value of bridging academic research and operational practice. A scoping review by Hill et al. (2023) mapped fire-related scholarship across disciplines and proposed a multidisciplinary model to facilitate systematic knowledge exchange. A pilot implementation demonstrated its utility in informing National Fire Chiefs Council policies, suggesting a blueprint for US fire departments to integrate evidence-based psychological insights into their organizational learning processes.

Conclusion

The limited integration of professional psychology within formal fire service systems reflects an opportunity for growth in policy and practice. As fire and EMS personnel continue to face increasing demands, including exposure to trauma, operational pressures, and organizational stressors, the need for culturally competent, specialized psychological support becomes more evident. Recognizing fire service psychology as a key stakeholder can facilitate more informed decision-making, promote ethical care, and bolster the overall resilience of personnel. Other high-risk professions have successfully incorporated behavioral science to enhance performance and well-being, offering a model from which the fire service can benefit. Advancing this interdisciplinary collaboration is a strategic step forward and an ethical commitment to the long-term health and effectiveness of the fire service and the communities it serves.

References

Centers for Disease Control and Prevention. (2023, April 7). QuickStats: Rates of death due to unintentional injury from fire or flames — United States, 2021. *MMWR, 72*(14), 550. https://www.cdc.gov/mmwr/volumes/72/wr/mm7214a5.htm

O'Brien, P. & Campbell, D. (2021). *Wildland firefighter psychological and behavioral health: Preliminary data from a national sample of current and former wildland firefighters in the United States*. 6th Annual Human Dimensions Conference of the International Association of Wildland Fire.

Taylor, J. A., Lee, J., Shepler, L. J., Davis, A. L., Zohar, D., & Resick, C. R. (2019). Development and validation of the fire service safety climate scale. *Safety Science, 118*, 126-136. https://doi.org/10.1016/j.ssci.2019.05.007

World Health Organization. (2023, October 13). *Burns: Fact Sheet*. https://www.who.int/news-room/fact-sheets/detail/burns

Preface

I've had the privilege of working closely with members of the fire service, an experience that has brought profound professional satisfaction and enduring personal connections. What began as an extension of my work with trauma-affected populations, including inmate-patients, law enforcement, and military personnel, gradually evolved into a deep and unexpected commitment to the fire service. Along the way, I encountered challenges I hadn't foreseen, but each has contributed to meaningful growth, both personally and professionally. Within this field, I discovered a powerful opportunity to apply psychological science in ways that directly enhance the health, safety, and longevity of firefighters.

This book seeks to capture the current state of fire service psychology, acknowledging its many strengths while also identifying areas where growth is needed. My hope is to support the continued development of the field, supporting the way for future generations. I envision a future where students, early-career professionals, committed clinicians, and fire service leaders of all ranks collaborate in a thriving, inclusive community, bringing together multidisciplinary perspectives from both psychology and the fire service.

While professional goals and contributions are significant, the greatest fulfillment in my life has come from the love of family and the support of friends. I am deeply grateful to those who have stood by me throughout this journey (Mark, Michele, Nana, Tracey, Scott, Shaun, and many others). To my family—John, Blake, Archer, and Shelby—you are my greatest joy. I love you today and always. And to my higher power, you are love, present in everything. I see you.

South Pasadena, CA Kristen Wheldon

Limitations in Research and Field Development

Given the limited presence of professional psychology within fire and emergency services, relatively few articles address the psychological needs of firefighters and their families. To bridge this gap, the Fire Service Psychology Association was established in 2017 to promote cultural competence among mental health professionals, provide education and support to fire departments regarding the psychological needs of firefighters and emergency medical providers, and encourage research focused on this unique first responder population. These efforts aim not only to improve health, safety, and longevity within the fire service.

Many people group members of the fire service into the classification of "firefighter" without acknowledging or understanding the variation in ranks, agencies, or assignments within the field. Although each department may have created different rank distinctions within their agencies, the fire service follows a general paramilitary structure. Therefore, the ranks commonly include positions such as recruits, probationary firefighters, firefighters, engineers, captains I or II (also known as lieutenants), battalion chiefs, assistant chiefs, and a Fire Chief. Recruits are individuals who are in the academy but have not yet graduated. Probationary firefighters have finished the academy but are still being evaluated for performance. Upon completion of probation, they are appointed as members of the department and promoted to firefighters. Engineers receive special training to operate an apparatus (vehicles) and should pass testing protocols to earn the position. To become a captain, the firefighter should complete a test and demonstrate through interviews that they would be an asset to their department in a leadership role. Captain IIs, battalion chiefs, and assistant chiefs should follow similar testing and interview processes as they move through the ranks. In many departments, the fire chief is ultimately responsible for appointing the assistant chiefs. In many cases, the Fire Chief is typically appointed by the mayor or city council. There are specialized positions within many agencies as well which may include arson investigators, fire marshals, fire inspectors, hazardous materials (HazMat) technicians/teams, technical rescue specialists, dive/water rescue teams, training officers, safety officers, public information officers (PIOs), emergency management coordinators, logistics/equipment officers, and tactical medics. Note, incident commanders are most often battalion chiefs who oversee multi-unit emergency operations. Whereas company officers at the rank of captains or lieutenants often lead crews and manage daily station operations.

Some firefighters work for wildland agencies, whereas others work for municipal organizations. This distinction is typically made on the basis of the geography of the area. Wildland firefighters protect life and property against wildfires. They function primarily during the fire season, and few are maintained year-round. Municipal firefighters are typically employed full time in densely populated areas and focus their duties on structure fires while also serving as emergency medical service (EMS) providers.

Given the role of fire prevention efforts within fire departments, there has been a significant shift in the specific job duties of firefighters across the United States. Most fire service agencies do not employ members who simply fight fire. Many firefighters now offer emergency medical services, and (in some agencies), this has become their primary function. Today, we see more Emergency Medical Technicians and Paramedics than ever.

Some of the research collected and referenced throughout the document has come from international sources. The fire service abroad may reflect significant cultural differences and the practical application of firefighting methods. Therefore, consideration of each international source could be critically assessed for variability and generalizability to populations within the United States.

References

Murphy, S. L., Kochanek, K. D., Xu, J. Q., & Arias, E. (2024). Deaths: Final data for 2021. *National Vital Statistics Reports, 73*(8). National Center for Health Statistics. https://doi.org/10.15620/cdc/158787

Centers for Disease Control and Prevention [CDC], 2023. https://search.cdc.gov/search/?query=fire%20death&siteLimit=NCHS&dpage=1

Contents

Chapter 1
Introduction

Throughout my professional career, I have come to deeply appreciate the importance of understanding the unique psychological variables of different populations, as they are the consumers of psychological services, and our effectiveness can have a profound impact on their lives. This is true for students who may receive educational accommodations on the basis of assessment findings, an accused individual who may receive mental health diversion programs instead of incarceration, or an applicant who is applying for a safety-sensitive position. With that said, in 2025, fire and emergency services were not formally recognized as a special population by the American Psychological Association (APA, n.d., 2023). While many departments may use the services psychologists provide, there have been no standards of practice formally created or evolved for the population. This study attempts to capture the current state of fire service psychology, recognizing that the field is in development and that there are limitations in our conceptualization of the population's unique needs. The author's hope is that this literature review and reflection of practical application highlight the areas of strength but also of weakness so that other professionals can seek to fill in the gaps and ultimately establish an ongoing and evolving discipline explicitly dedicated to the health, safety, and longevity of our fire service and emergency medical providers.

My journey into the fire service psychology world began through my connection to the broad scope of forensic psychology, where there were established practicums, internships, and postdoctoral opportunities to evolve not only as professionals but also to contribute to the discipline as a whole. The term "forensic" is related to the legal system. The legal system involves law enforcement, corrections, courts, and other government processes and functions. Currently, within the umbrella of forensic psychology, there is a special consideration for the psychological needs of law enforcement officers, and owing to the perceived connection between police and fire service populations, this is where the field of fire service psychology currently lives and hopefully evolves.

K. Wheldon, *Fire Service Psychology*,
https://doi.org/10.1007/978-3-032-02126-7_1

The Umbrella of Firefighting, Emergency Medical Services, and Fire Prevention

Firefighters, by definition, are known to "fight" fire. However, fire departments do not strictly engage in fire suppression activities. They have expanded their operations to include various prehospital medicine services, including basic life support (BLS), advanced life support (ALS), and even mobile integrated healthcare (MIH) units or community paramedicine programs (Choi et al., 2016). Additionally, some departments have integrated units to assist with the community's behavioral health needs, alongside other community risk reduction and fire prevention activities.

Since the late 1960s and early 1970s, there has been a significant shift in the role of the firefighting community. Once focused solely on fire prevention and suppression, departments have expanded their roles to include providing emergency medical services. This systemic evolution started with the inclusion of unstandardized medical responses focused primarily on transport rather than treatment in the 1960s and later included paramedics (Sanko et al., 2020). Several departments have recently advanced prehospital emergency care systems by adopting nurse practitioners.

Allied professionals (especially those in mental health disciplines) should understand the various roles and responsibilities a firefighter may play depending on their department, rank, license type (emergency medical technician, paramedic, or nurse practitioner), and assigned role within the team. These distinctions affect the level of service, team dynamics, position of power (subordinate vs. supervisor), and agency culture. There are "single-function" roles in different organizations where the department member may operate within emergency medicine without ever adopting the firefighter role. These variations lead to subcultures or ingroup/outgroup dynamics that have the potential to lead to conflicts (Brewer, 1999). Similarly, allied professionals should recognize the intersection between these variables and racial, gender, and age dynamics. These variations are often specific to each region because of differences among departments across the country. Fire departments may operate under volunteer, paid-on-call, municipal, wildland, or combination models. Importantly, many fire departments now require applicants to have either an emergency medical technician (EMT) or paramedic license upon hiring. As a result, candidates should be prepared to provide emergency medical services, even if it is not their preferred duty, to have the opportunity to fight fires. Interestingly, many organizations seeking applicants highlight firefighting responsibilities while downplaying the EMS role, even though EMS calls make up most of their community responses.

The way EMS services are structured often places varying levels of responsibility on providers on the basis of their scope of practice, and added responsibility can shape how they see themselves and others, especially when facing death. For example, if a paramedic and an EMT respond to a call that tragically results in a child's death, the paramedic might feel a heavier burden of responsibility. This sense of weight often stems from their broader scope of practice and the internalized belief that their advanced training could be enough to save lives (Crowe et al., 2020). How providers integrate the reality of death into their personal and professional worldview can affect whether they experience heightened moral distress or even moral injury, particularly when grappling with what they feel they could have done, also known as an act of omission (Lentz et al., 2021). One way to support providers in these painful moments is to help them reframe their role: reminding them that while professionals bring knowledge, skill, and ability to every situation, they are stewards of the moment, not controllers of the outcome. We influence outcomes; we do not control them. Moreover, even when we intervene exactly as we could, we do not always obtain the results we hope for.

Just as mental health professionals possess different knowledge, skills, and abilities that define their scope of practice, emergency medical providers also have distinct roles and specific skills that they are authorized to perform. Emergency medical technicians (EMTs) are trained to deliver basic life support (BLS) services, including cardiopulmonary resuscitation (CPR), wound care, and patient stabilization during transport (National Highway Traffic Safety Administration, 2021).

On the other hand, paramedics are equipped to provide advanced life support (ALS), which allows them to administer medications, perform intubations to clear airways, and carry out other advanced medical procedures. On a typical medical response team or "rescue," at least one EMT and one paramedic are usually assigned to the ambulance. Importantly, some agencies operate their rescue units, whereas others partner with private ambulance services for patient transport. Some fire departments have also introduced nurse practitioner (NP) units into their emergency medicine systems. Nurse practitioners have a broader and more independent scope of practice than EMTs and paramedics do, enabling them to conduct field assessments, make diagnoses, prescribe medications, and manage more complex medical cases directly in the field.

Emergency medical services (EMS) were historically incorporated into fire departments following the launch of a research initiative in Pittsburgh. The first paramedic-staffed emergency medical services (EMS) system, called "Freedom House," was created as a community project intended to take Black individuals from impoverished communities and empower them with the knowledge, skills, and abilities to perform as paramedics. These professionals were trained under the supervision of medical doctors and, importantly, demonstrated the ability of underserved populations to perform advanced life support skills (Edwards, 2019). This community project was developed to support social justice within public service. After the program was deemed successful, political influence ultimately reduced funding. They resulted in the allocation of funding to other public service agencies, including law enforcement agencies and fire departments, which assumed their duties.

The Freedom House Ambulance Service, operated by Pittsburgh's Black community members in the 1960s, played a critical and often under-recognized role in shaping modern emergency medical services (EMS). As one of the first programs to train paramedics under the supervision of physicians, Freedom House demonstrated the viability of structured prehospital care and contributed significantly to the development of national EMS standards (Edwards, 2019). Before this innovation, emergency medical transport was often conducted by firefighters, police officers, or mortuary personnel—individuals who lacked formal medical training and operated without standardized treatment protocols. The focus during that era was rapid transport rather than on-scene stabilization or care (Lerner et al., 2001). The widespread adoption of EMS practices in the following decades was likely influenced by multiple factors, including advancements in trauma medicine, the integration of combat medicine principles from military contexts, and increased public awareness driven by cultural phenomena such as the 1970s television series Emergency! (Webb & Chertok, 1972–1977).

As emergency medical services have evolved to meet the changing needs of their communities, many departments have incorporated nurse practitioner units into their prehospital care models. This significant shift, which began in the 2010s, reflects broader public health and safety initiatives to improve population health outcomes, reduce strain on emergency systems, and deliver more proactive, integrated care. These developments are often the result of collaborative efforts among fire departments, healthcare providers, and local governments seeking innovative solutions to address gaps in emergency medicine and overwhelmed hospital systems (Sanko et al., 2020). In addition to reducing unnecessary emergency department utilization, these models have expanded to include telehealth capabilities and direct linkages to community resources, such as behavioral health and social services. Most recently, the District of Columbia Fire and Emergency Medical Services (DC FEMS) further advanced prehospital care by launching its Whole Blood Program. This groundbreaking initiative, introduced in 2024, enables paramedics to administer low-titer type O whole blood at the scene of traumatic injury, a practice previously limited to hospital settings, demonstrating the fire service's expanding role in delivering life-saving interventions before patients even reach definitive care (DC Fire and Emergency Medical Services Department, 2024).

Reactive to Proactive Models: Community Risk Reduction

Community risk reduction (CRR) originated within fire and emergency services as a strategic shift from a reactive emergency response to proactive risk mitigation. Historically, fire departments focused on responding to incidents; however, the increasing complexity of community risk necessitated a more comprehensive approach. The CRR emerged as a framework emphasizing the identification and prioritization of local risks, followed by the implementation of targeted strategies to reduce these risks through education, engineering, enforcement, emergency response, and economic incentives (Walker, 2022).

In the United States, the formalization of the CRR was influenced by the development of standards such as the NFPA 1300, which provides guidelines for community risk assessment and reduction planning. Additionally, initiatives such as the Vision 20/20 Project have played a pivotal role in promoting CRR by encouraging fire departments to integrate data-driven risk analysis into their operations (Rowan-White & Williams, 2024). The integration of the CRR into fire service culture has been further supported by research highlighting its effectiveness in reducing fire incidents and enhancing public safety (Rowan-White & Williams, 2024).

Internationally, similar approaches have been adopted. For example, the United Kingdom's Integrated Risk Management Planning (IRMP) process aligns with CRR principles by assessing community risk and allocating resources accordingly. Furthermore, public health models have influenced CRRs by emphasizing the importance of prevention and community engagement in addressing health and safety risks (Shaw, 2012). Overall, the evolution of the CRR reflects broader recognition within the fire service of the need to proactively address the underlying causes of emergencies, thereby enhancing community resilience and safety.

Department of Justice

While there may be commonalities between law enforcement and other first responder groups, one significant difference is the role of the Department of Justice (DOJ). The DOJ is a federal agency with regulatory authority over local law enforcement organizations throughout the state. According to the Department of Justice, "The mission of the Department of Justice is to uphold the rule of law, to keep our country safe, and to protect civil rights" (U.S. Department of Justice, n.d.). Functionally, the Justice Department, led by the United States Attorney General, consists of over 40 distinct component organizations and a workforce exceeding 115,000 employees. From its headquarters at the Robert F. Kennedy Building in Washington, D.C., the Department operates field offices across all the U.S. states and territories and in more than 50 countries worldwide.

Per the U.S. Department of Justice website, the agency has five strategic goals: upholding the rule of law, keeping our country safe, protecting civil rights, ensuring economic opportunity and fairness for all, and administering just court and correctional systems. These strategic goals include protecting our democratic institutions, promoting good government, protecting the right to vote, combating discrimination and hate crimes, reforming and strengthening criminal and juvenile justice systems, expanding equal access to justice, advancing environmental justice and tackling climate crises, administering an equitable and efficient immigration court system, maintaining a safe and humane prison system, and reinvigorating antitrust enforcement and consumer protection.

United States Fire Administration

The United States Fire Service has no equivalent body to the Department of Justice. The United States Fire Administration was established for data and research purposes but was not designed to have regulatory authority. The United States Fire Service is not a collective organization or body of fire service agencies. Most departments act as their sovereign entity, beholden only to the "Authorities Having Jurisdiction" (AHJs) and rarely have direct connections with the USFA. These variables directly impact the standardization of practices within fire and emergency services. This is significant because there is no unifying body driving the direction of the fire service concerning best practices or policies (U.S. Fire Administration, n.d.). Even if the USFA creates documentation encouraging such practices, there is no authority to ensure that those intentions are implemented at the local level.

To understand the function of the U.S. Fire Administration (USFA), it is important to conceptualize both the context in which it was developed and the developmental process of the agency itself. In the 1940s, during the presidency of Harry S. Truman, the U.S. government began to recognize the need for a more coordinated federal effort to address fire prevention and safety, especially as urbanization and industrialization continued to increase the risks of large-scale fires (Truman, 1947). Although the concept of a national fire safety organization emerged, significant action to address the issue at the federal level did not occur until the following decades.

Although there was no unification or standardization, in the 1940s, there was basic acknowledgment at the federal level that the United States had a "fire problem." In 1973, a national commission was established to examine safety in the United States, which led to the release of a report titled "America Burning." The document highlighted that the United States faced one of the most severe fire problems among industrialized nations, concerning high rates of fire-related deaths, injuries, and property damage. This study demonstrated the limitations of current fire safety measures, prevention education, and firefighting resources (National Commission on Fire Prevention and Control, 1973). The report included information about fire safety awareness, fire prevention, firefighting resources, urban fire risk, and legislative and policy recommendations. The document provided recommendations to address these significant fire safety issues, including creating a federal agency to address fire prevention, safety, and education. This report ultimately led to Congress passing the Federal Fire Prevention and Control Act of 1974, which established the National Fire Prevention and Control Administration (NFPCA). Soon after, in 1978, Congress decided to rename the NFPCA the United States Fire Administration (USFA). The following year (1979), President Carter placed the USFA under the newly created Federal Emergency Management Agency (FEMA) through Executive Order 12127 (Carter, J., 1979). The FEMA subsequently developed the dual responsibilities of emergency management and civil defense (Carter, J., 1979).

As of early 2025, the United States Fire Administration (USFA) is a division of the Federal Emergency Management Agency (FEMA), which falls under the direction of the Department of Homeland Security (United States Fire Administration, n.d.). The USFA is focused on improving fire prevention and safety through education, research, and training. The primary goals of the USFA website include data collection and analysis, education and training, public awareness campaigns, and support for fire departments. Data collection and analysis function to gather and analyze fire incident statistics to understand current trends and improve fire safety practices. The education and training function of the USFA involves offering training programs to firefighters, emergency responders, and the public, which are intended to enhance both preparedness and fire safety (United States Fire Administration, n.d.). Public awareness campaigns are meant to improve prevention and safety measures. Finally, the USFA offers support for fire departments by providing resources, especially for those in rural or underserved communities (United States Fire Administration, n.d.).

Almost a decade and a half after the establishment of the USFA, in 1992, Congress developed the National Fallen Firefighters Foundation (NFFF) through Title XII in an effort to honor and remember America's fallen firefighters. The nonprofit was created after the nation acknowledged the sacrifices made by firefighters who died in the line of duty and subsequently began to provide support to families and departments.

The law tasked the foundation with organizing the National Fallen Firefighters Memorial Service, held annually at the National Fire Academy in Emmitsburg, Maryland, where the official national memorial is located. Initially established in 1981, this memorial became the symbolic and functional center of NFFF's work.

The NFFF not only honors those lost but also provides emotional and financial support services for surviving family members, such as grief counseling, scholarships, and peer support networks. In addition, it collaborates with fire service organizations to reduce firefighter fatalities through training, research, and the promotion of best practices. A notable initiative is the "Everyone Goes Home" program, which was intended to improve firefighter safety and prevent future line-of-duty deaths.

The term line-of-duty death (LODD) can carry heavy psychological weight for firefighters, often aligning their deaths with the kinds of sacrifices seen in military or police fatalities. These deaths occur in battle or at the hands of an adversary. Historically, a LODD was narrowly defined in the fire service as death occurring during active fire suppression. Over time, this definition has expanded to include fatalities from heart attacks within 24 h of a shift, occupational cancers, and, more recently, suicide (United States Fire Administration, 2022).

Understanding what qualifies as a line-of-duty death (LODD) in fire and emergency services has expanded significantly to better reflect the complex physical and psychological risks that firefighters face. For example, the Hometown Heroes Survivors Benefits Act of 2003 presumes that heart attacks or strokes occurring within 24 h of engaging in non-routine, stressful, or strenuous on-duty activities qualify as LODDs, allowing affected families to receive federal death benefits

(U.S. Congress, 2003). This presumption reflects strong evidence linking acute physical stress to cardiac events among firefighters.

Many states have enacted presumptive cancer laws recognizing specific cancers as occupational diseases for firefighters (LeMasters et al., 2006). Reinforcing this perspective, the World Health Organization's International Agency for Research on Cancer (IARC) formally classified firefighting as a Group 1 carcinogenic profession in 2022, citing sufficient evidence that occupational exposures during firefighting are carcinogenic to humans (IARC, 2023). This global acknowledgment underscores the serious health risks that firefighters face even beyond immediate hazards.

Amid growing concerns about the mental health crisis among first responders, recent federal policy initiatives have expanded support. In 2022, the Biden Administration extended the Public Safety Officers' Benefits (PSOB) Program to include deaths by suicide, provided that the suicide was the direct result of duty-related trauma, such as posttraumatic stress disorder (PTSD) or acute stress disorder. While this policy change represents an important step in acknowledging the psychological sacrifices of public safety personnel, it also introduces potential ethical concerns. Specifically, there is a risk of unintentionally valorizing suicide by equating it with deaths incurred during acts of physical bravery, potentially reinforcing dangerous narratives around PTSD and martyrdom.

Wingspread Conferences

Given that there is no overarching governmental regulatory authority, fire and emergency services are shaped by the influence of stakeholder groups, often called the "Nine Sisters." These groups often congregate to produce literature on the current state of affairs in fire and emergency services and to advocate for the needs of fire and emergency services. This phrasing, "nine sisters," is an informal but widely recognized reference, reflecting that participants were present at the Wingspread Conference and mentioned in the corresponding documents. The Wingspread Conference became a series of influential gatherings within the fire service community beginning in 1966. The goal was to bring together fire service leaders, experts, and policymakers to address critical issues facing the fire service and to develop strategies for improving fire prevention, firefighting, and emergency services.

This conference series is named after the Wingspread estate in Racine, Wisconsin, where the first meeting was held. The Johnson Foundation sponsored it, and the outcomes of these conferences have significantly impacted fire policy and practice in the U.S. The conference goals include identifying emerging issues, encouraging strong leadership and management practices, strategically planning fire responses, establishing multidisciplinary approaches to solve fire-related challenges, and providing a conference report that summarizes discussions and offers recommendations to address current and anticipated fire-related problems.

Wingspread Conferences are seen as key leadership platforms in fire and emergency services, helping guide policy decisions and fostering improvements in fire safety and emergency services over the years. As of 2024, six widespread conferences have been held within the fire service community:

- *Wingspread I (1966):* The original conference where leaders gathered to address emerging fire service issues and set the stage for future conferences.
- *Wingspread II (1976):* A follow-up conference to assess progress and address new challenges.
- *Wingspread III (1986):* Continued discussions focused on fire prevention, leadership, and growing urban challenges.
- *Wingspread IV (1996):* Emphasis on the evolving role of fire and emergency services in emergency medical services and other nontraditional areas.
- *Wingspread V (2006):* Addressed twenty-first-century challenges, such as terrorism and natural disasters, and integrated new technologies into fire service operations.
- *Wingspread VI (2016):* Focused on modern leadership, the future of fire prevention, and community risk reduction strategies.
- *Wingspread VII (2026)*

Nine Sisters

The Wingspread Conference documents reference representatives from national fire service organizations ("Nine Sisters"). These key stakeholders, which include national fire service organizations in the United States, often collaborate on firefighting and emergency response efforts. These organizations include:

1. *The Fire Department Safety Officers Association (FDSOA)* focuses on safety within the fire service.
2. *The International Association of Black Professional Firefighters (IABPFF)* advocates for the interests of Black firefighters.
3. *The International Association of Fire Chiefs (IAFC)* represents the leadership of fire service organizations (International Association of Fire Chiefs, n.d.).
4. *The International Association of Fire Fighters (IAFF)* serves as a labor union representing firefighters and paramedics (International Association of Fire Fighters, n.d.).
5. *The International Society of Fire Service Instructors (ISFSI)* concentrates on education and training for firefighters.
6. *The National Association of Hispanic Firefighters (NAHF)* represents the interest of Hispanic firefighters.
7. *The National Fallen Firefighters Foundation (NFFF)* honors fallen firefighters and supports their families (NFFF, n.d.).

8. *The National Fire Protection Association (NFPA)* is responsible for providing fire safety codes and standards (NFPA, n.d.).
9. *The National Volunteer Fire Council (NVFC)* represents volunteer fire and emergency service organizations.

In addition to representatives from the major stakeholder groups, Wingspread Conferences are attended by a select group of fire service leaders, experts, and policymakers. Attendees may include leaders of fire departments or emergency response agencies, academics and researchers, government officials and policy makers, private sector and industry representatives, and nonprofit and advocacy group members. The conference is considered invitation-only and highly selective, ensuring that those who attend are influential leaders who can shape future policies and practices within the fire service.

Recruitment and Retention

The concept of recruitment and retention in fire and emergency services should consider the complexity of the national fire service infrastructure. Most fire service departments across the United States rely heavily on a volunteer workforce. Over the past decade, suburban and rural populations have experienced significant growth, while the number of volunteer firefighters has decreased by more than 10%, highlighting the need for improved recruitment and retention strategies (Greene & Hendershot, 2017). The reduction in volunteerism can be tied to the values of the applicant pool. Firefighters' commitment to volunteer service appears to be shaped predominantly by a value-driven orientation, grounded in altruistic and community-focused motivations. However, differences in expected service duration are more closely linked to how volunteers perceive opportunities for personal growth and to how clearly they understand organizational objectives (Greene & Hendershot, 2017).

The recruitment of municipal or paid firefighters increasingly requires attention to both extrinsic and intrinsic factors that shape career decision-making. While intrinsic motivations such as a sense of duty and community service remain foundational, extrinsic rewards, including competitive pay, benefits, and work-life balance, are critical in attracting candidates, especially as they compare firefighting with other career options (Grant, 2008). Research indicates that intrinsic motivation strengthens the relationship between prosocial motivation and job performance, but when intrinsic motivation is lower, extrinsic factors become more influential in sustaining engagement (Grant, 2008). Furthermore, public sector research shows that when extrinsic rewards are perceived as limited, individuals often compensate with heightened intrinsic and prosocial motivation (Kroll & Porumbescu, 2017). Qualitative studies, such as those examining firefighter motivations in Trinidad and Tobago, also highlight the importance of job security and salary alongside intrinsic desires to help others (Salina & Wallace, 2025). These findings underscore the need for fire departments to frame firefighting careers competitively, emphasizing both the tangible and intangible benefits to appeal to a broad pool of prospective recruits.

Hiring Processes/Performance Standards

Given that the fire service is not beholden to a national fire service authority, the hiring practices of fire departments may vary depending on the location. While fire departments may not use universal hiring strategies, there are legal requirements that shape practices, although employment laws vary by state. The following is based on California law for demonstration purposes. Specific legal requirements could be explored state by state, and legal questions could be referred to legal counsel for accuracy and applicability.

In California, employees have the right to various legal protections from employers. These legal protections may be related to wage and hour requirements, discrimination and harassment, family and medical leave, workers' compensation, at-will or employment contracts, California labor codes, workplace safety standards, whistleblower protections, worker privacy, union rights, and severance and unemployment benefits. While these laws can be complex, employers should ensure compliance with legal requirements. Employees should be familiar with their employment rights and seek legal counsel when necessary (California Department of Industrial Relations [DIR], n.d.; California Chamber of Commerce, n.d.).

Hiring standards should be rooted in business necessity, not arbitrary standards. To prove business necessity, a job analysis should demonstrate that the standard used to qualify or disqualify someone translates into what would be required to do the job effectively.

Written Tests

Written tests are often used to determine a candidate's aptitude and ability to perform a job. Some tests may include questions related to fire safety, fire behavior, fire prevention, and emergency medical procedures (Firefighter Candidate Testing Center [FCTC], n.d.). They may also include assessments of mathematical and analytical skills, reading comprehension, situational judgment, problem-solving, critical thinking, and memory and retention skills (Public Safety Testing, n.d.).

Research related to written tests among firefighter applicants is limited. One study investigating the role of practice effects included repeat applicants who underwent the same cognitive and context judgment examinations multiple times, demonstrating that the results were impacted by practice effects. Specifically, practice effects were observed the first and second times a person took the examination in areas of abstract reasoning and mechanical comprehension (Dunlop et al., 2011). Fewer effects were observed on a timed test of numerical comprehension and an untimed test of teamwork (Dunlop et al., 2011). By the third time the test was performed in all categories, practice effects were more minor and nonsignificant (Dunlop et al., 2011).

Over the years, there have been concerns about fire department hiring practices, particularly with respect to discrimination and nepotism. To address these concerns, hiring authorities have begun to critically examine the most valid and equitable methods for evaluating candidates, focusing on predictors that are genuinely related to job performance. One study by Barrett et al. (1999) reviewed the use of written tests for firefighter selection and reported that the strongest predictors of actual job performance were composite tests measuring both cognitive and mechanical abilities. In contrast, other commonly used variables, such as personality assessments (e.g., evaluations of conscientiousness, emotional stability, and agreeableness), biodata inventories (personal history and life experiences), situational judgment tests (responses to hypothetical job-related scenarios), and interest inventories (preferences and values), tended to have weaker predictive validity. While frequently included in selection procedures, these additional components often lack clear job-related justification and could introduce bias or adverse impacts (Barrett et al., 1999). Therefore, all components of the firefighter selection process must be grounded in business necessity, supported by job analyses, and directly linked to measurable job performance outcomes.

Given these findings, there is a strong rationale for exploring the development of more structured psychological screening protocols within the fire service, similar to those established for peace officers under California's POST (Peace Officer Standards and Training). POST mandates formal psychological evaluations to assess traits such as impulse control, emotional regulation, judgment, and stress tolerance, which are likely critical for effective performance in firefighting (California Commission on Peace Officer Standards and Training [POST], 2022). However, applying similar standards to fire and emergency services requires careful research and job-specific validation to ensure that the criteria used do not inadvertently exclude qualified candidates or admit those who may not be well suited to the unique demands of the role (Barrett et al., 1999).

While widely used tools such as the MMPI-3 and CPI have been normed for firefighter populations and are common in public safety evaluations (Ben-Porath & Tellegen, 2020), there are no formal statewide or national psychological screening standards or guidelines specific to firefighter selection. This lack of a standardized framework distinguishes firefighting from law enforcement, where protocols such as POST contribute to consistency in hiring and enhanced safety for both personnel and the communities they serve (POST, 2022).

This discrepancy highlights the need for fire and emergency services to consider developing an evidence-based psychological evaluation model tailored to their specific operational demands. Such tools could be legally defensible, grounded in validated job analysis, and designed to predict performance and support long-term wellness and resilience (Barrett et al., 1999). Advancing this conversation could significantly strengthen the legal and ethical framework of the firefighter selection process.

In summary, while written tests remain a staple in the firefighter selection process, the effectiveness and fairness of these assessments depend on their alignment with actual job demands. Research has underscored the predictive value of cognitive and mechanical components (Barrett et al., 1999). However, it also cautions against overreliance on less validated measures, which may introduce bias or lack demonstrable relevance to firefighting duties. Additionally, findings related to practice effects suggest that repeated exposure to cognitive testing can influence outcomes, raising further considerations for equitable administration (Dunlop et al., 2011). As fire and emergency services evolve, refining selection instruments through rigorous job analysis and incorporating validated psychological screening, similar to practices in other public safety sectors, can enhance performance prediction and workforce stability. Establishing comprehensive, evidence-based testing standards is important to ensure that hiring practices reflect operational realities while promoting diversity, legal defensibility, and the long-term success of fire service members.

Physical Fitness Evaluations

Under the authority having jurisdiction (AHJ), each city, county, state, or federal department may have different assessment requirements for hiring a firefighter. To standardize the process, the National Fire Protection Association (NFPA) uses a consensus committee to establish fitness standards and guidelines for candidates and incumbents. The most recent version of these documents was published in 2022 (National Fire Protection Association [NFPA], 2022b, 2022c). The NFPA 1582 is titled "Standard on Comprehensive Occupational Medical Program for Fire Departments" and outlines the medical evaluations for candidates and incumbents to ensure health, safety, and effectiveness (National Fire Protection Association [NFPA], 2022b). The NFPA 1583 is not focused explicitly on candidates. However, candidates are expected to achieve and maintain the level of fitness to perform the functions of the job. NFPA 1583 is also called the "Standard on Health-Related Fitness Programs for Fire Department Members" and was meant to establish minimum requirements for developing, implementing, and managing health-related fitness programs for fire departments (National Fire Protection Association [NFPA], 2022c).

In 2021, Scarlett, Rogers, Adams, Dreger, and Petersen conducted a multiphase study to validate treadmill-based physical aptitude tests for firefighter candidates. The primary objective was to assess the validity and reliability of these assessments and establish performance standards grounded in empirical evidence and professional expertise (Scarlett et al., 2021).

The study was structured into three phases. First, 49 structural firefighters evaluated how well the test activities reflected the real-world physical demands of firefighting. In the second phase, 23 participants completed the treadmill tests three times to assess reliability over time. In the final phase, an expert panel of 25 firefighter supervisors employed the bookmark method to determine cutoff scores, combining independent assessments with group discussions to set minimum performance standards (Scarlett et al., 2021). The results demonstrated strong evidence of both validity and reliability, and the use of an expert panel further strengthened the scientific credibility and operational relevance of the revised tests (Scarlett et al., 2021).

Diversity Considerations

Despite the rigorous methodology, Scarlett et al. (2021) did not report demographic characteristics, such as gender, ethnicity, or body composition, of the expert panel in their study on the applicability of physical fitness standards in the hiring process. The absence of diversity within expert panels is a notable concern. Research has shown that homogeneous panels, particularly those lacking variation across gender and physical profiles, may inadvertently establish standards that favor the dominant group's capabilities and disadvantage underrepresented populations (Schenk & Johanson, 2021).

Non-inclusive physical testing standards can create unintended barriers to entry, disproportionately affecting women and smaller-framed individuals, even when such differences are unrelated to actual job performance (Hulett et al., 2008; ideas42, 2022). This effect not only reduces workforce diversity but also impedes efforts to create fire and emergency services that are more reflective of the communities they serve.

Research further underscores that diverse expert panels, comprising individuals with various backgrounds, experiences, and perspectives, are better equipped to develop fair, representative, and job-relevant testing standards. Panels that include diverse experiences are more likely to recognize hidden biases and ensure that physical standards accurately reflect important firefighting tasks without unnecessarily excluding qualified candidates. Promoting demographic and experiential diversity within expert panels supports the development of firefighter physical aptitude tests that are both scientifically robust and socially equitable (Hulett et al., 2008). An inclusive approach promotes equal opportunity, improves operational effectiveness, and strengthens public trust in firefighting.

With the development of a complex human experience through biological, psychological, and social influences, people naturally develop biases toward groups and individuals who are part of those groups. One primary responsibility of firefighters is to make life-or-death decisions on the basis of a collective understanding of which lives matter most. Individuals are inherently biased due to the complexity of their psychological interpretations of certain groups identified as "others." However, individuals' prejudices, if they are in direct conflict with the institutional culture of the fire service, may mitigate discriminatory behavior (Scarborough, R. C., 2017). Therefore, to objectively evaluate discrimination in fire and emergency services, the focus needs to be less on the individual and more on the culture itself (Scarborough, R. C., 2017). This does not mean that there could be no individual consequences for individual behavior, but strategic efforts could address the "big picture."

Legal challenges to hiring and promotion decisions are not unfamiliar to the fire service. A notable example is Ricci v. DeStefano (2009), a landmark U.S. Supreme Court case that addressed the intersection of race, employment practices, and civil rights within a fire department context. The case emerged when the New Haven Fire Department (New Haven, Connecticut) administered a promotional exam for lieutenant and captain positions, which yielded racially disparate outcomes: White and Hispanic candidates scored significantly higher than African American candidates did. The city discarded the exam results because of potential lawsuits alleging disparate impact discrimination. However, White and Hispanic firefighters who performed well sued, claiming that the city's actions violated Title VII of the Civil Rights Act of 1964, prohibiting employment discrimination on the basis of race (McCormick, 2012).

In *Ricci v. DeStefano*, 557 U.S. 557 (2009), the Court held that the city's decision to discard the test results was based on racial disparities, without a "strong basis in evidence" that the test was itself discriminatory, thereby violating Title VII. Writing for the majority, Justice Kennedy stated, "Fear of litigation alone cannot justify an employer's reliance on race to the detriment of individuals who passed the examinations and qualify for promotions."

The framing of Ricci often focused primarily on the underrepresentation of Black and Latino men in supervisory roles, yet critical perspectives noted that such framing ignored the compounded exclusions faced by women of color within the New Haven Fire Department (McCormick, M. L., 2012). Intersectional analyses reveal how the systems of race and gender discrimination together create even more profound disparities, disparities that simple race-conscious or colorblind frameworks fail to address (McCormick, M. L., 2012).

This historical context offers a critical lens for evaluating firefighter physical aptitude tests validated by Scarlett et al. (2021). While their study sought to establish valid and reliable standards for assessing firefighter candidates, the expert panel responsible for setting performance cutoff scores was composed entirely of professional firefighters whose demographic diversity was not reported. Given the well-documented historical lack of diversity in fire and emergency services, it is reasonable to infer that the panel likely reflected a predominantly White, male perspective.

When a demographically homogeneous group develops physical standards, there is a risk that those standards may unconsciously reflect the physical experiences, body types, and assumptions of the group. Research shows that rigid, narrowly constructed physical ability tests can create barriers to entry for underrepresented groups, particularly women and people of color, whose physiological profiles may differ from the dominant group's norms. These barriers are not only exclusionary but also undermine efforts to build fire service organizations that reflect the diversity of the communities they serve.

Moreover, the Ricci case illustrates how initiatives intended to address racial inequity can themselves be weaponized through narratives of "reverse discrimination," especially when institutional Whiteness is normalized as a neutral baseline (McCormick, M. L., 2012). This dynamic highlights the importance of embedding intersectional perspectives into the development and validation of hiring and testing standards. A diverse expert panel, informed by multiple identities and experiences, is important to ensure that physical aptitude tests are equitable, defensible, and truly reflective of the broad range of individuals capable of performing the important functions of firefighting. Ultimately, ensuring diversity among candidates and among those setting standards is necessary to advance fairness, equity, and operational excellence within the fire service.

Legal Challenges to Written and Physical Hiring Standards in Fire and Emergency Services

Over the past several decades, numerous legal cases have challenged the fairness and legality of the written and physical tests used by fire departments in hiring decisions. While facially neutral, plaintiffs have often alleged that these testing practices have had disparate impacts on protected classes under Title VII of the Civil Rights Act of 1964, particularly related to race and gender (Civil Rights Act, 1964). This section summarizes major cases and research findings where courts determined specific written or physical assessments unlawfully excluded qualified candidates and highlights broader legal developments influencing firefighter hiring practices.

One of the most prominent cases is the United States and Vulcan Society v. City of New York, where the U.S. Department of Justice and the Vulcan Society sued the FDNY over its written entrance exams (United States v. City of New York, 2010). The court reported that these exams were not sufficiently job related and disproportionately excluded Black and Hispanic candidates. Disparate impact and intentional discrimination claims were upheld, leading the city to agree to extensive remedies, including nearly $128 million in back pay and reforms to its hiring process (Vulcan Society v. City of New York, 2012).

Similarly, in Lewis v. City of Chicago (2010), the Supreme Court addressed a written hiring examination used by the Chicago Fire Department. Although the city may not have intended to discriminate, setting a cutoff score of 89 significantly disadvantaged African American applicants. The Court held that the city's use of the cutoff score constituted a new discriminatory act each time it was applied, thereby violating Title VII's disparate impact provisions (Lewis v. City of Chicago, 2010).

Legal challenges to written firefighter exams have not been limited to allegations of racial discrimination. Cases such as the Boston Chapter, NAACP, and Beecher (1974) further established that exams should be job related and validated, leading to consent decrees requiring remedial hiring practices for minority applicants (Boston Chapter, NAACP v. Beecher, 1974). A broader issue underlying many of these cases is the composition of the groups responsible for designing testing standards. Research suggests that homogeneous panels, those lacking diversity in race, gender, or experience, are more likely to introduce biases into the development of hiring criteria, intentionally or unintentionally (Hulett et al., 2008; ideas42, 2022). These biases can affect what is deemed "important" for the job, potentially resulting in written or physical exams systematically disadvantageous to otherwise qualified applicants from underrepresented groups (Hulett et al., 2008).

The tension between avoiding disparate impacts and avoiding intentional disparate treatment was highlighted in Ricci v. DeStefano (2009). In the City of New Haven case, they discarded a promotional exam because of concerns about racial disparities in results. However, the Supreme Court ruled the city's refusal to certify the exam results, motivated by race, resulted in intentional discrimination against high-scoring candidates, most of whom were White and Hispanic (Ricci v. DeStefano, 2009). The decision emphasized that employers should have a "strong basis in evidence" to believe that they would be liable for disparate impacts before discarding otherwise valid test results (Ricci v. DeStefano, 2009).

More recently, the U.S. Department of Justice brought suit against the City of Durham, North Carolina, alleging that its firefighter written test had a significantly disparate impact on Black candidates and lacked sufficient job relevance (United States v. City of Durham, 2024). The city settled, agreeing to end the use of the exam and providing retroactive hiring opportunities and monetary relief to affected applicants.

Research shows that written cognitive exams often create a "diversity-validity dilemma." While tests are strong predictors of training and job performance, they also tend to adversely impact racial groups (Ployhart & Holtz, 2008). Therefore, fire departments should continuously validate, revise, or supplement written exams with other assessment tools, such as structured interviews or job simulations, to ensure that hiring processes remain lawful and fair (Ployhart & Holtz, 2008).

In summary, legal precedents firmly establish that firefighter written and physical examinations should be demonstrably job related and validated. Failure to account for how homogeneous groups' design standards may inadvertently embed bias further complicates this landscape. Ensuring diverse perspectives in test development is necessary for creating equitable hiring practices that can withstand legal and ethical scrutiny.

Occupational Medical Evaluations in the U.S. Fire Service

Firefighters are exposed to numerous health risks, including the negative impacts of shift work, exposure to carcinogens, strenuous physical activities, and frequent exposure to potentially traumatic events. The evidence suggests that these risks contribute to increased rates of cancer, behavioral health issues, and a heightened risk of duty-related cardiovascular events among firefighters (Jahnke et al., 2016). Given these occupational hazards, there is a growing awareness of the importance of implementing annual medical evaluations for all firefighters (Tobia et al., 2024).

The fire service currently relies on committee consensus to determine what could be included in occupational medical evaluations. Committee members represent a range of stakeholders and are not necessarily required to have medical expertise. Although subject matter experts may participate, there is no formal requirement for medical qualifications. NFPA 1583 currently outlines occupational medical standards. While this consensus-driven process ensures diverse inputs, it may underrepresent evolving scientific findings if expert input is limited, raising concerns about the influence of group dynamics over evidence-based decision-making.

Chapter Review—Assignment: Fire Service Psychology Case Analysis and Professional Proposal

Conceptual Integration (Short Essay: 750–1000 Words)

Fire and emergency services have evolved from primarily reactive fire suppression roles to multifaceted public health agents engaged in a variety of roles, including fire prevention, fire suppression, emergency medical services (EMS), community risk reduction (CRR), arson investigation, and behavioral health response. Yet, they are not recognized as a special population within the American Psychological Association (APA); therefore, there are no specific practice guidelines.

- Discuss the implications of this absence of recognition on psychological service delivery, using at least two distinct psychological subfields that may overlap with the population (e.g., forensic psychology, health psychology, sports psychology, organizational psychology).
- Compare the current status of fire service psychology to that of law enforcement and military psychology, identifying structural and policy differences that may hinder or help professionalization for the fire service.
- Conclude by explaining how these differences shape the ethical responsibilities of psychologists and other mental health professionals working with this population.

In your response, cite evidence from the chapter and at least three additional scholarly (peer-reviewed journal) sources to justify your rationale. Address relevant legal, ethical, and organizational implications of your conceptualization.

Chapter 2
Firefighter Development

Firefighters are individuals shaped by distinct life experiences, personal goals, and motivations. The reasons that draw a person to the fire service offer insight into their values and aspirations. Over time, however, integration into the fire service culture fosters an evolution of identity, as individuals adapt to the group's social norms, expectations, and traditions. This transformation reshapes how firefighters perceive themselves and their interpretation of the world around them. Repeated exposure to potentially traumatic events, coupled with the demands of shift work, can profoundly affect mental health, lifestyle choices, family relationships, and one's connection to the broader community. Throughout their careers, firefighters progress through defined transitional periods, marking professional achievements, leadership responsibilities, and their standing within the department. These milestones help shape career paths and broader perceptions of oneself, others, and the communities one serves. Ultimately, many firefighters face a final transition through retirement, whether through medical separation or after a long career. This transition marks a profound shift in identity, as individuals step away from the rhythms, roles, and responsibilities that have defined much of their adult lives.

What Draws Someone to the Fire Service?

There has been limited research on what drives people to pursue a career in firefighting. However, it is known that fire service is viewed as a helping profession. One hypothesis is that people join the firefighting profession because they value service to others. By definition, emergency services are provided in response to a request from someone in the community, and assistance is given as soon as that request is made. This concept aligns with the empathy–altruism hypothesis, which suggests that people may help others out of genuine concern rather than self-interest (Batson et al., 1991). Another possible explanation is that firefighters may have higher rates

K. Wheldon, *Fire Service Psychology*,
https://doi.org/10.1007/978-3-032-02126-7_2

of childhood trauma, which has been associated with elevated risk for posttraumatic stress responses following critical incidents, and some may cope with these early experiences by seeking control or structure in their adult lives (Komarovskaya et al., 2014).

Given the number of applicants received per job opening, career firefighting may be considered a prestigious employment opportunity in American culture. The average salary for firefighters varies, considering that many departments utilize volunteer resources. In California, entry-level career firefighters earn between $65,000 and $95,000 annually (LAFD Job Bulletin, n.d.). With opportunities for advancement within the ranks and over time shifts, these numbers can quickly inflate an income to a figure well over six figures.

Some firefighters spend considerable time at the firehouse, depending on the call volume of a particular station. The flexibility of adjusting call volume creates a dynamic work environment. Furthermore, within some departments, firefighters may be permitted to take on additional shifts at various stations throughout their city or county. This not only creates an opportunity to increase income but can also help firefighters get to know other members within the organization. Note that a firefighter's work schedule and shifts can vary greatly, given the differences between voluntary, career, municipal, and wildland agencies.

Depending on the number of resources (engines, ambulances, trucks, etc.) available at a specific fire station, the facility can house anywhere from 6 to 12 people at a time. These individuals maintain work schedules alongside the same team, and this frequent contact can create a sense of cohesion and camaraderie. The social nature of this dynamic can serve as a strong motivator when considering a career as a firefighter. Social identity theory suggests that a person's self-concept is derived primarily from group membership, reinforcing feelings of belonging, pride, and loyalty (Tajfel & Turner, 1979).

Society often defines success on the basis of our ability to earn tangible rewards, attract a partner, or leave a legacy through the stories others tell about our lives. Many cultures have created shared narratives that demonstrate how society values the contributions of specific individuals, whether through public service, military service, charitable contributions, or heroic acts. We may also remember events of great tragedy where we have lost a significant number of civilians within a community system. Because firefighters are often seen as heroes in the community, people are more likely to express admiration through behaviors such as community members standing with respect to a firefighter entering the room after a wildfire. These expressions may also be reflected in community events, such as parades that invite fire trucks to participate or when residents bring food or baked goods to stations. For those considering a career in firefighting, this kind of appreciation can serve as a powerful motivator to join. It may also affect current firefighters, who can grow accustomed to and become influenced by the ongoing social recognition they receive. As admiration for firefighters grows, individuals may start to see themselves as special community members. This experience can make it difficult for them to adjust to everyday life shifts, especially when family or friends do not show the same level of gratitude or adulation. As a result, a firefighter may feel overlooked or unappreciated. This emotional dissonance may be linked to a fragility of self-esteem when social roles shift, a phenomenon supported by role theory and identity disruption frameworks (Thoits, 2013).

Hagiography originated in the Catholic Church and refers to the reverence or idealized portrayal of saints. Similarly, firefighters are often highly revered and admired within their communities. Within the collective identity, society may be less likely to hold firefighters accountable when they behave poorly, as it can be incongruent with the expectations of how a firefighter should behave. For example, there have been cases in which firefighters have engaged in domestic violence but rather than condemning the act of domestic violence or centering the experiences of the victims, the narrative often shifts to emphasize the firefighter's mental health and the toll of their profession. The concept may reflect moral licensing, where past heroic or virtuous behavior grants leniency or justification for morally questionable actions (Miller & Effron, 2010). Similarly, there may be situations where a firefighter dies while engaging in unnecessary risk-taking behavior, but the focus becomes on hagiographic themes rather than denouncing maladaptive behavior.

Our society's interpretation of honor and death can have an impact on a firefighter's relationship with their mortality. For example, with consideration for Japanese samurai, the honor of death is of utmost importance. In that culture, for example, death is the appropriate response to shame or dishonor (Benesch, O., 2014). In the U.S. Marine ideology, sacrificing life is the ultimate honor on the battlefield. Some may argue that life has no purpose without something worth dying for (Grossman, D., 2014). This ideology may not prioritize longevity as the goal of a well-lived life. These ideas reflect the cultural worldviews described in terror management theory, which posits that humans seek symbolic immortality through honor, heroism, or social legacy to manage the anxiety of inevitable death (Greenberg et al., 1997).

Purpose in life may not need to be directly translated into the risk of death. The battlefield may be different from the fireground. Countries need soldiers to be prepared to fight and possibly die. In that context, however, the relationship with death is the perception of protecting one's own family or country. The fire service is not a battlefield. It is a strategic engagement with chemistry and physics. Anticipating and managing fire occurs long before ignition. We can shift our ideology to celebrate the firefighters who carry wagons full of smoke detectors into underserved communities and help disadvantaged or Disabled community members install new ones or replace batteries. We can celebrate that community risk reduction ultimately saves lives through sprinkler advocacy. This reorientation aligns with contemporary shifts in social recognition theory, where value is placed on acts of visible bravery and quiet, systemic contributions that improve collective safety and well-being (Honneth, 2007).

A potent mix of identity, community validation, and cultural narrative shapes legacy in the fire service. Social psychology suggests that while these motivations can be noble and deeply human, they can also lead to emotional vulnerability, idealized perceptions, and resistance to accountability. A healthier, future-forward legacy might honor preventive action, inclusivity, and community engagement just as much as physical risk and sacrifice.

How Does the Fire Service Influence the Individual?

From a social psychology perspective, environments can significantly influence an individual's values, thoughts, emotions, and behaviors. With respect to fire and emergency services, we consider agencies to be closed systems. Individuals are frequently changed by inclusion in this system (Ashforth & Saks, 1996). Given the hierarchical structure of fire and emergency services, firefighters have advanced through these ranks. Therefore, it is uncommon for individuals who have not been in the department for many years to have leadership roles. As such, there is a developmental process that occurs over time, which shapes the ideology of the individual firefighter to mirror that of the larger group.

Within the closed system of a fire department, some firefighters may serve in agency roles that are typically industry-specific within civilian workforces. Given access to these assignments, many firefighters may struggle to appreciate the subject matter expertise of civilian employees. Furthermore, given the unique physical and cognitive standards required to achieve membership as a sworn firefighter, some firefighters may discount the value of civilian employees because they have not "earned" their place within the department. Similarly, in some agencies, EMS providers work alongside firefighters without attending a firefighter academy. Although working for the same agency and serving similar functions, these distinctions can cause dissension among the ranks. This concept reflects group identification processes in which individuals prioritize membership and loyalty to their "in-group" and may view outsiders, even those within the same agency, with skepticism or exclusion (Tajfel & Turner, 1979).

The closed system of some fire service agencies can create barriers for fire departments to employ civilians, who may be the most qualified for positions. It can also create conflict between civilian and sworn counterparts in departments. With respect to mental health providers, these belief systems can generate distrust, given that most mental health professionals have not also served as firefighters. Finally, given the specific laws and ethics of professional psychology, some fire departments may be resistant to their employees being governed by an outside agency, which may challenge traditional organizational processes. These patterns may be understood through system justification theory, which suggests that individuals within structured institutions often defend and rationalize existing norms, even if these norms limit innovation or inclusion (Jost & Banaji, 1994).

Closed systems often classify behavior, whether overtly or subtly, as either acceptable or unacceptable. In turn, these dynamics create a unique culture of how fire department personnel interact with each other and the public. Although societal changes and public standards require agencies to adopt them, fire and emergency services may be resistant and slow to change, given their closed-system nature. This resistance can be linked to cultural lag, where traditional organizational values fail to keep pace with evolving societal norms (Ogburn, 1922).

This dynamic is evident in how firefighters experience and respond to their public image, particularly when operating in contexts unrelated to fire. Park and Fletcher (2018) reported that the U.S. firefighters often experience public confusion over their role when wearing station uniforms outside of emergency settings, resulting in what the authors call a "confused public identity." Firefighters in the study reported feeling misunderstood and encountering safety risks when civilians misinterpreted their presence or authority in public spaces. This misalignment between public perception and occupational identity reinforces the internal culture of fire and emergency services, where strong in-group cohesion and distrust of outside interpretation are common. These findings illustrate how even symbolic elements, such as uniforms, can amplify a firefighter's sense of cultural separation from the broader public and contribute to the defensive preservation of identity norms within the closed system (Park & Fletcher, 2018).

Given the predominance of males in the firefighting profession, traditional masculine cultural views are often amplified, and emotional content is suppressed. Personality traits, although established in early childhood, may be influenced by the traditions of the fire service. Although evidence suggests that emotional intelligence may contribute to mental health and life satisfaction, without acceptance from culture, many firefighters will not have access to this education or the opportunity to develop such skills. The suppression of emotional expression and help-seeking is consistent with research on gender-role socialization, particularly in male-dominated professions, where conformity to masculine norms is associated with greater psychological distress and reduced emotional insight (Addis & Mahalik, 2003; Wong et al., 2017).

In conclusion, just as firefighters may be drawn to fire and emergency services owing to their unique personality traits, they are also influenced by culture. Closed systems establish overt and subtle rules regarding which behaviors are deemed acceptable. Changes in society may take a substantial amount of time to be accepted and adopted within the fire service.

African American Firefighters

Since the inception of the United States, African Americans have faced challenges associated with racism and discrimination. As a microcosm of the greater social context, African Americans within fire and emergency services have had to navigate the complexities of institutional barriers, discriminatory policies, and complicated interpersonal dynamics. The struggle for equality has spanned generations. In 1818, Black citizens in Philadelphia, after being excluded from predominantly White fire departments, created the African Fire Association. This foundational effort and subsequent battles highlight the persistence of racial exclusion and mirror the broader racial tensions in American society (Bonilla-Silva, 1997).

The civil rights movement and subsequent legislation helped secure legal access to public service jobs. However, legal inclusion has not eliminated the lived experience of exclusion. African Americans in fire and emergency services continue to face systemic discrimination, often hidden in hiring practices, promotion opportunities, and workplace culture. A review of modern legal cases reveals repeated claims of discrimination across fire departments nationwide (Varone, 2022a, 2024a). These lawsuits suggest that while overt racism may be less familiar, institutional and aversive forms of racism remain deeply embedded in the culture and policies of some fire agencies (Dovidio & Gaertner, 2000).

One example is Bey v. City of New York, where Black firefighters with Pseudofolliculitis Barbae challenged the department's clean-shave policy. This case highlights how ostensibly neutral policies can disproportionately affect minority employees, particularly when they ignore racial and cultural differences. The case illustrates an how workplace rules can impact racial inequality, even when they appear objective on the surface.

From a social psychology lens, these dynamics are consistent with system justification theory, which posits that advantaged and disadvantaged groups often unconsciously defend the legitimacy of existing social arrangements, even when harmful (Jost & Banaji, 1994). In fire service, this may manifest as resistance to changing traditional policies or challenging long-held norms, especially when change is perceived as undermining group cohesion or authority.

Despite the increased representation of African Americans in fire departments, tokenism often limits their full inclusion. According to Kanter (1977), token members in an organization may be hypervisible yet isolated, excluded from informal networks, and held to different standards. This concept is captured by social identity theory, which suggests that dominant group members (e.g., White male firefighters) may unconsciously protect their in-group status by marginalizing or undermining outgroup members (Tajfel & Turner, 1979). For Black firefighters, this may result in exclusion from meaningful mentorship, internal advancement, and a sense of cultural belonging.

Very few psychological studies have explored the internal emotional experiences of African American firefighters; however, the few that have done so present significant findings. Arbona et al. (2016) explored the intersection of PTSD, depression, and substance use among African American male firefighters. The results revealed that symptoms of emotional numbing and dysphoric arousal were strongly related to depression and alcohol dependence. These findings suggest that racial minority firefighters may experience dual exposure to stress, the traumatic nature of the work itself and the added burden of navigating a workplace where they may not feel entirely accepted.

This dual exposure is further complicated by societal expectations to remain emotionally stoic, particularly in male-dominated professions. African American men in fire and emergency services may feel pressured to suppress emotional expression due to both cultural and professional norms. This experience can make it difficult to access mental health support, further reinforcing psychological distress (Wong et al., 2017).

The experience of African American women firefighters presents another layer of complexity. In their 1997 study, Yoder and Aniakudo reported that Black women in fire and emergency services frequently reported hostility, exclusion, and a lack of mentorship. These women, referred to as "outsiders within," often experience the burden of intersectional discrimination, facing challenges not only in terms of race but also in terms of gender. According to Cole (2009), intersectionality is key to understanding how social structures compound disadvantages for individuals with multiple marginalized identities. This compounded isolation increases stress and potentially limits professional growth and psychological safety.

The social psychology literature suggests that these patterns are not the result of isolated incidents or "bad actors," but part of a broader system that maintains group hierarchies, often unconsciously. As Sidanius and Pratto (1999) explain in social dominance theory, institutions are often organized to preserve the power and status of dominant groups. In fire service, this may mean that long-standing policies, cultural expectations, and informal norms work together to preserve the status quo, even at the cost of equity and inclusion.

Veterans in the Fire Service

Veterans bring extraordinary value to fire and emergency services, offering a wealth of skills, leadership experience, and resilience cultivated through military training and service. Their commitment to missions, teamwork under pressure, and operational discipline align naturally with the demands of emergency response environments. Many veterans embody selfless service and adaptability ethos, which enrich firehouse culture and operational effectiveness. However, the transition from military to civilian first responder roles can also present unique psychological challenges. Experiences of combat exposure, cumulative trauma, and the military's ingrained stoicism around emotional expression may create vulnerabilities when compounded by the stressors of the fire service. Research suggests that firefighters with prior military experience may be at greater risk for mental health challenges than nonveteran firefighters. For example, veterans have reported higher rates of sleep disturbances, depressive symptoms, and posttraumatic stress symptoms (Bartlett et al., 2018). However, the effect sizes in the study were small, indicating that while veteran status may confer elevated risk, these differences are not uniformly predictive of worse outcomes across the board. This suggests the importance of exploring additional factors, such as social support, trauma exposure, and the occupational environment, that may mediate or moderate the mental health outcomes of veterans in fire and emergency services.

A study by Bartlett et al., (2019), focused on occupational stress and functioning in this population. The results indicated that veterans in the fire service group not only reported higher occupational stress but also demonstrated greater levels of functional impairment. Importantly, veteran status serves as a moderator in the relationship between occupational stress and overall functioning, suggesting that while firefighters may be impacted by job stress, veterans may be more susceptible to adverse effects owing to their unique histories and cumulative exposure to trauma.

These findings echo broader concerns raised in a scoping review of PTSD in public safety and military populations. Obuobi-Donkor et al. (2022) found that PTSD in firefighters and military personnel often coexists with other conditions, such as depression and anxiety, and that prior trauma exposure and inadequate social support can exacerbate these outcomes. This dual burden of trauma, both military and occupational, underscores the need for tailored mental health approaches for veterans in fire and emergency services.

Addressing these concerns proactively is critical. Karicofe (2024) advocated for integrated mental health programs that mirror the proactive wellness models used in the military. His research suggested that embedding behavioral health services within the department, offering peer support teams, and incorporating early intervention screening tools can help reduce stigma and promote access to care. These strategies may be particularly effective when adapted to meet the specific needs of veterans, who may already be familiar with structured mental health programs from their military service.

Together, these studies support a growing consensus that veterans in fire and emergency services are a distinct subgroup, resulting in both resilience and vulnerability. Their experiences warrant consideration for policy development, wellness programming, and leadership training. Understanding how veteran identity intersects with fire service culture can help departments better support these individuals while leveraging their strengths.

Women in the Fire Service: A Review of Barriers, Culture, and Mental Health Outcomes

Women have historically been underrepresented in fire and emergency services, despite demonstrating the resilience, courage, and leadership qualities necessary for emergency response professions. Through inclusion, the profession benefits from diverse thought, experience, and problem-solving approaches, which can strengthen organizational adaptability and operational effectiveness. However, the path for women into and through fire and emergency services has been, and remains, marked by significant barriers. Recruitment challenges often begin early, shaped by cultural messaging and societal expectations around gender roles, whereas workplace experiences further influence whether women stay and thrive in the profession. Understanding women's experiences with fire and emergency services is a matter of equity, organizational health, and future sustainability. A comprehensive exploration should include both the factors that encourage women's entry into the field and those that impact their retention and well-being once they are there.

Early Gender Socialization and Career Perception

From a macro cultural perspective, occupational gender stereotypes begin to form at an early age and can contribute to later gender imbalances across various professions. In 2024, researchers in Britain and Argentina conducted a study asking children aged 6–7 years in Britain and 10–11 years in Argentina to draw figures representing various occupations, including dancers, nannies, firefighters, and pilots. The children were interviewed to understand their interpretations of each image's gender. The findings revealed that pronounced gender stereotypes were established in both countries, especially concerning women-dominated occupations. With respect to age, girls appeared to have more rigid gender views than boys did. The results highlight the pervasive and culturally consistent nature of occupational gender stereotypes, which could influence children's future career aspirations (Vivaldi & Rose, 2024).

Question: What is a firefighter?
"A firefighter is a man who has shirts and firefighter helmets, and they squirt water on the fire."
Archer (Age 5)
"A person wears a firefighter suit."
Shelby (Age 3)

Creating a culture that accepts women in the fire service begins long before an adolescent explores career aspirations. Whereas traditional gender expectations have historically limited children's ability to foster personal freedom in career choice, children's literature and educators can create a safe environment for facilitating discussions about gender roles, equity, and the complexities of identity (Lara & Leija, 2014). This concept was captured in a fourth-grade bilingual class, where a teacher, Mr. Paredes, used a book called "Max, the Stubborn Little Wolf" by Marie–Odile Judes to introduce a conversation about whether men, women, or both could choose those careers. The story was about a wolf who aspired to be a florist, whereas his father insisted that he choose a more traditional, masculine role as a hunter. While the students agreed that careers could be accessible to both genders, there was a specific focus on firefighting, which the class decided was "too dangerous and too hard" for women (Lara & Leija, 2014). While this classroom exercise may not be common in classrooms across the country, the theme suggests that children form conclusions about which jobs are appropriate for different genders in elementary school. Therefore, efforts to diversify the workforce must be developed in school-based programs and other fire safety themes.

Koeppel et al. (2022) emphasized the importance of early career encouragement, noting that girls often receive less encouragement to pursue physically demanding or traditionally male-dominated roles. This absence of support can restrict the fire department's talent pipeline, indicating that diverse efforts might start with school-based programs that promote gender equity across all professions.

Historical Overview of Women in Firefighting

Although women remain underrepresented in fire and emergency services today, their contributions span more than two centuries. One of the earliest documented women in the field was Molly Williams, an African American woman who served with Oceanus Engine Company No. 11 in New York City during a severe blizzard in 1818 (Smith, 1978). Her presence on the fire lines during a time of public health crisis and social inequality represented a bold challenge to prevailing gender and racial roles (Moseley, 2017).

In the 1820s, Marina Betts of Pittsburgh also gained recognition for her role in early fire response, actively participating in bucket brigades and compelling male bystanders to assist. Her actions illustrated women's capacity to assert leadership and responsibility during emergencies (Floren, 2002). Similarly, Lillie Hitchcock Coit, a well-known fire supporter in San Francisco during the mid-nineteenth century, attended numerous fire calls and was later honored as an honorary member of Knickerbocker Engine Company No. 5, demonstrating early public acknowledgment of women's contributions (Smith, 1978; Floren, 2002). These accounts are further supported by the U.S. Fire Administration's report Emerging Health and Safety Issues Among Women in the Fire Service (USFA, n.d.), which emphasizes that, despite legal and social constraints, women participated in volunteer fire service in meaningful ways.

The late nineteenth and early twentieth centuries saw sporadic but significant integration of women into fire service roles. In 1895, Carrie Rockefeller became a member of Engine Company No. 1 in West Haven, Connecticut. By 1915, female support roles within volunteer fire company were documented Silver Spring, Maryland, operating for more than a decade and setting a precedent for female involved fire protection (Floren, 2002).

The onset of World War II marked a turning point in women's involvement. In the United Kingdom, the Auxiliary Fire Service (AFS) was established in 1938, and later, the National Fire Service (NFS) brought thousands of women into key support roles, including communications, logistics, and apparatus operation. Although typically not engaged in direct suppression, their work was integral to the country's wartime resilience.

In the United States, women stepped into roles left vacant by enlisted men. At facilities such as the Pearl Harbor Naval Shipyard, women such as Katherine Ah Lan Lowe trained in fire hose operation and equipment handling, supporting military readiness at home (National Park Service, 2023). The American Women's Voluntary Services (AWVS) trained more than 325,000 women for civil defense, including firefighting, ambulance operations, and emergency medical response (Yellin, 2004).

During this period, all-female fire crews were employed at military installations, including Scott Field and the Savanna Ordnance Depot in Illinois. Simultaneously, the U.S. Forest Service and Forest Fire Fighters Service began recruiting women for wildland fire suppression, and all-women crews operated in California and Montana as early as 1942 (Floren, 2002). These developments demonstrated women's ability to meet the physical and operational demands of firefighting, effectively challenging gender-based assumptions. However, academic evidence for long-led all-female support units is sparse; as the U.S. Fire Administration report notes, many "all-female volunteer fire companies" in the 1910s are mentioned in summaries but lack detailed archival or peer-reviewed documentation (USFA, n.d.).

In the postwar era, formal entry points into professional fire service roles expanded. Sandra Forcier was hired in 1973 as a Public Safety Officer in Winston-Salem, North Carolina, becoming one of the first women paid specifically for firefighting duties (Floren, 2002). In 1974, Judith "Judy" Brewer became the first full-time career firefighter in Arlington County, Virginia, a pivotal moment in fire service history (Floren, 2002).

In the late 1970s, additional female trailblazers were observed. Toni McIntosh, hired in 1976, became one of the first African American women in the fire service, joining the Pittsburgh Fire Department. Similarly, Genois Wilson joined the Fort Wayne Fire Department in 1975, where she later developed one of the nation's first fire safety programs for deaf children (Floren, 2002).

A landmark moment came in 1982, when Brenda Berkman, following a successful legal battle, joined the New York City Fire Department (FDNY) alongside the first class of female recruits. This integration into one of the country's largest and most visible departments marked a major advancement in public acceptance and institutional inclusion (Floren, 2002).

Over the ensuing decades, women progressively assumed leadership roles within the fire service. A notable milestone occurred in 2002, when Rosemary Cloud became the first Black woman to serve as a fire chief in the United States, leading the East Point Fire Department in Georgia (Floren, 2002. Presently, federal civil rights legislation prohibits gender-based employment discrimination, providing women with legal protections and enabling their advancement across both urban and rural fire departments.

Despite these advancements, the contributions and experiences of women, especially early pioneers, are still largely absent from the historical record. Documenting and highlighting these accounts is necessary for developing a more accurate and complete history of the fire service and for supporting current efforts to advance equity and diversity in the profession.

Workplace Challenges and Cultural Barriers

Hollerbach et al. (2017) conducted focus groups and interviews with 73 female firefighters across the U.S., identifying six key challenges: exclusion in a male-dominated culture, harassment, injury risks related to ill-fitting gear, inadequate training, and the need to rely on endurance and technique rather than brute strength. These barriers might not only affect operational performance but also potentially hinder both morale and retention.

Sexual harassment remains a pervasive problem in society as a whole and represents a specific challenge in the context of fire and emergency services. According to Hom et al. (2017), 21.7% of female firefighters reported sexual harassment, whereas 20.3% experienced other forms of threats or intimidation. Such behavior can lead to an overall toxic work environment, leading to psychological distress and career dissatisfaction. Yoder and McDonald (1998) reported that women who frequently experienced sexist behavior reported greater workplace stress and felt undervalued by peers. They were also more likely to experience "token stress," a condition associated with being among the few women in a male-dominated workplace.

The IAWFES has identified several institutional barriers, including inadequate facilities, a lack of pregnancy-related policies, and gear designed on the basis of male anatomical standards. Similarly, Park and Langseth-Schmidt (2016) reported that female firefighters reported significantly lower satisfaction with the fit and comfort of their uniform pants, which had a negative effect on their performance. These design issues affect safety and contribute to feelings of exclusion and marginalization.

Gender-Specific Psychological Variables

Mental health is a critical yet often overlooked aspect of the well-being of female firefighters. Stanley et al. (2017) investigated the relationship between PTSD symptoms and suicide risk, identifying cognitive anxiety sensitivity (AS) as a major contributor. Women with higher levels of cognitive AS were more likely to report suicidal ideation and behavior. A follow-up study revealed that suicidal ideation increased significantly after women entered the fire service, indicating the psychological toll of their professional experiences.

Hom et al. (2018) reported that exposure to suicide among peers was strongly correlated with increased psychiatric symptoms. With respect to females, women who reported the death of a colleague by suicide presented higher levels of depression and anxiety. These findings underscore the need for proactive mental health resources tailored specifically for female firefighters.

Haddock et al. (2017) explored substance use among female firefighters and reported that nearly 40% engaged in binge drinking. Research has indicated that problem drinking is linked to higher rates of both posttraumatic stress and depression, as well as increased injury rates and reluctance to recommend the profession to other women. Similarly, Gulliver et al. (2019) reported that women's alcohol consumption increased over time, with higher rates of binge drinking by the end of their third year of service.

Reproductive Health Concerns

Reproductive health is another area where gender disparities manifest. Jung et al. (2021) conducted a comprehensive study on miscarriage risk among female firefighters and reported that they had a 2.33 times higher age-standardized incidence of miscarriage than nurses did. The risk was particularly high among volunteer and wildland firefighters. Factors such as shift schedules, fire exposure, and physically demanding duties contributed to these outcomes.

The lack of formal policies addressing reproductive health and pregnancy in many fire departments further exacerbates these risks. IAWFES has called for improved disclosure protocols and policy updates to provide accommodations and protection for pregnant firefighters. Without these measures, women may feel compelled to hide pregnancies or leave the profession entirely after becoming pregnant.

Representation, Leadership, and Media Influence

The leadership culture within fire departments often fails to recognize or support the contributions of women. Bendersky (2012) argues that the firefighter archetype should be redefined to include qualities such as empathy, communication, and collaboration, which are often socially coded as feminine. Support for diverse policies increases when these traits are recognized as key components of effective firefighting.

Media representation plays a role in the conceptualization of women in the firefighting profession. While many may believe that there is value in acknowledging women who are the first to serve a particular function within the firefighter ranks, Pompper (2021), from a media-studies perspective, suggests coverage that spotlights 'firsts' can unintentionally reinforce tokenism. Applying that lens to firefighting media helps explain how narratives may create the perception that women are exceptions rather than peers. This framing may contribute to the public perception that women are less capable or deserving of their roles. If there is a critique of the work, the focus becomes more on the gender of the individual rather than the work itself.

In wildland firefighting, informal workplace dynamics often reinforce deeply embedded gender inequities. These dynamics include unspoken norms, social rituals, and interpersonal interactions that may appear neutral but subtly uphold a masculine culture. Eriksen (2019) reported that women in these settings frequently rely on humor as a coping mechanism to navigate everyday challenges and tensions. While humor can serve as a form of resistance and solidarity, it also tends to obscure underlying discrimination, making it harder to confront exclusionary behaviors directly. This dynamic can inadvertently normalize sexist attitudes and reinforce patriarchal norms, as women may feel pressured to "go along to get along" rather than challenge problematic conduct.

In addition, Reimer and Eriksen (2018) reported that female leaders in such environments often face skepticism about their authority and capabilities. They are caught in a double bind: efforts to increase gender diversity in leadership are sometimes perceived as compromising competence, leading to a false dichotomy between merit and inclusion. As a result, women leaders may be viewed as symbolic or token appointments, regardless of their qualifications, and must continuously prove their legitimacy in ways that their male counterparts do not. These intersecting dynamics (informal cultural expectations and structural biases) create significant barriers to full inclusion and equitable advancement for women in wildland firefighting.

Furthermore, union contracts play an often unseen but practical role in shaping how workers balance the competing demands of their professional and personal lives. With respect to female firefighters, these contracts often reflect dominant gender norms within a profession. In a comparative study of nurses and firefighters, Crocker and Clawson (2012) reported that firefighter contracts, shaped within a male-dominated occupation, tend to emphasize equitable access to overtime and fairness in scheduling rather than prioritizing work–life balance. In contrast, nurse contracts, which reflect caregiving responsibilities more typically in a female-dominated field, include detailed provisions for vacation time, mandatory overtime limits, and predictable schedules. As a result, the firefighter contract structure reinforces a breadwinner model that supports uninterrupted full-time labor, placing women at a disadvantage when balancing caregiving responsibilities (often gender normed in society as a whole) and professional obligations (Crocker & Clawson, 2012).

This structural imbalance may contribute to the higher divorce and stress rates observed among female firefighters. As women in the fire service juggle the same high-risk, trauma-exposed roles as their male counterparts do, they often do so without the contractual support that accommodates family responsibilities. The lack of flexibility in scheduling and the absence of protection against excessive overtime can exacerbate family strain and burnout, particularly for individuals with caregiving responsibilities at home. Given the gendered assumptions of union negotiations, female firefighters may feel marginalized or underrepresented, which can contribute to lower retention and job satisfaction (Crocker & Clawson, 2012). These findings underscore the need for more inclusive labor policies that reflect the diverse needs of the workforce and actively promote work-life balance for different genders.

Broader Implications for EMS and Policy Development

Rudman et al. (2023) conducted a comprehensive scoping review of diversity and inclusion within the EMS workforce, revealing persistent underrepresentation of women and minority groups in key areas such as leadership roles, equitable compensation, and opportunities for advancement. These structural disparities not only reflect ongoing gender and racial inequities but also contribute to a workplace culture that may hinder the retention and progression of underrepresented individuals.

The review underscores the necessity of evidence-based policy development to support recruitment, retention, and the cultivation of a more inclusive professional environment.

However, policy reform alone is insufficient without attention to the social dynamics that affect employee well-being. Craig and Jacobs (1985) reported that women often rely on close, same-sex friendships and familial relationships as sources of emotional support during periods of psychological distress, with reciprocal support being a critical factor in maintaining mental health. This suggests that beyond formal policy change, workplace interventions should also incorporate structured peer-support networks. By institutionalizing these systems within EMS departments, organizations can provide accessible, culturally attuned mental health resources that reflect the ways in which women tend to seek and sustain emotional support.

Together, these findings point to the importance of addressing both structural and interpersonal dimensions of inclusion. Effective strategies must go beyond representation and equity metrics to foster environments where women not only advance but also feel supported, connected, and psychologically safe.

The lived experiences of women in fire and emergency services are complex and multifaceted. As Felicia and Mau (2022) illustrate through literary analysis, cultural narratives often reinforce patriarchal themes, contributing to emotional suppression and professional isolation. This psychological burden can deter women from remaining in the profession, exacerbating the retention issue.

The underrepresentation of women in fire and emergency services is not a reflection of their ability but rather the result of deeply embedded cultural, institutional, and psychological barriers. From early gender socialization to workplace discrimination, inadequate gear, mental health risks, and reproductive health challenges, women face a multitude of obstacles throughout their careers. Research indicates that these barriers are not only unjust but also detrimental to workplace safety, team cohesion, and public trust. Notably, studies have shown that psychological safety and diversity are critical factors that enhance team learning, efficacy, and overall performance, underscoring the importance of inclusive and supportive work environments (Edmondson, 1999; Fyhn et al., 2023).

Addressing these challenges requires a coordinated, multilevel approach. Policy reforms should encompass inclusive training practices, reproductive health protocols, accessible mental health resources, and family-supportive workplace policies. However, meaningful change also depends on leadership that is actively committed to equity, representation, and accountability. Recruitment efforts must start early—long before the academy—by introducing gender-equitable narratives in schools and reshaping perceptions about who belongs in the fire service. Ultimately, diversity is not only a moral imperative but also a practical imperative. An inclusive fire service is more adaptable, more effective, and better equipped to serve the diverse communities that rely on it.

Firefighter Personality

It has become increasingly common for people to combine police and fire department personnel into a single unit, often referred to as first responders. With this combination, it is assumed that police and fire personnel are similar in terms of skills, abilities, personality characteristics, community relationships, and duties. As a result, mental health resources are often provided via a "one-size-fits-all" approach. Without recognition, there are distinct differences between these groups; mental health providers are not given the tools necessary to understand the unique needs of firefighters or their families, and the recipients of the services are not provided with adequate and specialized care. Psychological research on firefighters is limited, and there is a notable lack of representation from the field of psychology within fire departments across the United States. However, the need for psychological services has become increasingly apparent; owing to the delay in research studies, fire service psychology lags behind advances made with military and police populations.

The American Psychological Association (APA) recognizes personality as individual differences in patterns of thinking, feeling, and behaving. The study of personality focuses on variations in individual characteristics and how these characteristics combine to form an individual's personality. Little research has been conducted on the personality profiles of firefighters, and much of what is available has been conducted overseas. A person's personality is formed in childhood and reinforced by the environment until a specific navigation strategy is established. Individuals within systems can form group personality dynamics, also known as cultural norms, which influence how group members ultimately behave.

Occupational choice frameworks have shown that personality influences person–job fit, successful job performance, and work role functioning (Tokar et al., 1998). Therefore, personality can be responsible for an individual's pursuit of the firefighter profession and for how successfully the person performs his or her duties. In 1990, Mitchell and Bray proposed that emergency personnel choose their career because they have significantly different personalities than the general population does. Specifically, they suggested that first responders have a high need for stimulation, engage in frequent risk-taking behavior, are highly dedicated, and feel compelled to assist others (Mitchell & Bray, 1990). However, research regarding the "rescue personality" has provided mixed results.

Studies assessing firefighter personalities frequently utilize a measure called the NEO (Neuroticism–Extraversion–Openness to Experience) Personality Inventory (NEO-PI-R; Costa & McCrae, 2008), a 240-item self-report measure of the five-factor domains of personality. Specifically, this measure explores rates of neuroticism, extraversion, openness to experience, agreeableness, and conscientiousness. Six subscales, within each of the five factors, assess more specific facets of each domain (Costa & McCrae, 2008). With respect to neuroticism, the aspects of anxiety, anger/hostility, depression, self-consciousness, impulsiveness, and vulnerability are explored. In the domain of Extraversion, the NEO-PI-R identifies six facets: warmth, gregariousness, assertiveness, activity, excitement-seeking, and positive emotions. The Openness to Experience factor includes the facets of fantasy, aesthetics, feelings, actions, ideas, and values. For Agreeableness, the six facets are trust, straightforwardness, altruism, compliance, modesty, and tender-mindedness. Finally, the domain factor of conscientiousness includes competence, order, dutifulness, achievement striving, self-discipline, and deliberation.

One study investigating Mitchell's description of the personality of a first responder did not support the "rescue personality" hypothesis (Wagner, S. L. et al., 2009). Two groups, one comprising paid firefighters and the other comprising a random sample, reported similar levels of characteristic openness to experience, characteristic conscientiousness, type A behavior (dominance), and tolerance for risk-taking behavior (Wagner et al., 2009). In the same study, firefighters reported higher levels of characteristic extraversion than did the comparison group (Wagner et al., 2009). Another study that explored the personality profiles and psychophysiological response patterns of police and firefighter recruits (Salters-Pedneault, K. et al., 2010) found that police recruits scored higher on gregariousness, dutifulness, deliberation, and facets of conscientiousness than their firefighter counterparts did (Salters-Pedneault et al., 2010). Both police officers and firefighters scored higher on excitement-seeking, a facet of extraversion, than did the general population (Salters-Pedneault et al., 2010). In this study, physiologically, firefighters presented higher heart rates and skin conductance (SC) levels than did the general population and police recruits did (Salters-Pedneault et al., 2010).

Many fire departments offer emergency medical services (EMS). However, not all EMS providers serve in a firefighting capacity. Private agencies, other than fire departments, may offer ambulatory services, depending on the service location. Additionally, the frequency of EMS calls among fire personnel may vary depending on the agency's location and population density. Therefore, a study exploring the "rescue personality" of the EMS profile may or may not apply to firefighters, depending on their agency. This study aimed to investigate the personalities of EMS providers via the NEO-PI-R with a sample of 171 EMS providers. The findings revealed that they scored lower on neuroticism and openness but higher on conscientiousness, risk-taking, and competition-seeking than did a normative sample (Klee, S., & Renner, K., 2013). The study also revealed that EMS personnel had lower agreeableness scores and no differences in extraversion (Klee, S., & Renner, K., 2013). Tenure was not associated with personality, except for extraversion, which preliminarily supports a predisposition model. There were no significant differences between participants who were volunteers and those who were career EMS providers (Klee, S., & Renner, K., 2013).

Historically, the personality profile of firefighters has been minimally examined in professional psychology. In 1956, a psychological research study was used to explore the validity of the Minnesota Multiphasic Personality Inventory (MMPI) Scales of responsibility and dominance. Those scales are no longer included in the updated versions of the MMPI. However, the findings at the time reflected that each scale failed to yield mean values for male firefighters. However, the study demonstrated that the mean values of the MMPI responsibility and dominance items were slightly higher than those obtained from the original sample of high school and college students (Olmsted, D. W., & Monachesi, E. D., 1956). In 2001, Liao et al. examined 171 firefighters over a 12-year period to assess the correlates of incentives between demographic, personality, and economic variables and workplace injuries. When these findings are considered, distinguishing between the duration of an injury and the occurrence of an injury is essential. Research suggests that female firefighters are more likely to be injured on the job than male firefighters are, and those injuries are correlated with the MMPI scales Conversion Hysteria, Psychopathic Deviance, and Social Introversion (Liao et al., 2001b). Demographically, injury duration is significantly correlated with age, tenure, marital status, type of injury, gender, and wage variables (Liao et al., 2001b). There also appeared to be an interaction effect between marital status and gender. Finally, the MMPI-2 scale for psychopathic deviation and schizophrenia are significantly related to injury duration (Liao et al., 2001b).

The MMPI-3 has been increasingly applied in the psychological evaluation of firefighter candidates, exploring behavioral and emotional risk factors relevant to public safety work. In a study by Whitman et al. (2023), MMPI-3 scores from 237 firefighter applicants were analyzed in conjunction with psychosocial history data to assess their predictive validity in pre-employment evaluations. The study revealed that the MMPI-3 scale was significantly associated with key clinical concerns such as impulse control, substance use, and interpersonal functioning, issues that are particularly pertinent to the demands of firefighting. Interestingly, firefighter candidates tended to present lower and less variable MMPI-3 scores than did the general population, reflecting a potential self-favorability bias common in high-stakes assessments (Whitman et al., 2023). These findings support the practical utility of the MMPI-3 in identifying candidates requiring further evaluation or support before entering the fire service.

In Korea, job stress and posttraumatic stress disorder (PTSD) were examined via the MMPI-2 and medical surveillance over 5 years. Findings have suggested that greater age and job duration are related to higher rates of PTSD. However, it is possible that age and job duration are directly related to the amount of cumulative trauma exposure. With respect to the MMPI-2, higher PTSD risk was associated with higher scores on the masculinity–femininity scale and social introversion for both high and low job stress levels. These findings may suggest that adherence to traditional gender norms, specifically related to emotionality, may increase the risk for PTSD.

With respect to the relationship between burnout and PTSD, research suggests that symptoms may vary depending on personality traits (Jo et al., 2018). Specifically, one study conducted in South Korea revealed that burnout was a significant predictor of PTSD symptoms. In general, having a sense of calling for firefighting may be considered positive (Jo et al., 2018). However, research suggests that the more a firefighter feels compelled to perform his or her duties, the greater the risk for PTSD if they are burned out or exhausted (Jo et al., 2018). If a firefighter is burned out, their sense of calling for work should not be encouraged (Jo et al., 2018).

In efforts to understand occupational burnout among firefighters in France, some researchers have taken a closer look into the “Big Five” personality traits (openness, conscientiousness, extroversion, agreeableness, and neuroticism), occupational burnout, and the mediating role of achievement goals in this relationship (Vaulerin, J. et al., 2016). Note that a person's intrinsic motivation characteristically defines mastery approach goals, whereas mastery avoidance is particularly related to extrinsic motivation strategies. The findings revealed that neuroticism was positively correlated with three dimensions of burnout, both directly and through mastery avoidance goals (Vaulerin, J. et al., 2016). Additionally, research has suggested that mastery approach goals mediate the relationships between physical fatigue and conscientiousness, as well as between openness to experience and physical fatigue (Vaulerin, J. et al., 2016).

To understand neuroticism within the firefighter personality, one study explored a group of Greek firefighters to understand the psychological consequences of a 2007 wildfire, which led to 43 fatalities, including 3 firefighters (Psarros et al., 2018). These firefighters were interviewed and asked to complete various questionnaires and inventories. The findings indicated that 18.6% of the firefighters met the diagnostic criteria for PTSD. Specifically, fear of dying during a fire and insomnia, as well as increased neuroticism and depression, increase the likelihood of PTSD (Psarros et al., 2018). Among those studied, career firefighters had a 70% lower likelihood of developing PTSD than did seasonal employees (Psarros et al., 2018).

Emotional expression, as it relates to the "Big Five" personality trait of openness, may be culturally influenced by fire and emergency services. Specifically, the hypermasculinity of firefighter culture does not promote the exploration of emotional content. Despite the high-stress nature of the work, the understanding of the role of social interaction and emotional perception within firefighter populations remains limited (Farnsworth, J. K., & Sewell, K.W., 2011). One study conducted in the United States revealed that fear of emotion was the strongest individual predictor of PTSD and a moderator of the relationship between PTSD symptoms and social interactions (Farnsworth & Sewell, 2011).

A study conducted in Croatia explored a group of firefighters' psychological responses to stress via instruments such as the COPE questionnaire, the Perceived Stress Scale (PSS-10), the State-Trait Anxiety Inventory (STAI-X1 for anxiety as a condition and the STAI-X2 for anxiety as a personality trait), and the Beck Depression Inventory (Lalić et al., 2007). These findings suggest that firefighters do not experience significant adverse stress effects. While the urban firefighters experienced slight state anxiety, medium trait anxiety was persistently observed across the different groups. While depression levels were significantly different between the groups, they were not significantly different from those of the general population. Ultimately, this research revealed that firefighters have a certain amount of "working anxiety," which may be intrinsic to their personality and may allow for optimal functioning within challenging work environments (Lalić et al., 2007).

In conclusion, further research into the personality structure of firefighters may provide valuable insights into ways to prevent adverse psychological outcomes. This information may also assist with recruitment efforts to create a more diverse workforce within the fire service. Finally, with a better understanding of the personality traits that contribute to pursuing and maintaining a career in fire and emergency services, treatment providers can become more culturally competent and provide better care to this population.

Family Considerations in the Fire Service

The consequences of cumulative trauma exposure, vicarious trauma, ambiguous loss, and transitions appear to be significant challenges for firefighters, as they create and maintain intimate partner relationships and families. However, research suggests that male firefighters are divorced at a similar rate to men in the general population (Haddock et al., 2016b). Statistics concerning the marriage and divorce rates among firefighters in the United States indicate that 45% of male and 64.3% of female firefighters between the ages of 19 and 29 have never been married. The same study revealed that 77% of male firefighters are married, whereas 57.5% of men in the general population are married. On the other hand, 42.6% of female firefighters are currently married, whereas 55.4% of the general female population is married. The divorce rates indicate that 11.8% of the male firefighters are currently divorced, whereas 9.4% of the men in the general population are divorced. Compared with women in the general population, female firefighters are statistically more likely to be divorced at a rate of 32.1%, which reflects a rate of 10.4%. One-fourth of the firefighters in the study reported having been divorced at some point. Among married firefighters, the divorce rate was higher for females (27.3%) than for males (19.6%). When all firefighters were examined, the prevalence of ever having been divorced was substantially greater among female firefighters (40%) than among male firefighters (24.4%) (Haddock et al., 2016b).

Many fire departments maintain a system where firefighters work 24-h shifts. During this time, they should adhere to the social demands of the firehouse, manage the duty of incidents, whether fire-related or emergency medical, and respond to an unpredictable and increasingly frequent call volume. The transition from firefighters to civilians can pose challenges for family life. One of these considerations may be the transfer of firefighters' reactions to dangerous and traumatic events to their families. A study conducted in New South Wales with volunteer firefighters reported that 56% had been seriously threatened at some point in their careers, with 26% experiencing the threat within the past year (Bryant & Harvey, 1995). Another study conducted in Australia reported that 85% of firefighters reported having been exposed to one critical Incident within the last two months including mass casualties, deaths, and direct exposure to bodily harm (MacDermid et al., 2019). Canadian public safety personnel experience regular exposure to potentially traumatic events including violence, threats of violence, fires, explosions, and are at higher risk of developing subsequent mental health disorders (Carleton et al., 2018a, 2018b). These cumulative exposures can pose unique challenges, as these stressors can spill over into other aspects of their lives.

Few studies have explored the relationship between job stress and the quality of marital interactions. According to police samples, studies indicate that job stress can cause spouses to feel more negatively toward the relationship (Roberts & Levenson, 2001). Research on couples within a community sample has shown that emotional exhaustion and negative emotional states are often associated with a partner reporting higher levels of family conflict (Bodenmann et al., 2007). Furthermore, when report experiencing higher levels of job stress, their wives spouses often exhibit greater levels of autonomic arousal during conversation (Levenson, 2001).

The evidence suggests that job stress related to the firefighting profession may have a direct effect on the health of their children, their partners, and their marital satisfaction. Pfefferbaum et al. (2002) explored posttraumatic stress symptoms experienced by the wives of firefighters involved in the 1995 Oklahoma City bombing. Fifty percent of these women reported bomb-related PTSD symptoms, 37% reported permanent changes in their relationship, and 7% reported temporary changes in their relationship related to the bombing (Pfefferbaum et al., 2002). Another study assessed traumatic stress in the children of emergency medical technicians who were involved in rescue efforts during the September 11, New York Twin Tower bombing. The findings suggested that 18.9% of the children had a high prevalence of probable PTSD (Duarte et al., 2006).

According to family stress theory, stress and distress occur when internal or external events disrupt the family's equilibrium. The level of stress a family experiences depends on several factors, including how they manage boundaries and roles, how they communicate, how they perceive and interpret the event, the meaning they assign to the situation, the resources available to them, their coping strategies, and how family members interact with one another (Boss et al., 2016). Ambiguous loss occurs when there is uncertainty about a person's presence or absence in the family system. Importantly, this loss describes an incongruence between a family member's physical status in the family and their psychological presence. It can be experienced within firefighter families when a significant incident occurs and when the family is unsure of whether the firefighter is safe. Ambiguous loss can also occur if the firefighter is present but unable to engage emotionally or perform typical functions. Ambiguous loss can create ambivalent feelings toward the individual and a sense of detachment (Boss et al., 2016).

A healthy family transition into a firefighter culture and lifestyle involves good work-family fit. Families are typically satisfied and adapt when there is a balance between the demands and rewards of the work environment. These factors include consideration of work hours, financial benefits, social status, emotional and physical demands, management support for family responsibilities, and the capacities and needs/motivations of individuals within the family and family unit. Threats to this work-family fit include persistently high stress levels, traumatic situations, and poor organizational commitment to employees. Greene and Hendershot (2017) found that the satisfaction of volunteer firefighters is related to whether their role and reward expectations align with the realities of the of the organizational behavior of the agencies they work for.

Couples where one or more partners are in the firefighter profession face unique challenges, as the firefighter may be exposed to stressful life events. Therefore, individuals and their families should utilize effective coping strategies (Cutrona,

1996). To support firefighters and their families, a study was conducted to test the validity of the Couple Resilience Inventory among married or cohabiting firefighters (Sanford et al., 2017). This instrument measures relationship behavior in relation to a couple's ability to cope with employment in a stressful occupation (Sanford et al., 2017). The findings suggested that the measure was consistent with the theoretical model and supported instrument validity (Sanford et al., 2017).

Conclusion

Firefighter development is a dynamic and multifaceted process shaped by personal, organizational, cultural, and systemic factors. From initial motivations rooted in altruism, identity, or societal adulation to the evolving internalization of group norms and occupational identity, firefighters undergo profound transformations throughout their careers. These transformations are influenced not only by exposure to trauma and operational stressors but also by the institutional structures and social narratives that define the fire service. As demonstrated across gender, race, veteran status, and family dynamics, these influences intersect with broader systems of inclusion, identity, and psychological health. Structural inequities, traditional norms, and resistance to cultural change continue to shape the lived experiences of many people within fire and emergency services, often at the expense of psychological safety, professional equity, and relational stability. Recognizing these influences and incorporating interdisciplinary, culturally competent, and evidence-based practices will foster resilience, promote inclusive leadership, and sustain a healthy, diverse, and effective workforce. As the profession continues to evolve, a more holistic understanding of firefighter development, one that values prevention as much as heroism and reflection as much as action, will be critical to the long-term vitality of both individuals and the communities they serve.

Chapter Review—Assignment: Clinical Case Scenario: "Assistant Chief's Medical Retirement"

Learning Objectives

By the end of this activity, students will be able to:

- Analyze the psychological impact of occupational identity development in the fire service using relevant social and clinical theories.
- Evaluate the influence of cultural, structural, and systemic factors (e.g., closed systems, gender norms, racial identity) on the mental health and well-being of firefighters.
- Apply trauma-informed and culturally responsive frameworks to assess presenting problems in a first responder clinical scenario.

- Propose appropriate interventions and supports, including individual, systemic, and policy-level recommendations, for clients in fire/emergency services.
- Reflect on their own assumptions, biases, and clinical considerations when working with clients from high-stress, closed-system professions.

Client: Captain Marcus Davis, age 48, African American, recently medically retired after 25 years in the fire service.

Referral Reason: Marcus was referred to therapy by his primary care physician due to symptoms of depression, irritability, and difficulty sleeping following his recent retirement. He describes "feeling lost" and says he is unsure how to define himself now that he's no longer a firefighter.

Background: Marcus joined the fire department at 23, motivated by a desire to serve his community and to find a structured path following a childhood marked by family instability and exposure to violence. He excelled in his early years, earning respect from his peers and eventually rising to the rank of Assistant Chief. He was known for his dedication and leadership during high-intensity calls. Marcus also served two tours in Iraq prior to becoming a firefighter.

Throughout his career, Marcus experienced multiple traumatic events, including the loss of a close colleague in a structural collapse, responding to child fatalities, and witnessing a civilian suicide. He coped by "pushing through," staying physically active, and taking on extra shifts. Over time, he became a mentor to younger firefighters and took pride in maintaining the "brotherhood."

Two years ago, Marcus sustained a serious back injury while responding to a wildland fire. Despite multiple surgeries and physical therapy, he was unable to return to duty and was medically retired.

Presenting Issues:

- Marcus reports intense sadness, emotional numbness, and difficulty connecting with his family.
- He avoids former coworkers and has not attended any department events since retirement.
- He admits he drinks nightly to help with sleep.
- Marcus says he feels "forgotten" and worries his identity as a firefighter is slipping away.
- He expresses confusion about his role in his family, especially with his teenage son who is beginning to rebel.

Identity and Role Transition:

- How might Marcus' sense of self have been shaped by fire service culture?
- What challenges arise when a strong occupational identity is suddenly lost?

Cultural and Systemic Influences:

- How might Marcus' experiences as a Black firefighter and veteran have intersected with organizational culture and expectations?
- In what ways might his experiences reflect aspects of social identity theory or system justification theory?

Mental Health and Coping:

- How might Marcus' current symptoms relate to cumulative trauma exposure?
- What are potential protective factors and vulnerabilities tied to his coping style?

Family and Social Dynamics:

- How might the chief's occupational stress and identity loss affect his relationships at home?
- Are there any connections between this case and the concepts of ambiguous loss and family stress theory?

Treatment Planning:

- What culturally responsive strategies would you consider in helping Marcus rebuild identity and purpose outside the fire service?
- How might you approach his alcohol use, emotional suppression, and social isolation?

Review the Clinical Case Vignette Read the provided firefighter case study. Note the client's presenting concerns, career timeline, demographic background, and any relevant psychosocial or cultural dynamics.

Case Conceptualization (15–20 min)

- In small groups or individually, identify at least three psychological or social development themes from this chapter reflected in the case (e.g., role theory, ambiguous loss, trauma exposure, identity disruption).
- Use at least one theory (e.g., Social Identity Theory, System Justification Theory, or Cultural Lag) to interpret the client's symptoms or worldview.

Clinical Application (10–15 min)

- Identify key mental health concerns and risk factors presented in the case.
- Propose 1–2 potential therapeutic goals or interventions (e.g., EMDR for trauma, psychoeducation on ambiguous loss, culturally attuned narrative therapy).
- Consider how you would build rapport with considerations for the client's profession, culture, and identity.

Group Debrief/Reflection (10 min)

- Share takeaways with peers or submit a brief written reflection.
- Reflection: What assumptions might clinicians make about firefighters? How can we challenge these while providing effective, ethical care?

Chapter 3
Understanding Psychology and Its Application to the Fire Service

Psychology offers valuable insights into human behavior, emotional resilience, and decision-making under stress, which are key factors in working in fire and emergency services. However, despite its long-standing role in military and law enforcement communities, psychology remains underutilized and often misunderstood within the firefighting community. Historically, fire departments have relied on psychological insights drawn from other professions without fully accounting for the cultural, operational, and emotional complexities unique to fire and emergency service professions. The intentional application of psychological principles can facilitate effective trauma response, while also enhancing resilience, improving operational performance, and supporting sustained well-being throughout a firefighter's career. A precise understanding of the occupational hazards faced by firefighters, the culturally embedded coping mechanisms within firehouse settings, and the systemic barriers to accessing mental health resources is imperative for informing effective support strategies and policy development. By adapting psychological science to the specific demands of firefighting, fire and emergency services can lead to a stronger, safer, and more sustainable future for generations.

Fire service and EMS providers operate across local, regional, and national systems; however, the U.S. Fire Service lacks centralized regulatory authority. The U.S. Fire Administration focuses primarily on data collection, public education, research, and training initiatives, whereas standard setting remains the responsibility of local jurisdictions. Major fire service organizations, collectively known as the "Nine Sisters," advocate for the profession at the federal level; however, the psychology field remains notably underrepresented in these efforts. Although psychology is well regulated, its targeted integration into fire and emergency services remains unexplored, mainly raising ethical concerns when unvalidated psychological practices across fire and emergency medical service agencies are applied. While the National Fire Protection Association (NFPA) issues necessary operational standards, it does not have jurisdiction over psychological health and wellness practices. Recognizing fire service psychology as a national stakeholder is a necessary step for

K. Wheldon, *Fire Service Psychology*,
https://doi.org/10.1007/978-3-032-02126-7_3

advancing mental health support, ensuring adherence to ethical and legal standards, mitigating risk, enhancing performance, and promoting the overall well-being of fire service personnel.

Occupational Exposure

In 2020, fire departments across the United States responded to 26,959,000 incidents (U.S. Fire Administration [USFA], 2022). Notably, the majority of these calls, 64%, involved emergency medical services (EMS) and rescue operations, whereas only 4% were fire related. Residential properties were the most common setting for fire department responses, accounting for 55% of all incidents. Among these residential calls, 70% required EMS or rescue services, and only 3% involved active fires. Other significant categories included good intent calls (12%), false alarms (8%), and service-related calls (8%) (U.S. Fire Administration [USFA], 2022).

Temporal patterns in incident types revealed additional nuances. Fire-related calls were most frequent on Saturdays, whereas severe weather-related incidents peaked on Tuesdays and Thursdays. Monthly trends indicated heightened demand during January and July, with a noticeable drop in April (U.S. Fire Administration [USFA], 2022). Regionally, fire departments in the southern United States handled the most significant volume of calls (40%), reflecting the region's population distribution. Although EMS and rescue runs dominated nationally, the Northeast reported a lower percentage (50%) than other regions, partly because some fire departments in that area focus more strictly on traditional fire suppression roles. Aid-related calls accounted for 8% of all fire department runs, with mutual or automatic aid being more common in response to fires than to other incident types. Well-structured mutual aid agreements and practical collaboration help improve resource distribution and strengthen emergency response efforts (U.S. Fire Administration [USFA], 2022).

Exploring psychology within the context of firefighting operations highlights how both external circumstances and internal cognitive processes shape outcomes, whether through the strategic coordination of emergency responses or the navigation of shared emotional experiences. The frequency and nature of incidents play a critical role in influencing psychological responses, affecting not only individual resilience but also the collective performance and cohesion of teams operating under pressure.

Psychological Risk Factors for Occupational Exposure

Public safety personnel (PSPs), including police officers, firefighters, and paramedics, face heightened psychological risks due to routine exposure to potentially traumatic events. While it is well established that adverse childhood experiences (ACEs) contribute to poor mental health outcomes later in life, the specific mechanisms underlying this relationship remain poorly understood, particularly within public safety professionals (Roth et al., 2022). Chronic occupational exposures compound these vulnerabilities, increasing susceptibility to disorders such as posttraumatic stress disorder (PTSD), depression, and anxiety.

Recent research by Roth et al. (2022) sheds important light on this relationship by identifying moral injury (MI) and emotion regulation as key factors. In a study involving 294 Canadian and American PSPs between the ages of 22 and 65, participants completed self-report measures assessing ACEs, emotion regulation difficulties, and a range of adult mental health symptoms, including PTSD, dissociation, depression, stress, and anxiety. The participants also completed the Moral Injury Assessment for Public Safety Personnel, a tool specifically designed for the population's unique occupational experiences. Path analysis revealed that ACEs significantly predict adult psychopathology, with MI mediating this relationship and emotion regulation moderating it. In other words, higher levels of ACEs were linked to greater mental health symptoms, mainly through the development of moral injury. Moreover, strong emotion regulation skills served as a protective factor (Roth et al., 2022). This study is notable for being the first to demonstrate MI as a bridge connecting early adversity to later psychological distress in PSP, offering critical implications for targeted interventions.

Complementary findings from other studies underscore the complexity of this vulnerability. Haim-Nachum and Levy-Gigi (2021) investigated how cognitive flexibility, specifically, the ability to update negative associations in light of positive experiences, moderates PTSD symptom development following adult trauma exposure. In a sample of firefighters, individuals with diminished updating capacity presented stronger links between ACEs and PTSD symptoms, suggesting that an inability to reframe or adjust to previous negative experiences exacerbates psychological risk (Haim-Nachum & Levy-Gigi, 2021). Importantly, those who struggle to integrate positive corrective experiences into their worldviews remain more vulnerable to PTSD when confronted with new trauma.

These findings highlight a critical intersection between developmental history, occupational exposure, and psychological processing skills. Among PSP, early adversity sets a foundation of risk. Nevertheless, moral injury and deficits in emotion regulation and cognitive updating significantly shape whether this risk manifests as mental health symptoms later in life (Roth et al., 2022; (Haim-Nachum & Levy-Gigi, 2021). Understanding these mediating and moderating factors provides a more precise roadmap for future research and intervention efforts aimed at protecting the psychological health of trauma-exposed workers.

Identified Psychological Needs

Firefighters face various psychological challenges shaped by occupational and relational factors. Recent research has highlighted the importance of relationship satisfaction with mental health outcomes among firefighters. In a study involving 200 married or cohabiting firefighters, Zegel et al. (2024) reported that those reporting dissatisfaction in their romantic relationships presented significantly higher levels of all measured mental health symptoms. Using the Couples Satisfaction Index-4 with a cutoff score of 13.5, the study demonstrated that relational strain can amplify psychological vulnerability within this population (Zegel et al., 2024).

In addition to relational factors, firefighters are at substantial risk for psychological maladaptation through pathways such as burnout, compassion fatigue, and vicarious trauma. While much of the existing research uses quantitative methods to document these outcomes, Stout and Kostamo (2021) adopted a qualitative approach, employing photovoice as a digital storytelling tool to explore firefighters' lived experiences. In their study of seven firefighters from a large metropolitan department, participants submitted photographs and engaged in open-ended interviews, offering insights into the psychological landscape of their careers (Stout & Kostamo, 2021).

Two main themes emerged from their narratives. The first contributors to stress included traumatic incident exposure and the cumulative effects of sleep deprivation and fatigue from shift work. The second, stress mitigation, highlighted firefighters' reliance on mentoring relationships, therapeutic interactions with dogs, and lifestyle practices, such as exercise, adrenaline-driven activities, and striving for a work–life balance (Stout & Kostamo, 2021). These findings emphasize the importance of proactive stress management strategies and suggest that fire departments could reevaluate operational factors, such as shift scheduling, while fostering environments that support healthy coping mechanisms (Stout & Kostamo, 2021).

These studies illustrate that psychological wellness among firefighters is influenced not only by the inherent stresses of the job but also by the strength of personal relationships and the availability of adequate stress-mitigation resources.

Hostility

Understanding how personality traits influence mental health outcomes is critical in addressing psychological risks among firefighters. Wagner and Pasca (2022) explored the relationship between hostility and world assumptions, hypothesizing that greater hostility is associated with more negative beliefs about world benevolence, world justness, and self-worth. Drawing from a larger study involving 186 paid professional firefighters from British Columbia, Canada, participants completed questionnaires designed to assess these psychological constructs (Wagner & Pasca, 2022).

The findings supported this hypothesis: hostility was significantly correlated with negative perceptions of world benevolence and lower self-worth, even after controlling for neuroticism as a potential confounding variable (Wagner & Pasca, 2022). Interestingly, no significant associations were found between these psychological measures and years of service, suggesting that hostility and world assumptions may be more rooted in individual cognitive frameworks than in cumulative occupational exposure (Wagner & Pasca, 2022). Notably, world benevolence and self-worth were important predictors of mental health outcomes within the firefighter sample.

These results suggest important clinical and occupational implications. Reducing hostility and promoting more positive world assumptions could serve as valuable strategies in mental health interventions for firefighters. Programs focused on cognitive reframing and emotional regulation may help mitigate risk factors for psychological distress, supporting more resilient and adaptive worldviews among those serving in high-stress environments (Wagner & Pasca, 2022).

Anxiety

Public safety personnel (PSPs), including firefighters, correctional workers, paramedics, police officers, and public safety communication officials, routinely encounter potentially traumatic events and operate in environments marked by constant uncertainty. Research shows that Canadian PSPs screen positively for mental disorders at significantly higher rates than the general population does, underscoring the psychological burdens associated with these professions (Angehrn et al., 2020).

Two psychological factors, intolerance of uncertainty (IU) and anxiety sensitivity (AS), are known vulnerabilities that contribute to the development and persistence of mental health disorders. Angehrn et al. (2020) assessed IU and AS levels in a large sample of PSP participants ($n = 4304$; 33.3% women) and compared their results with those of normative clinical, community, and undergraduate populations. These findings revealed significant differences across groups, with PSP patients, regardless of whether they had a diagnosed mental disorder, reporting lower IU and AS scores than clinical samples did (Angehrn et al., 2020). Notably, PSP patients without mental disorders had the lowest levels of IU and AS among all the groups studied (Angehrn et al., 2020).

These results suggest that many PSPs may develop resilience or adaptive coping mechanisms that help manage the constant uncertainty inherent in their roles, even if they remain vulnerable to elevated rates of mental disorders overall. This study highlights important implications for PSP training and mental health interventions, suggesting that further strengthening uncertainty tolerance and addressing anxiety sensitivity could be critical components of effective support strategies (Angehrn et al., 2020).

The Injury Nexus: Linking Physical and Psychological Factors

Although firefighting is widely recognized as a physically demanding profession with a high injury rate, few studies have explored how physical exercise, burnout, and coping strategies contribute to injury risk. In a descriptive study of 220 male

French firefighters, Vaulerin et al. (2016a) examined the nature and location of injuries and their associations with physical exercise habits, burnout symptoms, and coping mechanisms. The results indicated that sprains were the most common injuries (98%), followed by tendinitis (40%) and muscle tears (30%), with over two-thirds of the injuries occurring at the ankle. Physical exercise and cognitive weariness emerged as risk factors, whereas problem-focused coping strategies appeared to protect against injury (Vaulerin et al., 2016a). These findings underscore the need for targeted prevention strategies that address physical conditioning, psychological resilience, and cognitive fatigue.

Similarly, a study by Kaikkonen et al. (2017) examined the physical and psychological demands of a firefighter's work shift, including the physiological load and psychological stress, over 24 h among Finnish firefighters. Using R-R interval recordings, which measure the time between successive heartbeats to assess heart rate variability, researchers have reported that even younger, fit firefighters temporarily experienced high physical loads and psychological stress levels during their shifts Although average heart rates and oxygen consumption remained moderate, peak exertions were substantial, suggesting that their relative workload may increase as firefighters age and that recovery may slow without appropriate management strategies (Kaikkonen et al., 2017).

In the context of wildland firefighting, unique occupational exposures and health risks were examined through the Wildland Firefighter Exposure and Health Effect (WFFEHE) study, a 2-year repeated-measures investigation conducted across six federal firefighting crews in Colorado and Idaho (Navarro et al., 2022). Researchers have assessed cardiovascular and pulmonary function, kidney health, workplace exposure, and noise-induced hearing loss through biomarkers, physical testing, and self-reported symptoms. Despite logistical challenges in collecting data in remote wildfire environments, the WFFEHE study successfully enrolled 154 participants, providing critical baseline data for understanding acute and subacute health risks among wildland firefighters, though many longitudinal findings are still emerging (Navarro et al., 2022).

These studies highlight the complex interplay between physical conditioning, psychological stress, occupational exposure, and injury risk in firefighting populations, as well as the need for multifaceted prevention and intervention strategies that address the physiological and psychological demands of firefighting across various service contexts.

Posttraumatic Stress Disorder

Firefighters are repeatedly exposed to potentially traumatic events, placing them at heightened risk for various psychological challenges, including depression and posttraumatic stress disorder (PTSD). Recent research has begun to examine how pre-employment experiences and structured interventions might influence psychological outcomes in this population. In a study of 35 male firefighter recruits from seven U.S. cities, Pennington et al. (2018) investigated the effects of disaster exposure prior to employment on depression and PTSD symptoms. The findings revealed that recruits with prior disaster exposure experienced a significant increase in depression symptoms over their first 3 years of service, even after controlling for social support and on-the-job trauma exposure. Interestingly, PTSD symptoms did not differ significantly between the exposed and non-exposed groups, reinforcing that prior disaster exposure did not immediately translate into PTSD, though it predicted greater long-term increase in depression symptoms. However, the long-term increase in depression among the exposed group indicates that early traumatic experiences may contribute to delayed or differently expressed psychological vulnerabilities. These results highlight the need for targeted early mental health interventions tailored to recruits with prior trauma exposure.

Efforts to proactively address psychological risk were also explored in a randomized controlled trial by Skeffington et al. (2016), which assessed the effectiveness of a resilience-focused training program (Mental Agility and Psychological Strength [MAPS]) aimed at the primary prevention of PTSD among career firefighter recruits in Western Australia. Although the intervention did not significantly affect mental health symptoms, social support, or coping strategies at the 6- and 12-month follow-ups, participants demonstrated greater trauma-related knowledge, demonstrating feasibility while highlighting challenges for program efficacy (Skeffington et al., 2016). These findings highlight the practical challenges of implementing preventive mental health programs in firefighter training environments, offering insights for future program refinement.

Post-disaster psychological impacts among active-duty firefighters were further demonstrated following the 2007 wildfires in Greece, a catastrophic event that resulted in 43 deaths, including 3 firefighters. Psarros et al. (2018) assessed 102 firefighters 1 month after the wildfires and reported that 18.6% met the criteria for PTSD. Risk factors associated with PTSD include fear of dying during firefighting operations, insomnia, depressive symptoms, and increased levels of neuroticism. Notably, permanent employment status functioned as a protective factor, with seasonal firefighters showing markedly greater vulnerability to PTSD symptoms (Psarros et al., 2018).

Together, these studies highlight the intricate relationships among personal history, occupational exposure, employment status, and mental health outcomes in firefighters. They underscore the importance of early identification of psychological risk factors, the integration of evidence-based resilience programs, and the need for ongoing mental health support tailored to preexisting vulnerabilities and the unique demands of the fire service profession. These results suggest that early disaster exposure does not guarantee immediate PTSD symptoms, but may predispose recruits to increases in depression over time, pointing to the importance of screening and early prevention interventions among new firefighters.

Empathy and Psychological Detachment

The emotional demands placed on firefighters extend beyond the immediate physical dangers of their work, influencing their psychological health in complex ways. In a study involving 186 firefighters from two urban centers, Wagner et al. (2019) explored the relationships among empathy, traumatic stress, mental distress, aggression, world assumptions, and personality traits. The findings revealed that both traumatic stress and general mental distress were linked to higher levels of emotional empathy. Emotional empathy, in turn, is associated with anger, aggression, self-worth, and broader worldviews related to benevolence and meaningfulness (Wagner et al., 2019).

Interestingly, among the Big Five personality traits, only neuroticism was significantly related to emotional empathy, suggesting a unique pathway through which specific personality characteristics may exacerbate vulnerability to distress in the firefighting population (Wagner et al., 2019). These results imply that while emotional empathy can foster meaningful social connections, it may also increase susceptibility to traumatic stress and psychological strain when firefighters are repeatedly exposed to human suffering. Recognizing the dual nature of empathy is imperative for mental health interventions meant for this population. Programs designed to support emotional regulation, build psychological resilience, and promote healthy processing of empathic experiences may help mitigate the cumulative burden of caring, ultimately supporting the mental well-being of firefighters.

Spirituality in Mental Health

First responders, including firefighters, law enforcement officers, correction officers, and paramedics, face elevated risks for both substance misuse and psychological distress. In a national study of 320 first responders, Kaufman et al. (2024) examined the co-occurrence of alcohol misuse and posttraumatic stress disorder (PTSD) alongside coping resources such as spirituality and religion (S/R) and other clinically relevant variables. The results indicated that nearly half of the participants (46.88%) met the criteria for both alcohol misuse and probable PTSD, underscoring the high comorbidity of these conditions within this population (Kaufman et al., 2024).

Further analysis revealed that individuals with comorbid alcohol misuse and PTSD reported significantly greater levels of negative religious coping, moral injury, and shame than those with either condition alone or neither condition (Kaufman et al., 2024). Additional correlations highlighted significant associations between alcohol misuse, PTSD symptoms, and factors such as positive and negative religious coping, moral injury, shame, guilt, and interest in receiving both general and spiritually integrated treatment services (Kaufman et al., 2024).

These findings point to the complex interplay between trauma, substance use, and spiritual or moral struggles among first responders. They also emphasize the potential value of incorporating spiritually integrated treatment options as part of comprehensive mental health support strategies for this uniquely vulnerable workforce.

Impact of Work Schedules

Unionization has long played a significant role in shaping the wages and working conditions of municipal employees, including those of firefighters. In a seminal study, Smith and Lyons (1980) reported that establishing firefighter union locals and implementing dues check-off systems were associated with increased wages and reduced working hours. Cities with growing populations and rising demand for fire and emergency services tend to see stronger union influence, although supply-side factors, such as firefighter availability, sometimes temper wage increases (Ichniowski, 1978; Smith & Lyons, 1980). These findings highlight the intricate interplay between municipal resources, labor organization, and service demands in shaping the working conditions of firefighters.

In addition to union-driven changes, shift schedules have become a growing focus of occupational health research. Some evidence shows that changing from Kelly-schedule to 48/96 improves sleep and well-being; however, chronic sleep debt persists under many schedules. Similarly, Billings et al. studied sleep–wake patterns among firefighters working 24/48 and 48/96 schedules and reported that firefighters consistently entered shifts with sleep deficits and continued to experience poor sleep across shifts, regardless of the schedule. These studies highlight that while modified schedules may offer some benefits, chronic sleep debt remains a persistent issue.

Firefighters' exposure to extended work shifts, high call volumes, and occupational hazards increases their vulnerability to physical and psychological health risks. Holland-Winkler et al. (2024) described the cyclical relationship between insomnia and mental health impairments in firefighters and noted that poor sleep exacerbates conditions such as PTSD, depression, and anxiety. Similarly, research by Huang et al. (2022) in Taiwan revealed that incomplete off-duty time was a significant predictor of poor sleep quality among firefighters, with longer hours on supposed off-duty days worsening sleep outcomes.

Shift work itself has broader health implications. A meta-analysis by Łagowska et al. revealed that shift workers, including firefighters, have significantly greater body mass indices (BMIs) than non-shift workers do, with long-term shift workers and male firefighters being particularly affected. Elevated cardiovascular risks were also documented by Choi et al., who reported a correlation between increased numbers of 24-h shifts and increased diastolic blood pressure among firefighters in southern California.

In addition to sleep and cardiovascular concerns, cancer risks associated with fire and emergency services have garnered increasing attention. Sidossis et al. reviewed the carcinogenic exposures that firefighters face from smoke, station contaminants, and occupational lifestyle factors, such as poor diet and disrupted sleep. They emphasized the urgent need for both occupational- and lifestyle-based prevention strategies to mitigate the elevated cancer risk in this population.

Other physiological stress studies, such as those by Rosalky et al., revealed that while work duration (short versus long bouts) did not significantly alter cortisol levels during live-fire exercise, psychological variables such as fear and anxiety still increased during extended bouts, reflecting the emotional load that firefighters carry even during controlled conditions. Finally, circadian disruptions caused by shift work remain an important concern. Kazemi et al. reported that slower shift rotations among Iranian petrochemical firefighters helped reduce melatonin disruption and nighttime sleepiness, suggesting that possible adaptations could improve shift workers' alertness.

This growing body of research highlights the complex ways in which organizational structures, shift designs, and occupational hazards intersect to impact the health of firefighters. While unionization has historically improved wages and hours, contemporary challenges such as chronic sleep loss, heightened cardiovascular risk, cancer exposure, and mental health burdens require multifaceted prevention and intervention strategies that are explicitly tailored to the unique realities of the fire service.

Adaptive and Maladaptive Coping in the Fire Service

Gallows Humor

Humor remains a critical yet often misunderstood coping mechanism within the fire service culture. Firefighters are generally hesitant to discuss their use of humor with outsiders, which limits a broader understanding of how humor functions in managing occupational stress. A study by Dangermond et al. (2022) examined the lived experiences of 72 Dutch firefighters across 37 stations, utilizing interviews and participant observations to investigate the role of humor in coping with critical incidents. The findings revealed that joking culture and joviality are integral parts of the fire service environment, fostering team unity but sometimes creating exclusion. The reception of jokes depends heavily on the joker, timing, content, and frequency of delivery. Dark humor, in particular, served a dual purpose, allowing firefighters to broach difficult emotions indirectly while strengthening group bonds. However, the absence of humor following specific critical incidents signals unspoken boundaries and highlights moments when crew leaders can more actively monitor their teams' coping processes (Dangermond et al., 2022).

In addition to humor, firefighters frequently contend with more serious psychological risks, including burnout, compassion fatigue (CF), and vicarious trauma (VT). Stout and Kostamo (2021) employed a photovoice methodology to capture the psychological realities of firefighters in a large metropolitan fire department in

Colorado. Two main themes emerged through photographs and in-depth interviews with seven participants: stress and stress mitigation. Contributors to stress included frequent exposure to traumatic incidents, fatigue from shift work, and chronic sleep deprivation. The participants described burnout as being linked to overwhelming job demands, role ambiguity, and strained workplace relationships. CF is tied to repeated exposure to others' trauma, whereas VT reflects more profound cognitive changes following traumatic encounters (Stout & Kostamo, 2021).

In contrast, firefighters identified several strategies to mitigate these stressors. Peer mentoring offered critical emotional and professional support, whereas therapy dogs and personal pets provided therapeutic relief. Physical activities, such as skiing and weightlifting, as well as other adrenaline-driven hobbies, served as outlets to maintain both physical and mental health (Stout & Kostamo, 2021). The participants emphasized that these individual strategies were helpful but also stressed the need for broader structural interventions, such as improvements in shift scheduling and sleep accommodations.

Taken together, these studies highlight that addressing occupational stress in firefighting requires both culturally attuned approaches, such as recognizing the protective function of humor, and systemic changes aimed at promoting mentorship, access to therapeutic resources, and sustainable work–life balance.

Pornography and Sexual Addiction as Coping Strategies for Stress and Trauma

A growing body of research suggests that problematic pornography use (PPU) and compulsive sexual behavior (CSB) can function as maladaptive coping mechanisms for managing stress, anxiety, depression, trauma exposure, and emotion dysregulation (Kraus et al., 2016; Vaillancourt-Morel et al., 2019).

For example, self-medication theories of behavioral addiction posit that individuals may engage in compulsive sexual behaviors, including excessive pornography consumption, to regulate negative affect and distract from emotional pain (Kraus et al., 2016; Reid et al., 2012). These behaviors serve as short-term relief mechanisms for psychological distress but often lead to negative consequences, including shame, impaired relationships, and functional impairment (Kraus et al., 2016).

An extensive study by Vaillancourt-Morel et al. (2019) revealed that individuals with a history of childhood interpersonal trauma were significantly more likely to report problematic pornography use. The study suggested that PPU may be a form of avoidant coping aimed at managing trauma-related emotional dysregulation. Similarly, Reid et al. (2012) identified emotion dysregulation and attachment insecurity as key predictors of hypersexual behavior, indicating that individuals may use sexual behaviors to modulate distressing emotional states resulting from early trauma or relational difficulties.

Moreover, Bőthe et al. (2019) demonstrated that stress, depression, and anxiety symptoms were positively associated with problematic pornography consumption, supporting the view that individuals may use pornography to cope with negative emotional experiences.

Pornography Addiction Among Firefighters: Current Research Status

At present, there is little to no peer-reviewed research specifically examining pornography addiction among firefighters. While substance use disorders (e.g., alcohol, drugs, etc.) and mental health concerns such as PTSD, depression, and anxiety are well documented in the firefighter population (Haddock et al., 2017), compulsive sexual behaviors, including problematic pornography use, remain an under-researched area. The lack of empirical studies focused on firefighters does not imply that the issue is absent. Research in related high-stress, trauma-exposed occupations, such as military personnel and law enforcement, suggests that individuals in these professions may engage in maladaptive coping mechanisms. It is possible that they may turn to compulsive sexual behaviors and problematic pornography use as is seen in the general population (Grubbs et al., 2015; Kraus et al., 2016). These behaviors are often conceptualized within the broader framework of behavioral addictions or compulsive sexual behavior disorder (CSBD), which was included in the ICD-11 by the World Health Organization (WHO, 2019).

Studies on the general population indicate that compulsive pornography use can be associated with stress, anxiety, trauma exposure, and emotion regulation difficulties (Kraus et al., 2016). Given that firefighters are routinely exposed to high levels of occupational stress and trauma, it is plausible that pornography use could emerge as a coping strategy, mirroring patterns observed in other high-risk groups. However, without targeted research, the prevalence, correlates, and impacts of pornography addiction among firefighters remain largely speculative.

In related professional settings, organizational policies have addressed inappropriate pornography use (e.g., accessing explicit material during work hours) from a disciplinary perspective. Nevertheless, there is a paucity of research examining this behavior through a mental health or addiction lens within fire service contexts.

Key points from the literature:

- Stress and Trauma: PPU and CSB are often linked to past trauma and current stress as maladaptive coping responses (Vaillancourt-Morel et al., 2019).
- Emotional Regulation: Difficulty managing negative emotions is a consistent predictor of compulsive sexual behaviors (Reid et al., 2012).
- Avoidance Coping: Using sexual behaviors to escape from distress rather than address underlying issues (Kraus et al., 2016).
- Short-term Relief, Long-term Harm: Although these behaviors offer temporary relief, they often result in additional psychological and relational difficulties (Bőthe et al., 2019).

History of Psychology in First Responder Agencies

The integration of professional psychology into first responder agencies can be traced back nearly a century, beginning with law enforcement. In 1916, Lewis Terman, Ph.D., a pioneer in intelligence testing, was commissioned to assess the suitability of police applicants for the San Jose Police Department. However, it was not until the mid-twentieth century that the relationship between psychology and public safety truly took root. The President's Commission on Law Enforcement and Administration of Justice (1967) formally recommended psychological testing to identify personal characteristics critical to practical police work. This recommendation catalyzed broader systemic changes, and in 1968, the Los Angeles Police Department (LAPD) hired Martin Reiser, Ed.D., ABPP, as the first full-time police psychologist at a major agency (Corey et al., 2011). Soon after, San Jose Police brought on Michael Roberts, Ph.D., ABPP, further solidifying the role of psychology within law enforcement agencies.

After the 1960s, psychological services within policing began expanding rapidly. The New York Police Department (NYPD) hired Dr. Sloussenburg in 1964, whose pioneering work in hostage negotiation helped create what became known as the "East Coast Model," emphasizing negotiation before tactical intervention (Bartlett et al., 2018). Meanwhile, the LAPD developed the "West Coast Model," which integrated negotiation strategies directly within tactical teams such as SWAT, blending psychology with operational planning (Bartlett et al., 2018).

Over the following decades, the role of psychologists in law enforcement expanded significantly. They became integral not only to selection and crisis negotiations but also to post-incident support, organizational consultation, and resilience training for officers (Bartlett et al., 2018; Sommerfeld et al., 2017). Today, psychology is deeply embedded in police operations, shaping everything from leadership development to wellness programs.

In contrast, fire and emergency services have historically lagged in this area. While law enforcement agencies have embraced psychological expertise to improve operational outcomes and officer well-being, firefighting organizations have been slower at incorporating psychologists into their ranks. The lack of integration has left a significant gap in mental health services tailored specifically for firefighters. This gap continues to affect the profession's ability to address psychological risk and resilience proactively.

Fire Service Culture and Mental Health Access

Firefighters often experience barriers to accessing mental health services due to cultural distrust, stigma, and limited exposure to the benefits of professional psychology. Despite rising awareness of mental health needs within the fire service, many departments remain resistant to embedding psychologists into their organizational structure. Studies have shown that training programs that integrate motivational interviewing and behavioral health education can increase firefighters' acceptance of mental health care and treatment engagement (Gulliver et al., 2016).

However, most fire departments lack full-time psychologists, and mental health interventions typically occur only after critical incidents. Consequently, psychology is often perceived as a reactive service rather than a proactive, performance-enhancing resource (Bastug et al., 2019; Meyer et al., 2021). Efforts to educate firefighters about practical psychological applications could reduce stigma and increase trust.

Mistrust and Traditional Masculine Culture in the Firehouse

The traditional masculine culture within the fire service further complicates access to mental health care. Firefighters report stigma about being perceived as weak, and fear of judgment, which may be amplified in male-dominated organizational cultures (Kim et al., 2018). Research indicates that the stigma surrounding psychological treatment may influence not only individual firefighters but also organizational attitudes, impacting concerns about job impact or career consequences thereby reinforcing reluctance to seek help (Kim et al., 2018; Bartlett et al., 2018). Exposure to culturally competent psychologists can mitigate mistrust; however, negative initial experiences with providers can leave lasting impressions that deter future help-seeking behavior (Sommerfeld et al., 2017). Recognizing this dynamic is crucial for developing effective and sustainable programs that support firefighter mental health.

Barriers to Treatment

Despite growing mental health awareness, stigma remains a significant barrier to care in fire and emergency services. Research in South Korea revealed that while 5.4% of firefighters met the criteria for probable PTSD, only 9.7% had received mental health treatment in the previous month. Among those who did not seek care, concerns about stigma (33.8%) and barriers to access (29.3%) were the most frequently cited reasons (Kim et al., 2018). Importantly, individuals with more severe PTSD symptoms expressed higher stigma concern and higher likelihood of seeking treatment with severity (Kim et al., 2018).

Similar dynamics exist in the U.S. fire and emergency services as firefightersirefighters who experience high PTSD symptoms combined with low distress tolerance are at the greatest risk for suicidal ideation and future suicide attempts (Bartlett et al., 2018). Addressing stigma, improving accessibility, and offering culturally competent psychological services are important factors in closing the treatment gap.

Fire Departments Across the United States

Some fire departments have implemented mental health support within their organizations. For example, the Austin Fire Department and Fairfax County Fire Department have historically held full-time psychologist positions and partnered with academic institutions to produce and disseminate research specific to firefighter populations. Similarly, the Houston Fire Department has full-time psychologists, collaborated with a research team from Houston State University, and developed an active peer support team (Houston Fire Department, n.d.). These models demonstrate that large departments can successfully integrate mental health services, provide direct care and training, and contribute to research in the broader field of mental health.

Peer Support Teams in the Fire Service

Peer support programs have emerged as critical components in addressing the mental health needs of firefighters, who are routinely exposed to traumatic events and high-stress environments. Originally pioneered in military contexts, peer support teams are increasingly being adopted by fire departments as an effective strategy for early psychological intervention, emotional support, and the promotion of posttraumatic growth (Sattler et al., 2014). These teams operate within the organizational structure to provide culturally appropriate support that aligns with the values and communication styles of firefighters.

Key Components of Effective Peer Support

Successful peer support initiatives are grounded in several best-practice components. These include the careful selection and vetting of peer supporters, comprehensive and ongoing training, structured deployment procedures, systematic after-action reviews, and the collection of non-identifiable outcome data to inform program improvements (Sattler et al., 2014; Money et al., 2011). Peer supporters should receive specialized training in active listening, crisis response, confidentiality, and appropriate referral practices.

Bartone and Dooley (2021) underscore the importance of incorporating psychological hardiness (defined by the attributes of commitment, control, and challenge) into peer support frameworks. Hardiness serves as a protective factor against the negative psychological effects of trauma and stress and can be cultivated through structured group interactions and shared meaning-making (Bartone, 2004). These findings suggest that fire departments and mental health professionals should design peer interventions not only to mitigate distress but also to foster long-term resilience and adaptation.

Psychological Outcomes and Benefits

Empirical evidence supports the efficacy of peer support in enhancing mental health outcomes for first responders. Access to social support, internal locus of control, and participation in post-incident interventions have been shown to mitigate post-traumatic stress symptoms and promote psychological recovery (Sattler et al., 2014). Firefighters with strong coping resources who engage in peer support report higher levels of posttraumatic growth, a construct associated with positive psychological change following adversity (Bartone et al., 2018).

Programs such as the Tragedy Assistance Program for Survivors (TAPS) offer a model for integrated, trauma-informed peer support. This model provides layered care, including peer mentoring, bereavement-specific interventions, and connections to professional services as needed (Dooley et al., 2019). These structures reinforce the importance of flexible, scalable interventions that can adapt to the severity and nature of firefighters' psychological needs.

Addressing Variability in Help-Seeking Behaviors

Despite these benefits, help-seeking behaviors among firefighters remain highly individualized. Research by Tamrakar et al. (2020) identified five distinct help-seeking profiles among UK firefighters, ranging from exclusive reliance on family members to preferences for informal peer networks and limited engagement with formal psychological services. These findings emphasize the need for a nuanced approach in designing support services. Fire chiefs and mental health professionals should ensure that peer support systems offer multiple access points and modes of engagement to accommodate varying preferences and cultural attitudes toward mental health.

Moreover, attention to demographic factors such as gender is essential. Bartone and Roche (2024) reported significant sex differences in coping strategies and psychological hardiness among West Point cadets, indicating that gender may also influence how firefighters perceive and utilize peer support services. Program developers should be mindful of these differences in recruitment, training, and outreach to ensure inclusivity and effectiveness.

Implications for Practice

For psychologists and fire chiefs, the integration of peer support teams within fire departments offers a promising avenue for proactive mental health care. These programs should be embedded within a broader organizational culture of wellness, stigma reduction, and psychological safety. Regular evaluation, supervision by licensed mental health professionals, and collaboration between behavioral health experts and fire leaders are essential for sustaining effective peer support.

In conclusion, peer support teams represent a vital, evidence-informed strategy for addressing the complex psychological needs of firefighters. When carefully implemented and continuously evaluated, these programs can increase resilience, facilitate recovery, and reduce barriers to care, ultimately contributing to the overall readiness and well-being of fire service personnel.

Employee Assistance Programs

Employee assistance programs (EAPs) connect firefighters with mental health providers who accept their insurance. However, distrust in EAPs mirrors broader skepticism toward psychology in the context of fire and emergency services (Sommerfeld et al., 2017). Many firefighters question the confidentiality, cultural competence, and effectiveness of Employee Assistance Program (EAP) services, leading to underutilization even when services are technically available.

Chaplains in the Fire Service

Chaplains have long provided emotional and spiritual support within fire departments. Given their historical role, some chaplains may be threatened by the increasing inclusion of mental health professionals. As departments expand their behavioral health services, professionals should acknowledge the contributions of chaplains and foster collaborative, rather than potentially competitive, relationships between chaplains and mental health professionals (Davidson et al., 2020).

Performance Psychology and Firefighter Training

The relevance of psychology to fire and emergency services extends beyond crisis intervention to performance optimization. Social facilitation, social inhibition, and social loafing are critical for understanding how firefighters perform during training and operations.

Social facilitation improves performance during familiar tasks when others are present, whereas social inhibition can impair performance on new or complex tasks under observation. Structuring firefighter training to minimize social inhibition through small-group practices and supportive environments can enhance skill acquisition. Awareness of social loafing, where individuals contribute less in group settings, highlights the importance of assigning clear individual roles and fostering a culture of accountability. Tailoring training programs to leverage social and performance psychology principles can enhance both individual performance and team cohesion in fire and emergency services.

Integration of Psychology in the Fire Service

The integration of psychology into fire and emergency services remains underdeveloped compared with its role in law enforcement. Persistent cultural stigma, traditional masculine cultural norms, limited access to culturally competent providers, and distrust of mental health services continue to pose challenges. However, the increasing visibility of firefighter mental health needs presents an opportunity to advance fire psychology as a distinct field of study and to serve firefighters with specific focus.

Efforts to normalize mental health support, expand training programs, enhance peer support structures, and embed psychologists within fire departments will reduce psychological suffering and optimize operational performance and team functioning. Addressing these needs requires a systemic, culturally informed approach that recognizes the complex realities of firefighting in the modern era.

Transitional Considerations: Retirement and Medical Discharge

Transitioning out of fire and emergency services represents a major life event with significant psychological implications. Unlike many other professions, firefighters often develop a strong occupational identity, where their role as first responders becomes deeply intertwined with their sense of self and social belonging (Haslam et al., 2008). Therefore, career transitions such as retirement, medical discharge (due to duty-related or non-duty-related injuries), involuntary resignation, or voluntary separation can pose substantial challenges to their psychological well-being (Regehr & Millar, 2007). Despite its importance, there remains underdeveloped empirical research examining these transitions within the firefighter population.

Evidence from international emergency service populations suggests that a career as a first responder has a long-term impact on health and quality of life. A study by Bracken-Scally (2014), focusing on retired ambulance and fire personnel in Ireland, revealed that, compared with the general population, life as a first responder was associated with significantly greater levels of posttraumatic stress disorder (PTSD) symptoms and lower self-reported quality of life. This study emphasized that years of service and cumulative trauma exposure were key factors contributing to these adverse outcomes, suggesting that the psychological effects of emergency service work often persist beyond active duty (Bracken-Scally, 2014).

Transitioning out of the fire service often involves losing role identity, disrupting social networks, and adjusting to new life structures. Firefighters leave behind not only the operational demands of their role but also the camaraderie and team cohesion, which are central to their occupational experience (Haslam et al., 2008). For veterans, the retirement transition may be further complicated by feelings of involuntariness, physical limitations, and financial uncertainty, increasing susceptibility to depression, anxiety, and diminished self-worth (Oster et al., 2017).

Theoretical frameworks, such as role-exit theory (Ebaugh, 1988), provide a valuable lens for understanding these transitions. Role-exit theory posits that leaving a role central to one's identity involves a complex psychological process that, if not supported, can result in identity crises and emotional distress (Ebaugh, 1988). The theory may be particularly relevant for firefighters, whose occupational identity is often deeply embedded within personal and community narratives (Brough et al., 2016).

Research has shown that PTSD symptoms may intensify after retirement in emergency service personnel, as leaving operational duties reduces avoidance opportunities and allows unresolved trauma to surface (Bracken-Scally, 2014). Research highlights the need for targeted interventions that not only address the long-term psychological impact of a firefighting career but also support the broader lifestyle and identity adjustments associated with this significant life transition. From a prevention standpoint, supporting firefighters during these transitions aligns with tertiary and quaternary prevention efforts. Proactive strategies such as pre-retirement planning, peer support groups for retirees, and access to specialized mental health services can mitigate the psychological risks associated with retirement and medical discharge (Brough et al., 2016; McLennan & Birch, 2022). These initiatives could be tailored to address the unique stressors and experiences of first responders, ensuring that interventions are culturally competent and grounded in evidence-based practices.

In summary, the psychological impact of transitioning out of fire and emergency services, whether through retirement or medical discharge, represents a critical yet underexplored dimension of firefighter behavioral health. Integrating transitional support structures into comprehensive mental health frameworks is important for promoting adaptive adjustment, preserving quality of life, and mitigating the long-term effects of occupational stress and trauma.

Role of Emotional Intelligence and Proactive Coping in Firefighter Behavioral Health

In high-risk, high-stress occupations such as firefighting, individual psychological resources play a significant role in buffering against the adverse mental health outcomes associated with repeated trauma exposure and occupational stress. Among these resources, emotional intelligence (EI) and proactive coping have emerged as critical protective factors influencing psychological resilience and overall well-being.

Emotional intelligence refers to an individual's capacity to recognize, understand, regulate, and manage their own emotions and those of others. This self-regulatory capacity is particularly relevant in firefighting, where managing emotional responses during high-pressure situations is important for personal well-being and effective team functioning. Similarly, proactive coping involves anticipating potential stressors and engaging in goal-directed behaviors to prevent or mitigate their impact, fostering control and reducing psychological distress (Aspinwall & Taylor, 1997).

Research suggests that emotional intelligence and proactive coping are important factors influencing firefighters' quality of life and resilience across their careers (Wagner, S. L., & Martin, C. A., 2012). Emotional intelligence is defined as a person's level of emotional self-awareness, motivation, self-regulation, and ability to effectively empathize and demonstrate proficiency in relationships (Wagner, S. L., & Martin, C. A., 2012). Proactive coping is defined as efforts undertaken in advance of a potentially stressful event to prevent it or to modify it before it occurs (Aspinwall & Taylor, 1997, p. 417). One study examined the coping strategies employed by first responders in military and emergency services, including those in ambulatory, fire, and police services (Arble, E., & Arnetz, B. B., 2017). The findings suggested that approach coping behaviors were directly related to better subjective reports of well-being, whereas avoidance coping styles reflected fewer reports of well-being (Arble, E., & Arnetz, B. B., 2017). Similarly, research suggests that work-recovery strategies can moderate the relationship between occupational stress and mental health symptoms among firefighters (Sawhney et al., 2018). Specifically, researchers have reported that strategies such as spending time with coworkers and supervisors, exercising, relaxing, engaging in other mastery experiences, and participating in recreational activities help moderate the effects of work stress and mental health outcomes (Sawhney et al., 2018).

A study by Wagner and Martin (2012) specifically examined the roles of emotional intelligence and proactive coping in predicting mental health outcomes among professional firefighters. The study assessed 94 firefighters and a comparison group of 91 nonemergency workers via validated measures, including the Impact of Events Scale-Revised (IES-R), the Symptom Checklist 90-Revised (SCL-90-R), the Emotional Intelligence Scale, and the Proactive Coping Scale. The findings indicated that, within the firefighter group, emotional intelligence was a significant negative predictor of self-reported traumatic stress symptoms ($\beta = -.198$), suggesting that greater emotional intelligence was associated with reduced trauma-related distress (Wagner & Martin, 2012). Furthermore, proactive coping was found to negatively predict various mental health symptoms, including obsessive–compulsive tendencies ($\beta = -.192$), depression ($\beta = -.220$), and anxiety ($\beta = -.295$), underscoring its role in promoting psychological resilience (Wagner & Martin, 2012).

Interestingly, the comparison group demonstrated a broader influence of emotional intelligence, with significant negative associations observed with interpersonal sensitivity, depression, anxiety, and hostility. However, proactive coping in this group predicted only a reduction in psychoticism-related symptoms (Wagner &

Martin, 2012). These differential findings suggest that within fire and emergency services, proactive coping may serve as a more targeted buffer against specific stress-related symptoms. Moreover, emotional intelligence plays a broad role in supporting emotional regulation and stress management among firefighters and the general population.

In the United Kingdom, to best understand the coping strategies employed by firefighters after a perceived stressful event, some researchers categorize methods as emotion-focused, problem-focused, or both emotion-focused and problem-focused (Young, P. M. et al., 2014). Their findings suggested that half of the total coping strategies quoted by participants fell into the problem-focused category, where one-third of the responses were categorized as strictly emotion-focused, and 17% were considered both (Young, P. M. et al., 2014). Given the anticipatory quality prior to arriving at an incident, participants shared that they tended to use more problem-focused methods en route and during early operational tasks (Young, P. M. et al., 2014). Emotion-focused strategies are typically employed during periods of fatigue and exhaustion and in the aftermath of an incident (Young, P. M. et al., 2014). Both strategies were found to be used after the incidents (Young, P. M. et al., 2014). Therefore, postvention was found to have value in supporting firefighters in these strategies to address critical incidents (Young, P. M. et al., 2014).

Emotional intelligence and proactive coping are relevant across multiple levels of behavioral health prevention in fire and emergency services. At the primary prevention level, training programs designed to enhance emotional intelligence and develop proactive coping skills can serve as foundational interventions, equipping firefighters with tools to manage stress before it escalates into clinical concerns. In the context of secondary prevention, fostering these competencies can aid in the early recognition and self-management of emerging psychological symptoms, reducing the need for more intensive interventions. Additionally, integrating emotional intelligence and proactive coping strategies into tertiary prevention efforts may improve treatment engagement and recovery outcomes for firefighters already experiencing mental health challenges.

In summary, emotional intelligence and proactive coping are pivotal individual-level factors that can mitigate the psychological impact of occupational stressors in fire and emergency services. Their inclusion in comprehensive mental health promotion strategies offers a proactive, strengths-based approach to enhancing firefighter resilience and reducing the burden of trauma-related and stress-induced mental health disorders.

Organizational Stress: The Impact of Workplace Factors on Firefighter Well-Being

While much attention to firefighter behavioral health has focused on operational stressors such as trauma exposure, there is growing recognition of the profound influence of organizational stressors on firefighter well-being. Organizational stress refers to the strain arising from workplace structures, cultures, and interpersonal dynamics, which is distinct from the inherent dangers of emergency response work. Factors such as workload, work patterns, interpersonal conflict, role ambiguity, and perceived lack of support can significantly affect psychological outcomes, including anxiety, depression, burnout, and overall job satisfaction (Armstrong et al., 2016; Payne & Kinman, 2019).

Using a job demands-resources (JD-R) framework, Payne and Kinman (2019) conducted a comprehensive study to assess the organizational hazards that impact firefighter well-being. The JD-R model posits that while job demands (e.g., workload, emotional strain) can deplete energy and lead to strain, job resources (e.g., role clarity, support, job control) can buffer these effects, promoting engagement and well-being (Bakker & Demerouti, 2007). In their study of 909 firefighters across seven UK fires and rescue services, Payne and Kinman examined key variables, including workload, the work environment, relationship conflicts, job control, support, role clarity, and change management, alongside recovery strategies such as psychological detachment, affective rumination, and problem-solving pondering (Payne & Kinman, 2019).

The findings revealed that relationship conflicts and affective rumination were the primary risk factors for diminished well-being, particularly those associated with increased levels of anxiety and depressive symptoms. Conversely, role clarity, job control, and recovery strategies such as problem-solving, pondering, and detachment during off-duty hours are protective, enhancing work-related well-being (Payne & Kinman, 2019). Notably, several job resources (role clarity, support, and job control) were found to fall short of benchmarks established by the UK's Health and Safety Executive (HSE), indicating systemic gaps in organizational support within the fire service (Payne & Kinman, 2019).

These findings align with prior research, which emphasized that, compared with operational stress alone, organizational stressors may have a more pervasive and chronic impact on firefighter mental health (Armstrong et al., 2016). Chronic relationship conflicts, poor role definitions, and a lack of job control erode psychological resilience over time, often exacerbating the effects of acute trauma exposure (Bakker & Demerouti, 2007).

Importantly, interventions targeting organizational stress can serve as both primary and secondary prevention measures. By addressing modifiable factors such as enhancing role clarity, improving leadership communication, strengthening conflict resolution mechanisms, and promoting effective recovery strategies, fire service organizations can mitigate the cumulative impact of workplace stress on behavioral health outcomes. Encouraging firefighters to engage in problem-solving, an adaptive form of reflection focused on actionable solutions, while discouraging affective rumination, which is linked to emotional distress, represents a promising individual-level intervention strategy (Payne & Kinman, 2019).

Ultimately, the influence of organizational stressors on firefighter behavioral health is significant and actionable. A comprehensive approach to firefighter well-being should address not only the psychological impacts of operational hazards but also the systemic organizational factors that shape daily work experiences.

Occupational Exposures: The Role of Sleep and Fatigue in Firefighter Behavioral Health

Firefighters are routinely exposed to a wide range of occupational demands and stressors, including direct and indirect encounters with potentially traumatic events, shift work, and physically taxing environments. These factors significantly increase the risk of behavioral health challenges, such as posttraumatic stress disorder (PTSD), depression, anxiety, and burnout (Jahnke et al., 2019). However, recent research suggests that beyond trauma exposure, sleep quality, fatigue, and recovery experiences are critical determinants of mental health outcomes in this population (Kauffman et al., 2022; Zhang et al., 2023).

Sleep disturbances are pervasive in fire and emergency services and are driven by irregular shift schedules, nighttime emergency calls, and the physiological hyperarousal inherent in emergency response work (Barger et al., 2015). Poor sleep quality has been repeatedly linked to heightened psychological distress, often exacerbating posttraumatic symptoms and impairing daily functioning (Wolkow et al., 2019). In a large-scale study involving more than 3000 career firefighters from a metropolitan fire department in China, Zhang et al. (2023) employed network analysis to examine the interplay between sleep, recovery experiences, fatigue, and mental health. The findings revealed that sleep quality, rather than duration, was more strongly associated with mental health outcomes, emphasizing the importance of restorative sleep processes to firefighter well-being. Moreover, relaxation and mastery experiences, such as engaging in hobbies or skill-building activities, were found to buffer against declines in life and social functioning, further highlighting the protective role of effective recovery strategies (Zhang et al., 2023).

Expanding upon the impact of fatigue, a study by Kauffman et al. (2022) specifically examined the role of fatigue sensitivity in predicting mental health outcomes among trauma-exposed firefighters. Fatigue sensitivity refers to the degree to which individuals experience fatigue as distressing, threatening, or indicative of personal inadequacy (Kauffman et al., 2022). In their cross-sectional study of 107 trauma-exposed firefighters, the results indicated that fatigue sensitivity was a significant clinical correlate of PTSD, anxiety, and depressive symptom severity. Notably, these associations persisted even after controlling for factors such as years of service, sleep quality, and trauma load, suggesting that fatigue sensitivity independently contributes to psychological vulnerability (Kauffman et al., 2022). These findings underscore the importance of addressing not only the physical aspects of fatigue but also the cognitive and emotional appraisals, which may perpetuate distress and maladaptive coping (Kauffman et al., 2022).

These studies demonstrate that sleep quality, fatigue sensitivity, and recovery experiences are central to understanding how occupational exposures translate into mental health outcomes for firefighters (Kauffman et al., 2022; Zhang et al., 2023). Beyond trauma exposure, these factors act as mediators and amplifiers of stress responses, influencing both immediate well-being and long-term psychological resilience. Recognizing these relationships broadens the traditional trauma-centric perspective of firefighter behavioral health and suggests a more holistic approach to prevention and intervention.

To address these challenges effectively, fire service organizations should consider organizational interventions, such as optimizing shift schedules to promote sleep hygiene, implementing fatigue management training, and fostering a culture that prioritizes recovery experiences as integral to job performance (Barger et al., 2015; Jahnke et al., 2019). Concurrently, individual-level interventions targeting maladaptive fatigue sensitivity through cognitive–behavioral strategies or psychoeducation could serve as valuable adjuncts to traditional mental health services. Such multifaceted approaches are important for mitigating the cumulative impact of occupational exposure on firefighter behavioral health.

Workers' Compensation Systems

Understanding injury patterns among firefighters is fundamental for developing effective prevention strategies. A recent analysis of firefighter injury claims in Ohio using workers' compensation data from 2001 to 2017 revealed notable trends in injury frequency, causes, and diagnoses (Quinn et al., 2023). Over the past 16 years, the total number of claims has declined, but overexertion involving external sources has remained the leading cause of injury (Quinn et al., 2023). Differences emerged in the types of injuries associated with specific tasks, particularly between firefighting activities and patient care duties (Quinn et al., 2023). The study also noted possible seasonal patterns in injury occurrence, suggesting that prevention efforts could be optimized by aligning strategies with seasonal risks (Quinn et al., 2023).

The researchers identified a total of 33,069 claims, with the majority classified as medical-only (66.28%). Most claims were filed by males (93.81%) and were associated with individuals aged between 25 and 54 years (86.54%) (Quinn et al., 2023). Among tasks that could be categorized, injuries during firefighting operations accounted for 20.48% of claims, whereas patient care incidents accounted for 17.60% (Quinn et al., 2023). Overexertion and being struck by objects or equipment were the most common injury events, and the most frequent diagnoses were sprains of the back (16.02%), lower extremities (14.46%), and upper extremities (11.98%) (Quinn et al., 2023).

These findings provide a critical foundation for designing more targeted firefighter injury prevention programs. This study emphasizes the need for training initiatives specifically addressing common injury mechanisms. This also highlights the importance of more detailed data collection to enable rate calculations, which could further refine risk assessments and improve the precision of prevention efforts (Quinn et al., 2023).

Conclusion

The fire service exists at an intersection of physical danger, emotional complexity, and organizational challenges. However, psychology, a discipline uniquely positioned to address these domains, has only recently begun to find its position within this critical profession. Ultimately, the psychological well-being of firefighters is shaped by a complex matrix of operational stressors, relational dynamics, occupational culture, and systemic organizational factors. While the field has long recognized the risks of trauma exposure, emerging research highlights how factors such as moral injury, sleep deprivation, organizational betrayal emotional intelligence, coping strategies, and even shift schedules can influence mental health outcomes.

Despite compelling evidence supporting the application of psychological science to fire and emergency services, significant barriers persist. Cultural stigma, mistrust of mental health professionals, and traditional masculine norms continue to undermine both prevention and treatment efforts. Moreover, the absence of a centralized mental health regulatory framework in the U.S. fire service leaves departments without consistent guidance, allowing disparities in care, training, and psychological safety to flourish. The growing recognition of issues, including burnout, vicarious trauma, hostility, anxiety sensitivity, and maladaptive coping, including problematic substance and behavioral use, underscores the urgent need for culturally competent, evidence-based interventions that are explicitly tailored to the realities of firefighting.

The integration of psychological principles must extend beyond crisis response to encompass performance enhancement, organizational leadership, family system support, and transitional care for those exiting the profession. Emerging models, such as peer support teams, embedded psychologists, and proactive coping and resilience training, offer promising frameworks; however, scalability and standardization remain ongoing challenges. Similarly, leveraging emotional intelligence, addressing moral injury, and implementing proactive recovery strategies may provide a roadmap for early intervention and prevention.

Ultimately, a modern fire service must evolve to view mental health not as an ancillary concern but as a foundational pillar of operational readiness and human sustainability. Psychology offers more than just treatment; it also provides leadership, prevention, connection, and transformation tools. To realize this potential, fire service organizations must commit to systemic change that aligns with empirical evidence and the lived experiences of those who serve. Only then can we fully honor the psychological demands of firefighting with the same seriousness afforded to its physical risk.

Chapter Review—Assignment: Case Study Analysis—Mental Health Intervention in the Fire Service

Learning Objectives:

- By the end of this exercise, students will be able to:
- Analyze the unique psychological stressors experienced by firefighters.
- Identify evidence-based psychological concepts (e.g., moral injury, emotional regulation, and peer support) applicable to fire service settings.
- Evaluate the cultural and organizational barriers to mental health access within fire departments.
- Propose an intervention strategy informed by psychological theory and fire service culture.

Scenario:

You are a psychologist assigned to assist a mid-sized municipal fire department that has recently experienced the suicide of a firefighter after a series of critical incident responses. Department leadership is concerned about morale and mental wellness across shifts. They have requested your input to help them understand:

- What might have contributed to this outcome,
- What signs or risk factors they may have missed,
- And what they can do to prevent future crises.

Assignment: Write a 1000–1500 word response addressing the following:

(a) Risk Factor Analysis:

- Based on what you've learned, identify three key psychological risk factors firefighters face that may have played a role in this case (e.g., cumulative trauma, moral injury, stigma, and sleep deprivation).
- Reference at least two peer-reviewed studies from the chapter to support your analysis.

(b) Cultural and Organizational Considerations:

- Discuss how firehouse culture, masculine norms, and organizational structures might prevent firefighters from seeking mental health support.
- Incorporate relevant findings (e.g., stigma, leadership communication, and shift schedules).

(c) Intervention Design:

- Propose a realistic, evidence-informed mental health intervention for the department.
- Include elements such as peer support, embedded psychologists, training programs, or revised scheduling.

- Justify your approach using psychological theories or empirical evidence from the chapter.

Assessment Criteria:

- Critical thinking and application of psychological principles (30%)
- Use of evidence and integration of research (25%)
- Clarity and structure of writing (20%)
- Feasibility and creativity of proposed intervention (15%)
- APA formatting and professionalism (10%)

Chapter 4
Fire Service Mythology and Culture

The culture of American fire and emergency services is deeply intertwined with enduring mythologies that shape collective identity, institutional traditions, and individual behavior. Drawing on Jungian concepts of archetypes such as the hero and the warrior (Jung, 1959a, 1959b*), these myths provide a framework through which bravery, sacrifice, and solidarity are valorized. Firefighter culture often embraces narratives that foster cohesion and resilience while also reinforcing norms that may inhibit emotional openness, diversity, and critical reflection. Mythological constructs, from the heroic conquest of danger to the memorialization of fallen firefighters, play a pivotal role in how firefighters may interpret risk, loss, and honor. By critically examining the function of mythology within the fire service, professionals are made aware of variables impacting psychological well-being, organizational culture, and the evolving challenges of our modern fire service. By investigating the cultural narratives that have long defined firefighting, it becomes possible to identify pathways for preserving tradition while promoting emotional health, operational safety, and sustainable leadership.*

Fire Without Consciousness or Intent

In professions such as the military and law enforcement, the adversary is a conscious human being capable of intention, aggression, and strategic harm. These professions frame their conflicts through interpersonal dynamics rooted in will and decision-making. In firefighting, however, the "enemy" is fire, which is an unconscious, amoral force governed by physics, not volition. Despite this fundamental difference, fire is often anthropomorphized within fire service culture, described as "hunting," "attacking," or "devouring" (Desmond, 2007). This linguistic and symbolic framing reflects a psychological process known as projection, whereby individuals externalize internal fears, anxieties, and conflicts with outside objects or phenomena (Jung, 1959a, 1959b). By personifying fire as a malevolent opponent, firefighters unconsciously craft a narrative that transforms chaotic, impersonal danger into a familiar heroic struggle, shielding themselves from more profound existential anxieties associated with mortality and loss of control (Van der Kolk, 2014). Research on high-risk occupational identity suggests that this symbolic

K. Wheldon, *Fire Service Psychology*,
https://doi.org/10.1007/978-3-032-02126-7_4

externalization fosters bravery and group cohesion but may also subtly reinforce risk-taking behaviors (Wong et al., 2017) and suppress emotional vulnerability, increasing the risk for psychological distress (Stanley et al., 2017). Recognizing fire not as a conscious adversary but as an unconscious force, and understanding the psychological projections involved, offers a pathway toward fostering operational safety and emotional resilience.

Fire is a force without consciousness, yet it is often spoken of as a living, thinking adversary. Phrases such as "the fire is hunting for fuel" or "the flames devoured the structure" are common among firefighters. While powerful and poetic, these metaphors subtly shape how firefighters perceive both fire itself and their relationship to it. In effect, we humanize the fire, creating an adversary that should be conquered.

Carl Jung's theories on archetypes reflect an important psychological process. When fire is personified as a "red devil" or a "dragon," firefighters psychologically project onto it their internalized myths of battle and conquest (Jung, 1959a, 1959b; Moore & Gillette, 1990). The fire becomes something to fight, not merely a chemical reaction to control. This distinction is important because it may directly influence risk-taking behavior. The more a fire is seen as a conscious enemy, the more firefighters may feel morally compelled to defeat it rather than strategically manage it.

The visual iconography of fire and emergency services reinforces this adversarial framing of fire. Skulls, crossbones, dragons, and burning towers are common symbols on fire patches, shirts, and decals. However, rarely, if ever, do we see imagery honoring sprinkler systems or evidence-based fire suppression tactics. The cultural imagination of firefighting remains steeped in the narrative of heroic battle rather than strategic containment or commitment.

A poignant example of the cultural imprint of mythological symbolism can be seen in the aftermath of the September 11th attacks. The original FDNY Engine 10/ Ladder 10 patch, created in 1984, depicted a firefighter straddling the Twin Towers, each tower ablaze, a design meant to symbolize the company's proximity to and protection of the World Trade Center (FDNY Ten House, n.d.). After 9/11, however, this imagery took on a radically different meaning. Rather than symbolizing protection, the burning towers evoked profound collective trauma, irreversible loss, and vulnerability. Although there were calls to alter the patch to avoid memorializing destruction, Ten House ultimately chose to preserve it, reframing the symbol as a tribute to sacrifice and endurance (FDNY Ten House, n.d.). New generations of firefighters, many of whom were too young to remember the terrorist attacks directly, inherit the emotional weight of this symbol through storytelling, ceremonies, and institutional memory. The meaning they attribute to these symbols may profoundly shape their identity, sense of mission, and potentially their operational behavior on the fireground.

The decision to retain the original patch likely highlights a deeper psychological process that Carl Jung (1959a, 1959b) describes as an engagement with the collective unconscious. Images such as burning towers operate at an archetypal level, representing existential themes of destruction, death, and rebirth. In this light, the towers are not merely historical structures; they become mythic emblems of collective mortality and sacrifice. Keeping the original imagery reflects an unconscious attempt to integrate trauma into the cultural mythos, allowing firefighters to reaffirm courage and meaning in the face of existential chaos. Symbolic representations of loss are thus not passively received but actively reinterpreted through the communal psyche. In this way, the adaptation of fire service imagery after 9/11 illustrates the dynamic tension between honoring sacrifice and protecting the psychological resilience of the group, as well as an ongoing negotiation between memory, identity, and survival.

Firefighters today inherit not just a job but also a mythology. This mythology is emotionally powerful and socially binding. All the while, it can also subtly encourage cavalier risk-taking when a fire is perceived as an adversary to be vanquished rather than a hazard to be tactically neutralized. Understanding these dynamics does not require abandoning pride or tradition. Rather, it requires us to be intentional about the stories we tell and the symbols we elevate. If we continue to frame fire as a thinking, malevolent enemy, we risk perpetuating behaviors that place heroism over safety. If, instead, we can frame fire as an unconscious force, dangerous but predictable, we allow a new mythology to emerge, one where wisdom, strategy, and life preservation are the marks of true mastery and heroism.

The Hero Myth and the Fire Family

In Jungian psychology, the hero is one of the primary archetypes, representing the ego's journey toward growth and self-realization through overcoming obstacles (Jung, 1959a, 1959b). The warrior can be seen as a specific aspect or subtype of the hero archetype, focusing on courage, strength, discipline, and the defense of a cause. While all warriors are heroes, not all heroes are purely warriors. A hero's journey often involves multiple roles, such as lover, sage, or trickster, depending on the stage of their development. In myths and stories, the warrior embodies the hero's active and aggressive side, the part that faces enemies, conquers fears, and fights for ideals. At the same time, the broader hero archetype also includes personal transformation, sacrifice, and wisdom. Thus, the warrior is an important but specialized expression of the hero's greater quest.

Firefighter culture is deeply influenced by enduring mythology and folklore, which reinforce a collective identity rooted in bravery, sacrifice, and solidarity. The "hero" archetype is central to this mythology, represented by an idealized figure who fearlessly risks their life to protect others (Jung, 1959a, 1959b). The firefighter culture described here primarily draws from the hero archetype, emphasizing the ideals of bravery, sacrifice, and selfless service. Although elements of strength and resilience are present, traits associated with the warrior archetype, the dominant narrative focuses on protection and altruism rather than direct combat or aggression (Jung, 1959a, 1959b). This narrative is reinforced by media portrayals, departmental traditions, and societal reverence, shaping public expectations and firefighters' self-concepts. While the hero myth fosters pride and purpose, it also contributes to cultural norms that discourage vulnerability and emotional expression, particularly in male-dominated environments (Addis & Mahalik, 2003; Wong et al., 2017). It may also foster hostility toward female colleagues if they do not conform to male norms, distancing themselves from traditionally female-gendered identities.

Thus, the warrior is an important but specialized expression of the hero's greater quest. In fire and emergency services, these archetypal patterns extend beyond individual identity and are woven into collective cultural constructs. Complementing this mythos is the notion of the "fire family," a psychological framework rooted in shared danger and mutual trust. Like a band of warriors bound by loyalty and common purpose, the fire family reinforces the heroic ideals of bravery, sacrifice, and solidarity within a communal context (Tajfel & Turner, 1979). Firefighter folklore, including initiations, rituals, superstitions, and spiritual symbols such as Saint Florian and the Maltese Cross, anchor these ideals, providing emotional coping mechanisms and cultural continuity in high-risk occupations. However, as with the Warrior archetype's potential for rigidity and exclusion, the fireful family can also uphold narrow identity norms and resist change, creating barriers for women, mental health professionals, and others who challenge traditional narratives. Understanding the function of these myths within the fire service is, therefore, critical to supporting cultural change, emotional well-being, and organizational inclusivity.

Knights and Dragons: Archetypes in the Fire Service

Throughout history, mythological archetypes have offered powerful frameworks for understanding individual and collective struggles against adversity. Within the context of fire service, these enduring symbols continue to shape cultural identity and operational behavior. Among the most prominent is the warrior archetype, reflected in the imagery of knights confronting dragons. Narratives valorize courage, loyalty, discipline, and the defense of order against chaos. Rooted in Jungian theory (Jung, 1959a, 1959b), the warrior archetype operates as an unconscious blueprint, influencing how firefighters interpret danger, duty, and self-sacrifice. Firefighters are often cast as modern knights, embodying stoic resilience and an unwavering commitment to protect others. At the same time, fire is personified as a living, destructive force to be battled and subdued. This mythological framing may inspire bravery and loyalty, subtly reinforcing cultural norms that prioritize risk-taking, emotional suppression, and individual heroism over caution and strategic collaboration.

The warrior archetype, often reflected in the symbolism of knights and dragons, offers a psychologically rich framework for understanding firefighters' internal struggles in high-risk, male-dominated professions such as firefighting. The warrior archetype, grounded in medieval tales of honor, courage, and sacrifice, mirrors the idealized image of the firefighter, who is task-driven; committed to maintaining order through bravery, discipline, and loyalty; and characterized by selflessness and steadfastness in the face of danger. This archetype resonates with cultural expectations that firefighters be stoic protectors, often suppressing emotional expression in pursuit of a heroic identity (Moore & Gillette, 1990).

Fire is often equated with dragons, potent symbols of fire, danger, and destruction, mirroring the behavior of uncontrolled flames. In mythology, dragons breathe fire, destroy villages, and are nearly unstoppable, much like a fast-moving blaze. According to Jungian theory, such imagery arises from the collective unconscious, where dragons symbolize archetypal forces of chaos that the individual should confront to achieve growth and integration (Jung, 1959a, 1959b). By comparing fire to a dragon, firefighters use a psychological projection process, externalizing inner fears, dangers, and desires onto a tangible adversary. Thus, fire becomes not only a physical threat but also a symbolic mirror reflecting the internal struggle between order and chaos within the human psyche. This archetypal projection transforms firefighting into a profound symbolic act, where battling fire represents an unconscious battle against the darker, uncontrollable forces within oneself.

As Jung (1959a, 1959b) explained, archetypal projection can significantly influence behavior. In the context of the fire service, it may occur when firefighters frame their work in heroic, mythic terms and encourage a warrior mindset. When fire is perceived as a "beast" to be conquered, firefighters may unconsciously feel compelled to prove their courage by "slaying the dragon," often leading to elevated risk-taking. Moore and Gillette (1990) emphasize that the Warrior archetype valorizes disciplined action and stoic bravery, qualities that, when projected onto the fireground, can romanticize hazardous situations, elevate danger as an admirable pursuit, prioritize individual acts of heroism over collaborative efforts, and diminish the value placed on caution and tactical decision-making. In this way, while inspiring bravery, archetypal imagery may inadvertently reinforce behaviors that increase operational danger (Jung, 1959a, 1959b).

While mythological projections, such as the dragon metaphor, foster courage and reinforce a heroic identity, they also heighten the psychological and operational risks associated with the excessive valorization of danger. Beyond the metaphor of battle, however, lies a deeper mythological narrative. Drawing again on Jung's (1959) insights into the collective unconscious, the Prometheus myth frames the relationship with fire as a fight and a sacred burden. Through this lens, the fire service's confrontation with danger becomes a story of heroism and enduring sacrifice, moral responsibility, and often unseen psychological costs borne by those who carry fire on behalf of others (Moore & Gillette, 1990).

Prometheus: The Sacred Burden of Fire

The Greek myth of Prometheus, who stole fire from the gods and endured eternal suffering for the sake of humanity, offers a mythological lens through which we can view the firefighter's relationship with danger, knowledge, and sacrifice (Hamilton, 1942). Firefighters, like Prometheus, may embrace the paradox of fire, as it is both the destroyer and the sustainer of life. By confronting fire, they confront the elemental force and the existential burden of responsibility for others' lives (Jung, 1959a, 1959b).

The Promethean figure positions the firefighter as a visionary rebel who willingly bears suffering in service to a collective good. However, Prometheus' punishment imposed by Zeus, being chained and endlessly tormented, also speaks to the psychological consequences of this sacred mission. In fire and emergency services, this burden may manifest as moral injury, guilt, or the silent endurance of cumulative trauma. On social media, PTSD is often discussed as a "badge of honor," symbolizing the epic battle and the sacrifices made for others over oneself (V., 2025).

In this mythology, fire is more than a physical phenomenon; it becomes a moral object. To bring fire under control, wrestling it from chaos and bending it toward human needs becomes a sacred act. In doing so, firefighters metaphorically share in Prometheus' guilt. The guilt stems from carrying an impossible responsibility and the persistent sense that, no matter how much is given, it is never enough.

Thus, the Promethean lens offers the profound insight that while heroism is revered, it is often paid for through hidden psychological costs. Prometheus does not suffer because he was weak; he suffers because he cared (Moore & Gillette, 1990). In this way, society has often tied mental health conditions such as post-traumatic stress and even suicide to the job as if it is a singular metaphoric exchange (a direct and inevitable consequence of the job itself), rather than a complex psychological process involving a plethora of risk and protective factors. This framing risks reducing complex psychological experiences to a symbolic "cost of heroism," rather than recognizing mental health conditions and subsequent behaviors as outcomes shaped by a constellation of individual, organizational, and cultural risk and protective factors (Kraft-Todd & Rand, 2019). Such oversimplifications obscure the nuanced realities of trauma exposure and coping, limiting our ability to design effective, empathetic interventions.

Valhalla: Death, Honor, and the Perpetual Order

Norse mythology gives us another powerful cultural metaphor through the myth of Valhalla, the great hall where fallen warriors reside, feasting and preparing for Ragnarök. In fire service, Valhalla's echoes resonate powerfully in how fallen firefighters are memorialized, honored, and mythologized (Lindow, 2001; Simek, 1993).

The ceremonial rituals following a firefighter's death, the sounding of the final bell, the procession of rigs, and the rows of dress blues transform the individual into a symbol, securing their place in the eternal order of the honored dead. Valhalla transforms tragedy into legacy. Death is not perceived as a hopeless loss but rather a sacred elevation giving meaning to danger and sacrifice, which allows the living to continue to risk their lives within a framework promising immortality through memory, honor, and a sacred bond.

This cultural myth serves critical psychological functions. It transforms grief into pride. It offers meaning in the face of perhaps even a senseless tragedy. It creates an infinite ceremonial bond. It also allows living people to continue to risk their lives, as death does not represent oblivion but rather exaltation, entry into a heroic pantheon. This can be especially relevant in cases of wildland firefighting, where an accident can lead to a greater number of fatalities since fire suppression activities occur within the context of a larger group spread over a greater distance.

While myths offer emotional meaning and collective solace, they can also blur important distinctions surrounding death. Fire service mythology, particularly archetypes such as heroes and warriors, often sanctifies all deaths equally, obscuring whether fatalities are preventable or inevitable (Jung, 1959a, 1959b; Jost & Banaji, 1994). This framing risks insulating the profession from examining systemic failures, strategic oversights, and untreated mental health conditions. Mythologies such as Valhalla imbue sacrifice with a sacred legacy, transforming loss into symbolic immortality (Lindow, 2001; Simek, 1993). Ceremonial practices such as memorial bell traditions further embed fallen firefighters within a continuum of reverence. While this cultural lens fosters unity and resilience, it may also condition members to accept death as a natural, sometimes even necessary, dimension of their role. To honor the dead with integrity, mythology must be accompanied by critical reflection, ensuring that reverence does not obscure the imperative for safety, accountability, and systemic change.

Fire and Faith: Biblical Imagery and the Moral Mythology of the Fire Service

Like much of the nation's public service tradition, American fire and emergency services have long drawn upon Judeo-Christian beliefs with cultural and spiritual foundations. For many firefighters, particularly in a workforce historically composed of White men, biblical imagery and language offer a powerful lens through which danger, sacrifice, and duty are interpreted. In this context, fire is not only a physical phenomenon but also a moral and spiritual phenomenon charged with symbolic meaning that reinforces archetypes of divine calling, heroic suffering, and ultimate redemption.

Fire as a Purifier and Judgment

The Bible portrays fire as both destructive and sacred, simultaneously representing a force of divine judgment and a holy presence. In the Old Testament, fire often signals God's power and purification: "For the Lord thy God is a consuming fire, even a jealous God" (Deuteronomy 4:24, KJV). "The fire shall ever be burning upon the altar; it shall never go out" (Leviticus 6:13, KJV). These passages resonate with the firefighter's intimate relationship with fire. Like biblical fire cleanses and tests, the fireground also demands purification through trials, both in terms of character and courage. Fire becomes a moral landscape where judgment and mercy meet, echoing the archetypal journey of the firefighter as a protector of life and property and as a guardian of sacred human dignity.

Confronting Hell: The Firefighter's Battle against the Infernal

In Christian ideology, fire is also intimately tied to the concept of hell, a place of torment and moral reckoning, often depicted as a fiery abyss ruled by the devil. While modern theology may nuance this imagery, the cultural language persists, especially in the symbolic frames often used by firefighters: "The Son of man shall send forth his angels… and shall cast them into a furnace of fire: there shall be wailing and gnashing of teeth" (Matthew 13:41–42, KJV). "And death and hell were cast into the lake of fire. This is the second death" (Revelation 20:14, KJV).

For many in the fire service, particularly those raised within Christian traditions, entering a burning structure can feel like stepping into a version of that mythic battle, a descent into chaos that mirrors biblical struggles against evil. It is common for fire to be referred to in near-spiritual terms: "fighting the devil's heat" or "holding the line at the gates of hell." Whether it is a metaphor or mindset, this language offers a moral framework for navigating danger and death.

Biblical Themes: Deliverance from the Flames

The stories of Shadrach, Meshach, and Abednego (Daniel 3:16—27) are among the most enduring biblical narratives of fire. Ordered to be burned alive for refusing to worship false gods, the three men are cast into a blazing furnace yet emerge unharmed, protected by divine presence: "Lo, I see four men loose… and the form of the fourth is like the Son of God" (Daniel 3:25, KJV).

This story of spiritual courage in the face of annihilation may resonate strongly with firefighters. It reflects the archetype of righteous warriors who walk through fire with bravery and faith. In this sense, the modern firefighter, even in a secular context, steps into a mythic lineage that echoes these sacred narratives: facing death not recklessly but with conviction in a greater good.

Satan, Sin, and the Fireground as Moral Theater

Scripture frequently associates fire with the punishment of Satan and the final triumph of good over evil: "And the devil that deceived them was cast into the lake of fire and brimstone… and shall be tormented day and night for ever and ever" (Revelation 20:10, KJV).

This portrayal turns fire into a weapon of divine justice, used not against the innocent but against the forces of corruption, evil, and deception. Within fire service mythology, this theme is echoed in how danger is faced, not as random chaos but as something to be resisted with moral clarity. The fire becomes the adversary, and the firefighter, consciously or not, often sees himself battling on the side of good, perhaps even in a cosmic sense.

Tradition, Identity, and Opportunity for Growth

Given that the American fire service remains predominantly White males (Danbold & Bendersky, 2020), and is often shaped by Judeo-Christian values, it is understandable that these religious and cultural narratives have deeply informed the profession's mythology. Moral clarity, the archetypes of protector and warrior, and the redemptive framework of sacrifice strengthen identity and purpose.

However, as the service becomes more diverse, including individuals of different races, genders, and faiths, there is a powerful opportunity to evolve the mythology to embrace a shared language of service, including additional interpretations inclusive of all those willing to face the risk of fire for the benefit of others.

Hagiography and the Construction of Heroic Identity

Within the American fire service, the memorialization of fallen firefighters frequently reflects elements of hagiography, a tradition rooted in the Catholic Church that idealizes the lives of saints as models of moral and spiritual excellence. This narrative framework emphasizes qualities such as bravery, sacrifice, and loyalty, often at the expense of acknowledging individual complexity, human fallibility, or the nuanced circumstances surrounding each death (Johnson, 2019). While concepts such as Valhalla highlight the internal, in-group cultural dynamics that shape how firefighters themselves interpret death, hagiographic practices illustrate how broader society responds to firefighter death. Through public monuments, ceremonial tributes, and collective storytelling, firefighters who died in the line of duty are often elevated to the status of moral exemplars, serving as enduring symbols of professional and civic virtue.

This hagiographic tendency serves important cultural functions. It binds the community together in shared reverence. It reinforces the values of sacrifice, loyalty, and courage. This ensures that the legacy of service is passed down through generations with honor and respect. However, as with all forms of mythology, there are inherent dangers. Idealization can lead to unrealistic expectations. Living firefighters may feel pressured to embody perfection, mask vulnerability, and deny struggles that deviate from a standard of stoicism and perfectionism (Thurnell-Read & Parker, 2008). Hagiography creates expectations that no human being can sustainably meet. Suppressing the complexity of the human experience by omitting struggles such as mental health challenges, suicide, substance abuse, organizational failures, or preventable accidents hinders honest engagement with the conditions that affect firefighter health and safety. The gap between myths and reality can erode mental health. When individuals inevitably fall short of the idealized image, they may experience shame, alienation, or a sense of unworthiness. When the complex nature of the firefighter experience is excluded from the fire service narrative, critical insights are obscured, and opportunities for growth, prevention, and systemic improvement are forfeited.

If we honor death without investigating context, we risk valorizing unnecessary loss. We reinforce the cultural expectation that sacrifice alone is the metric of honor, even when death results not only from valor but also from systemic issues left unaddressed (Jost et al., 2004; Teoh et al., 2019). While hagiography creates the opportunity to inspire and strengthen community identity, it should be balanced with a willingness to embrace the full humanity of the firefighter experience. In reimagining the mythology of fire and emergency services for future generations, it is imperative to honor not only how firefighters die but also how they live.

Firefighter Death, Memorialization, and the Myth of Mortality

In every culture, death demands meaning. In fire and emergency services, meaning is amplified through rituals, monuments, and storytelling that elevate the fallen into heroes, often regardless of the circumstances of their death (Johnson, 2019). This phenomenon parallels ancient hagiography, where saints were venerated less for the mundane details of their deaths and more for what their lives symbolized to the community they left behind.

Modern fire service memorialization practices, such as the Last Alarm, bagpipes, helmet ceremonies, and names etched in stone, serve to sanctify the memories of fallen firefighters (Johnson, 2019). These rituals provide the living with a sacred framework for processing grief, establishing continuity, and reinforcing the cultural values of bravery, sacrifice, and connection. Emotionally, they create communal spaces where loss is honored without the need for analytical dissection.

However, hagiography presents inherent dangers when it idealizes death to the point that critical discussions about cause, prevention, and context are marginalized (Dangermond et al., 2022). When every firefighter death is mythologized in the same way, regardless of the underlying factors, be it strategic failure, unsafe practices, suicide, or organizational breakdown, opportunities for learning and systemic improvement are lost.

In many cases, psychological studies have shown that behavior reinforced through honorific recognition is more likely to be replicated (Luthans & Stajkovic, 2003). If aggressive, risky behaviors are posthumously valorized without nuanced reflection, the next generation may inherit a distorted roadmap, equating recklessness with heroism. The fire service should thus grapple with a difficult but necessary tension: honoring sacrifice without sanctifying avoidable tragedy. It is important to differentiate between courageous sacrifice and systemic failure, reinforcing that true heroism includes operational excellence, risk assessment, and leadership accountability. Mythology should evolve not to strip death of meaning but to deepen it with wisdom and understanding.

Organizational Folklore, Humor, and Emotional Survival

The psychological outcomes of firefighters' exposure to potentially traumatic events, grief, injustice, and helplessness requires internal cultural mechanisms for processing pain. Humor, storytelling, and ritualized camaraderie form the informal folklore that sustains firefighters across generations.

In many stations, gallows humor operates as both a shield and a lifeline. It allows firefighters to speak the unspeakable, confront horror through satire, and collectively name their fears without vulnerability (Dangermond et al., 2022). Joking about death, injury, or loss does not necessarily signify disrespect; it often signals acknowledgment and a sense of survival.

However, like all cultural tools, humor should be used with care. While humor can create solidarity, it can also alienate those who process trauma differently, particularly recruits, other groups, or individuals with different emotional coping styles (Thurnell-Read & Parker, 2008; Eriksen, 2019).

Folklore, when rigid, can also reinforce unhealthy emotional norms, such as emotional suppression, masculinity scripts, or stigma against seeking help. Thus, while station humor remains critical to emotional survival, leaders should recognize the subtle signs when humor masks more profound, unaddressed trauma: prolonged silence, cynicism slipping into nihilism, or the sudden disappearance of humor altogether.

A mature fire service culture will not abandon its storytelling traditions, humor, or deep reverence for the connection that it fosters. Instead, it consciously adapts these practices to foster inclusion, psychological safety, and emotional honesty without losing the important spirit that makes firefighting culture unique.

European Roots, Franklin's Influence, and Fire Service Identity

The American fire service was never created in isolation; it emerged as a direct descendant of European firefighting models, particularly those evolving after the Great Fire of London in 1666 (Carp, 2001; London Fire Brigade, n.d.). Privatizing fire brigades under insurance companies, the emergence of fire marks, and the establishment of paid fire protection systems laid the groundwork for how Americans conceptualized fire protection as both a civic and commercial necessity.

Drawing from London's insurance brigade model, Benjamin Franklin helped launch America's first formalized insurance-based fire protection entity: The Philadelphia Contributionship in 1752 (The Philadelphia Contributionship, n.d.). Franklin's pragmatic, Enlightenment-era approach to communal safety combined fire protection with civic responsibility—a philosophical marriage that continues to shape the American fire service identity today.

Artifacts of this European lineage remain deeply woven into the fire service: the paramilitary rank structure, the use of fire marks as early symbols of coverage and community standing, and even the guild-like organization of volunteer companies into competitive and often politically charged fraternities (Carp, 2001; Merrimack, n.d.).

The rise of national organizations such as the National Fire Protection Association (NFPA) and the development of what became known as the "Nine Sisters" (key national fire organizations) further standardized and professionalized the fire service, pushing it beyond local rivalries toward a unified, evidence-based safety model.

Understanding this European inheritance is critical for understanding modern firefighting culture, not merely as a spontaneous American phenomenon but also as an evolving tapestry of global influences, adapted to local needs, mythologized through ritual, and continually reinterpreted across generations.

Shift Schedules and the Cultural Construction of Time

Although research consistently shows that shift schedules significantly impact firefighters' sleep quality, the U.S. fire and emergency services lack a federally mandated standard for work or rest hours, leading to wide variation across departments (Rajaratnam et al., 2011). Among the most common models is the 24/48 shift, where 24 h are on duty followed by 48 h off, which has evolved beyond a scheduling choice into a cultural cornerstone. While widely practiced, this model remains controversial because of its potential long-term effects on health, fatigue, and safety (Billings & Focht, 2016). It is often viewed as a badge of honor and a test of endurance, reinforcing shared identity, connection, and a sense of belonging. Enduring sleep deprivation, family disruption, and physical strain without complaints is often framed as a rite of passage and is deeply ingrained in the fire service ethos.

However, the cultural valorization of this schedule contrasts sharply with the empirical findings. Approximately 73% of firefighters report poor sleep quality (Barger et al., 2015). While Billings and Focht (2016) reported that the 24/48 model is associated with the best sleep outcomes compared with alternatives such as the Kelly schedule, it still presents challenges, especially for those working second jobs, who report significantly worse sleep, suggesting that cumulative work demands further diminish recovery and well-being (Barger et al., 2015; Billings & Focht, 2016). These findings underscore the importance of reconciling traditional practices with evidence-based scheduling, prioritizing firefighter health and operational effectiveness.

Growing research links traditional shift patterns to serious health consequences, including chronic circadian disruption, sleep deprivation, cardiovascular disease, mental health issues, and cognitive decline (Petruzzello et al., 2016; Smith et al., 2023). However, in a culture that equates endurance with strength, these outcomes are often interpreted as personal weakness rather than predictable physiological effects. Proposals for alternative schedules, such as 48/96 or hybrid models, frequently address cultural resistance rather than scientific scrutiny.

Within this narrative, the 24-hours shift symbolizes toughness, availability, and sacrifice. However, holding onto outdated models without regard for biological and psychological data may ultimately compromise the qualities of resilience, alertness, and courage the culture seeks to uphold. True cultural evolution will require integrating empirical evidence with fire service values, reframing rest and recovery not as indulgences but as critical tools for sustaining performance, sound decision-making, and long-term well-being.

Volunteers, Career Firefighters, and Cultural Fractures

The American fire service is not monolithic; it is an intricate ecosystem composed of career, volunteer, and combination departments, each with its own cultural myths, stresses, and identities. Volunteer firefighters, in particular, have historically embodied the mythos of the citizen-soldier: ordinary individuals are willing to make extraordinary sacrifices for their communities.

However, structural inequities complicate this narrative. Compared with their career counterparts, volunteer firefighters often face higher rates of depression, PTSD symptoms, and suicidal ideation, primarily driven by fewer resources, less formalized mental health support, and deeper barriers to care (Stanley et al., 2017). In volunteer organizations, loyalty to the community can sometimes create double-edged expectations: the notion that authentic service should come at the expense of personal well-being. Moreover, career firefighters benefit from stronger institutional support structures and face cultural pressures toward invulnerability, risk glorification, and peer comparison, which inhibit emotional openness. The tension between volunteer and career identities often extends beyond operational issues into questions of "who is a real firefighter," reinforcing hierarchical divides that complicate organizational belonging (Baigent,

2001; Carp, 2001). Recognizing these nuances is important. There is value in both volunteer and career firefighting roles, and specialization through professionalization plays a critical role in advancing the field. However, framing these roles as a simple dichotomy overlooks their complementary contributions and undermines the diverse strengths each brings to the fire service. Emotional wellness, risk mitigation, and professional dignity should become universal standards, regardless of paychecks or the organizational structure.

Cultural Competence, Organizational Safety Climate, and Modern Reform

One of the most pressing tasks facing fire and emergency services today is addressing how internal culture either reinforces or undermines safety behaviors. Decades of research show that a strong organizational safety climate, where leadership visibly prioritizes safety, listens to concerns, and models safe behavior, predicts reduced injuries, improved mental health outcomes, and decreased risk-taking (Hokmabadi et al., 2022).

However, many departments, consciously or not, still glorify risk-taking behaviors as part of a cultural ideal of bravery. Despite formal policies emphasizing safety, these behaviors are often reinforced through symbolic rewards, informal praise, heroic storytelling, or peer recognition.

As Jung and Chang (2020) aptly argue, cultural heroism and aggressive interior firefighting tactics are double-edged swords: they promote courage, but they can foster preventable fatalities if not checked by strategic thinking and organizational accountability.

Developing a truly resilient fire service culture requires more than updating policies—it means reshaping foundational norms. Evidence supports a holistic approach: reinforcing seatbelt compliance, rigorously managing carcinogen exposure (Smith et al., 2024), normalizing psychological help, and deploying data-driven tactics to assess and respond to risk.

Change should be emotionally resonant to be sustainable. Leaders should align new safety narratives with familiar archetypes, framing risk assessment and emotional intelligence not as weaknesses but as evolutions of the knightly virtues firefighters already honor: strength, wisdom, and loyalty to others.

Artifacts and Iconography in the Fire Service

In every mythology, physical artifacts serve as symbols that anchor cultural values in a tangible form. The fire service is no different. From the Maltese Cross emblazoned on helmets and patches to the polished brass bells and bugles displayed in firehouses, these objects are more than decorative; they are saturated with cultural meaning, signaling courage, sacrifice, and fraternity.

The Maltese Cross is the most universally recognized emblem within fire and emergency services. Originally associated with the Knights of St. John during the Crusades, the symbol represents bravery and protection in the face of overwhelming odds. For firefighters, wearing the cross is not just a tradition but also a daily affirmation of readiness to risk one's life for others. However, few may realize how the adoption of this medieval symbol reflects the fire service's deep-rooted need to connect contemporary acts of bravery to a mythic lineage of chivalric virtue.

Similarly, helmets are not merely protective gear but also artifacts of identity. Each helmet, scratched and smoke-darkened, becomes a personal ledger of experience and survival. Firefighters often inscribe names, slogans, or personal symbols inside their helmets, blending individual memory with collective tradition. A clean, untouched helmet can signal inexperience, whereas a weathered one, thick with the patina of years, quietly commands respect.

Badges, slogans, and patches offer additional layers of meaning. Units often design unique insignias featuring dragons, skulls, ladders, axes, and fire, a visual language steeped in themes of danger, mortality, and triumph. Firehouse walls are often adorned with plaques, memorial flags, or retired gear, creating sacred spaces of remembrance and belonging. These artifacts link each generation of firefighters to those who came before, reinforcing that today's actions are part of an unbroken heroic continuum.

Even everyday stationary objects carry symbolic weight, such as worn recliners in front of the TV, communal coffee pots, or ceremonial bells rung at funerals. They are the ordinary relics of an extraordinary life. Objects tell a story about community and resilience, and rituals make survival, loss, and legacy bearable.

Understanding fire and emergency services without artifacts would be similar to studying a religion without considering its icons. The objects with which firefighters surround themselves are not peripheral but central to how identity, memory, and mythology are constructed and maintained.

The Development of the "Nine Sisters" and the USFA

No discussion of American fire service mythology would be complete without exploring the creation of national standards and the organizations that embody collective identity today. Among them is the United States Fire Administration (USFA), which was formed in the wake of the 1973 "America Burning" report, a document that fundamentally reshaped the federal government's relationship to fire prevention and life safety (USFA, 2022).

The emergence of what many colloquially call the "Nine Sisters" (the major fire service organizations in the United States) represents a new layer of mythology: a national identity layered atop the local connection. These organizations, which include the IAFC, IAFF, NFPA, and others, serve as stewards of tradition, protectors of standards, and aspirational symbols of unity.

For example, the National Fire Protection Association (NFPA), with its red square and White flame logo, may evoke authority and trust. It is not simply a regulatory body but an archetype: the wise elder who gathers knowledge and shares it with the tribe. The standards it produces, such as NFPA 1710 on staffing and NFPA 1500 on occupational safety, have taken on a near-scriptural status within the fire service.

Similarly, the National Fallen Firefighters Memorial in Emmitsburg, Maryland, functions almost as a national shrine. The inscribed names, the eternal flame, and the ceremonial rituals reflect a distinctly American version of Valhalla, reinforcing narratives of sacrifice, immortality, and connection in death (Johnson, 2019).

However, while these institutions offer unity, they reflect the ongoing tension between tradition and transformation. The fire service remains deeply proud of its history but is challenged by the need to evolve its practices, leadership models, and inclusivity efforts. The mythology created by national organizations should therefore be reverent and dynamic, honoring the past without becoming shackled to it. The "Nine Sisters" test the fire service's belief in collective destiny, that firefighting is not merely a job but a calling woven into the nation's broader story of resilience, sacrifice, and hope.

Hagiography in the Digital Age

Fire service culture has long relied on storytelling to reinforce values, but the way we create and share these stories has evolved dramatically. In today's digital world, hagiography, the reverent portrayal of firefighters as flawless heroes, has found new platforms and amplified reach through social media, news coverage, and public memorials.

Platforms such as Facebook, Instagram, and YouTube now act as modern cathedrals where stories of sacrifice, bravery, and tragedy are curated and widely shared. When a firefighter falls in the line of duty, digital tribute quickly emerges: profile pictures change to mourning bands, flood timelines are posted with phrases such as "Never Forget," and hashtags such as #FallenHero or #LastAlarm trend across communities. These acts are not merely displays of grief but rituals, which are part of a larger myth-making process that sustains fire service identity (Johnson, 2019).

hagiography However, in the digital era, hagiographic portrayals often heighten the emotional weight that firefighters and society attach to both the memory of the fallen and the identity of the living. Today, firefighters grow immersed in images and stories that canonize prior generations, particularly surrounding events such as 9/11, where heroism is presented not only as an ideal but also as an expectation (Greenburg, 2001). This standard can create immense psychological pressure. Recruits may feel compelled to emulate the myth, pushing themselves into dangerous behaviors or internalizing feelings of inadequacy if they fall short of the idealized legacy (Stanley et al., 2017). This digital hagiography can be a double-edged sword. On the one hand, it powerfully cements community bonds, honors sacrifice, and reminds society of the important role of fire and emergency services. On the other hand, it can discourage honest conversations about the broader realities of firefighter life, including unsafe practices, psychological suffering, or structural failures, which sometimes contribute to tragedy. It becomes important, therefore, to ask ourselves: are we mythologizing firefighters in a way that strengthens their humanity, or are we unknowingly building a mythology that silences it?

Leaders, educators, and firefighters alike should grapple with this tension in shaping the next generation of fire service culture. We need myth, but we also need truth. Recognizing the full humanity of those we honor does not diminish their legacy; it deepens it, making the sacrifices more real, relatable, and ultimately more meaningful to those who carry on the profession.

Culture, Contamination, and the "Badge of Honor"

One of the more insidious ways that mythology impacts fire and emergency services is through the relationships among gear contamination, health risks, and cultural norms. Firefighters have long worn the soot and smell of fire like a badge of honor, a visible sign they have fought the "dragon" and survived. Nevertheless, what was once seen as a proud symbol of bravery is increasingly considered a silent, deadly threat to firefighter health (Wolffe et al., 2023).

Research has shown that exposure to carcinogenic fire byproducts involves not only firegrounds but also the very fabric of firefighting gear, apparatuses, and stations. The UK Firefighter Contamination Survey revealed that a lack of proper training regarding fire effluents was directly associated with unsafe practices, such as failing to clean personal protective equipment (PPE) or continuing to wear contaminated gear after incidents (Wolffe et al., 2023). Firefighters who endorsed the "badge of honor" mentality were twice as likely to engage in risky contamination behaviors as those who did not.

This is a prime example of how mythology, in this case, the story that visible dirt and soot equates to valor, can actively endanger firefighters rather than protect them. Cultural identity becomes so tightly woven with physical evidence of having "been through the fire" that questioning the practice feels like questioning someone's commitment to the fire service community.

The data paint a stark picture. The firefighters who view contamination as a badge of honor are as follows:

- More likely to eat without washing residue from their hands,
- More likely to report smoke particles in their noses and throats,
- More likely to notice the persistent smell of smoke on their bodies for days after an incident, and.

- Moreover, they are less likely to prioritize cleaning their gear and station (Wolffe et al., 2023).

All of these findings point to a severe occupational health crisis rooted not in negligence but in culture. Firefighters are not ignoring contamination because they do not care; they are doing so because, for generations, contamination has been culturally reframed as a visible mark of survival and toughness.

Altering these behaviors requires more than implementing formal policies; it necessitates a cultural shift that reexamines and reconstructs the foundational narratives shaping firefighter identity. Clean gear must be redefined as a marker of professionalism rather than perceived weakness, and decontamination practices should be understood not as optional routines but as important expressions of responsibility and acts of commitment to oneself, colleagues, and the communities served.

This issue extends beyond occupational safety; it involves reimagining the symbolic frameworks that guide firefighter behavior. Without such transformation, the long-term effects of toxic exposure, which might be seen as the metaphorical "dragon," risk undermining the very values the profession seeks to hold long after the flames have been extinguished.

Fire Service Mythology and our Relationship with Death

In ancient traditions, mythology was not merely entertainment; it was a matter of survival. Myths help communities understand the unknown, give structure to chaos, and prepare individuals to confront life's greatest inevitability, death (Campbell, 1949). The American fire service is no different. Our relationship with death is mythologized in ways that offer meaning, ritual, and collective identity but also invites complicated consequences.

Within the fire service, death is often treated with a sacred reverence. Fallen firefighters are memorialized through rituals that mirror religious rites, including the etching of names in stone, the playing of ceremonial bells, the sound of bagpipes, and the draping of the casket with the American flag (Johnson, 2019). These practices serve important psychological functions. They elevate sacrifice, bind survivors together, and help communities externalize their grief. In doing so, they reinforce the mythological narrative that dying in the line of duty is to achieve a form of immortality.

Hagiography, the idealized portrayal of individuals after death, plays a profound role here. As in medieval sainthood narratives, the details of how a firefighter dies are often less important than the fact that they died in the line of duty. The story becomes simplified, purified, and elevated. The risk, however, is that the myth can overpower reality. Death is often honored without examining the circumstances that led to it, whether it resulted from strategic miscalculations, cultural pressure to take unnecessary risks, or systemic organizational failures (Jung & Chang, 2020).

In doing so, we risk creating a mythology in which death itself becomes the final credential of valor, regardless of cause. The myth can subtly influence the perceptions of active firefighters regarding what constitutes bravery and the sacrifices expected. In the absence of critical reflection, younger generations may internalize the belief that dying in service is not only honorable but also expected, an expectation that carries immense psychological and ethical weight.

As we consider how to evolve the fire service culture, we must not abandon ceremonies, pride, or tradition. However, we should refine this myth. We should begin to distinguish between death as a tragic, sometimes preventable, outcome and behavior that embodies the highest ideals of fire service, wisdom, courage, discipline, and resilience.

Our relationship with death could not glorify sacrifice for sacrifice's sake. It could honor those who lived and served wisely, as well as those who employed strategies to preserve their own and others' lives as sacred trust. Only then can we craft a mythology that empowers the next generation not only to die bravely but also to live wisely, serve honorably, and lead the fire service forward.

The Knight, Dragon, and Fire Service: Risk-Taking, Masculinity, and Emotional Growth in the Fire Service

The mythological narrative of the knight facing the dragon provides a compelling metaphor for understanding the psychological and cultural dynamics at play within the fire service. The firefighter, much like the knight, is called to act with bravery, sacrifice, and honor, confronting not only external dangers but also internal fears (Moore & Gillette, 1990; Jung, 1959a, 1959b).

However, in many fire service cultures, the emphasis remains heavily weighted toward conquering the external dragon—the fire and the physical danger—whereas the internal dragons of trauma, fear, guilt, and grief are often left unaddressed (Desmond, 2007; Wong et al., 2017).

The traditional firehouse culture, steeped in masculinity and stoicism, valorizes outward acts of bravery but often stigmatizes emotional openness (Thurnell-Read & Parker, 2008). Culture is where mythology can both empower and imprison. While "knight" imagery fuels dedication and selflessness, it can also demand emotional suppression and perfection, and trait research increasingly connects this dynamic to burnout, depression, and suicidal ideation within the profession (Stanley et al., 2017).

The dragon, understood through a Jungian lens, represents external threats and the internal shadow—the unseen, unspoken vulnerabilities individuals should confront for proper psychological integration and growth (Jung, 1959a, 1959b). With respect to fire service, these internal dragons can manifest in various ways. Unprocessed grief after the loss of a civilian or a fellow firefighter often lingers silently, creating emotional wounds that may fester without acknowledgment.

Survivors' guilt may emerge following high-level incidents, burdening firefighters with feelings of responsibility for outcomes beyond their control. Moral injury can also occur, particularly when individuals are forced to act against their moral code or witness events that violate their deeply held values. Compounding these struggles is the internalized stigma against seeking psychological support, a stigma often reinforced by cultural norms that equate vulnerability with weakness. Additionally, organizational betrayals, in which firefighters feel abandoned, unsupported, or misled by their institutions, can deepen emotional injury, eroding trust and amplifying the internal struggle. Recognizing and addressing these internal dragons is critical for fostering resilience and supporting the psychological health of fire and emergency services.

Unfortunately, system justification theory and group identity research indicate that tightly bonded, high-risk cultures often resist acknowledging internal weaknesses because they fear that these will destabilize the collective identity (Jost & Banaji, 1994; Tajfel & Turner, 1979). In this context, emotional struggle can be mistakenly interpreted as a threat rather than a natural aspect of the human experience.

To promote resilience, fire service leaders should reframe emotional growth not as antithetical to bravery but as an evolution of it. Emotional intelligence, self-awareness, and vulnerability should be presented as new "armors," important tools for today's knights in an increasingly complex fireground environment (Festinger, 1957).

Without this cultural shift, the cost is clear: higher rates of psychological injury, burnout, and unnecessary operational risk (Petruzzello et al., 2016; Stanley et al., 2017). By integrating the mythic language firefighters already understand, knights, dragons, and quests, we can build bridges toward the necessary change. Myth, after all, is not static. It evolves.

PTSD: Not a Badge of Honor but a Call for Healing

Posttraumatic stress disorder (PTSD) should not be misunderstood as a badge of honor or an inevitable consequence of courageous service. Instead, it is a clinical condition reflecting chronic activation of the sympathetic nervous system, which is responsible for fight, flight, or freezing responses following trauma exposure (Bryant, 2019; Berger et al., 2012). When individuals experience trauma that is not fully processed, their bodies continue to signal danger even after the immediate threat has passed, resulting in persistent hypervigilance, emotional numbing, irritability, nightmares, and related health complications (Bartlett et al., 2018; Arbona et al., 2016).

Healing from PTSD is not about erasing memory or diminishing lived experience; it is about restoring regulation to the nervous system (Benight & Bandura,

2004). Evidence-based treatments such as Eye Movement Desensitization and Reprocessing (EMDR), Cognitive Processing Therapy (CPT), and Somatic Experiencing help guide the body and mind toward recognizing safety once again (Bryant & Harvey, 2012). In this sense, healing could be viewed not as a sign of weakness but rather as a restoration of strength, akin to a knight repairing his armor after battle and preparing himself for future quests.

Suppose that the goal of the fire service is to grow healthier and more resilient. In that case, it should reframe trauma recovery not as a hidden shame but as an important aspect of both personal and organizational development (Bartone, 2006). PTSD should not be considered an inevitable scar of duty; healing should be recognized as an accurate measure of survival and honor. Today's firefighters are called not only to battle external fires but also to confront and overcome the internal wounds left in the aftermath of service. Our conceptualization of heroism can conceptualize managing fires outside but also fires within.

Mythology and the Fire Service: Tradition, Risk, and the Path Forward

The culture of American fire and emergency services is profoundly shaped by enduring mythologies that celebrate bravery, sacrifice, and solidarity. Drawing on Jungian archetypes such as the Hero and Warrior (Jung, 1959a, 1959b), these narratives foster pride and reinforce norms that discourage emotional openness, limit diversity, and obscure systemic flaws.

Central to this culture is the personification of fire as a living adversary. This image encourages both courage and risk-taking while suppressing emotional vulnerability (Desmond, 2007; Stanley et al., 2017). Symbols such as dragons and devils externalize fear, framing fire as an enemy to be defeated rather than a hazard to be managed (Moore & Gillette, 1990).

Beyond the fireground, memorials, rituals, and storytelling elevate fallen firefighters to near-sainthood, reinforcing heroic ideals but sometimes stifling honest discussions about preventable deaths and systemic failures (Johnson, 2019; Dangermond et al., 2022). Artifacts such as the Maltese Cross, traditional helmets, and practices such as glorifying contaminated gear further entrench a culture that prioritizes a perception of strength over health and safety (Wolffe et al., 2023).

While mythology provides emotional survival and identity, it can mask hazardous norms and impede necessary cultural change (Hokmabadi et al., 2022). Drawing from Socratic philosophy, which posits that "no one errs willingly," it is clear that unsafe behaviors often reflect broader organizational and cultural conditions rather than simply individual failure. The Human Factors Analysis and Classification

System (HFACS) highlights how systemic influences shape frontline actions (Wiegmann & Shappell, 2003).

Unlike the military or law enforcement, fire and emergency services lack federally mandated safety standards and rely on local leadership and cultural shifts to drive reform. Reframing mythology is not about abandoning tradition but rather about aligning heroic narratives with modern understandings of safety, resilience, and emotional well-being. True honor lies not only in risking one's life but also in sustaining it, both physically and mentally, and within one's tribe.

Conclusion: Living Myth and Institutional Evolution

The mythology embedded in American fire service culture is both a source of cohesion and a potential constraint. These narratives have historically provided meaning, identity, and symbolic structure to the firefighter's role, grounded in archetypes such as the hero and the warrior, as well as figures drawn from biblical and classical traditions (Bartone, 2006; Dangermond et al., 2022). They assist in framing responses to danger, shaping perceptions of sacrifice, and reinforcing collective values. Mythology does not merely reflect tradition; it actively constructs behavioral norms, risk tolerance, and institutional expectations (Barton & Sutcliffe, 2009).

The anthropomorphization of fire, as an adversary, dragon, or infernal force, supports a narrative in which the firefighter is positioned as a righteous combatant, defending order against destruction. While this framing can inspire commitment and valor, it may also perpetuate patterns that elevate heroism over strategy, emotional stoicism over psychological resilience, and unquestioned sacrifice over systemic safety (Dangermond et al., 2022; Behnke et al., 2020). When cultural symbolism valorizes contaminated gear, idealizes preventable death, or equates trauma with honor, it can inhibit adaptation and obscure opportunities for reform (Bartlett & Schmitz, 2023).

Critical engagement with these mythologies is important for cultural sustainability. This engagement does not require the rejection of tradition but rather its intentional reinterpretation. As fire and emergency services become increasingly diverse and the demands of operational safety, mental health, and leadership evolve, the symbolic frameworks that once shaped identity must expand to accommodate contemporary realities (Bartone, 2006; APA, 2017). In this way, long-standing cultural narratives, whether rooted in chivalric, biblical, or civic imagery, can continue to serve as meaningful anchors, provided they are aligned with inclusive and evidence-based values (Sue, 2006).

The future of fire and emergency services requires technical proficiency, operational excellence, and cultural literacy. Leaders, educators, and practitioners must be prepared to revisit the stories that have defined the profession—not discard them but reframe them in ways that prioritize life, psychological well-being, and collective growth (Barton & Sutcliffe, 2009; Bartlett & Schmitz, 2023). Mythology can endure, but its highest function is not to sanctify risk but to support those who bear it.

Chapter Review

Assignment: Myth, Meaning, and Mental Health in the Fire Service

Learning Objectives

By the end of this activity, students will be able to:

- Identify key archetypes and mythological constructs (e.g., hero, warrior, Prometheus) that shape firefighter identity and behavior.
- Analyze how fire service mythology influences emotional norms, risk-taking, and organizational culture.
- Evaluate the psychological and organizational consequences of myth-driven behaviors, including emotional suppression, hagiography, and memorialization practices.
- Apply critical reflection to propose culturally sensitive reforms that integrate tradition with contemporary best practices in psychological health and operational safety.

Instructions for the Activity: Scenario-Based Analysis (Individual or Group Assignment).

You have been invited to consult with a large urban fire department following a recent LODD (line-of-duty death) incident. While the department has robust rituals to honor the fallen, internal reviews revealed that the death was likely preventable and involved excessive risk-taking and cultural resistance to safety protocols.

As part of your conceptualization, complete the following:

Assignment: Myth, Meaning, and Mental Health in the Fire Service

Learning Objectives

By the end of this activity, students will be able to:

- Identify key archetypes and mythological constructs (e.g., hero, warrior, Prometheus) that shape firefighter identity and behavior.
- Analyze how fire service mythology influences emotional norms, risk-taking, and organizational culture.
- Evaluate the psychological and organizational consequences of myth-driven behaviors, including emotional suppression, hagiography, and memorialization practices.
- Apply critical reflection to propose culturally sensitive reforms that integrate tradition with contemporary best practices in psychological health and operational safety.

Instructions for the Activity: Scenario-Based Analysis (Individual or Group Assignment)

You have been invited to consult with a large urban fire department following a recent LODD (line-of-duty death) incident. While the department has robust rituals to honor the fallen, internal reviews revealed that the death was likely preventable and involved excessive risk-taking and cultural resistance to safety protocols.

As part of your conceptualization, complete the following:

1. Part I: Archetype Identification and Analysis (Approx. 500–700 words)
    1.1. Select 2–3 archetypes from Chapter 4 (e.g., the Hero, the Warrior, Prometheus, or the Valhallan martyr).
    1.2. Explain how these archetypes shape behavior, identity, and expectations within the fire service.
    1.3. Use specific examples from the chapter (e.g., the 9/11 patch, hagiography, or dragon metaphors) to illustrate your analysis.
2. Part II: Myth vs. Mental Health (Approx. 500–700 words)
    2.1. Identify at least two unintended consequences of fire service mythology on psychological health (e.g., PTSD romanticization, emotional suppression, contaminated gear as honor).
    2.2. Use concepts such as projection, moral injury, or emotional numbing to support your evaluation.
    2.3. Reference relevant research or theoretical frameworks (e.g., Jungian psychology, social identity theory).
3. Part III: Culture-Conscious Recommendation (Approx. 400–600 words)
    3.1. Propose two specific, culturally respectful strategies to update or expand fire service mythology in ways that support psychological resilience, safety, and inclusivity.
    3.2. These can include reframing rituals, reinterpreting symbols, leadership messaging, or story-based training.
    3.3. Ground your suggestions in cultural change theory and/or empirical research.

Format & Submission Requirements:
Word Count: 1,400–2,000 total words
APA style for citations
Assessment Rubric

- Depth of archetype analysis—25%
- Critical application of psychological frameworks—25%
- Clarity and practicality of cultural reform recommendations—20%
- Integration of course content and readings—15%

Writing quality, organization, and APA style—15%

Chapter 5
Overcoming Resistance to Change in the Fire Service

*Resistance to change within the fire service is not merely an administrative hurdle but also a psychologically adaptive response to threats against core occupational values, bravery, loyalty, and control (*Oreg, 2006*). These values, long mythologized in the profession's heroic narrative, coalesce into a collective identity that shapes how firefighters perceive innovation, assess risks, and sanction behavior. Integrating psychological science offers a robust framework for navigating this resistance: social identity theory explains the role of group membership in self-worth (*Tajfel & Turner, 1979*), system justification theory illuminates why familiar but harmful practices persist (*Jost & Banaji, 1994; Jost et al., 2004*), and cognitive dissonance theory describes how conflicting beliefs provoke defensive reactions (*Festinger, 1957*). Rather than attempting to dismantle these cultural bedrocks, reframing concepts such as psychological safety, emotional intelligence, and behavioral health is a mission-critical competency. By embedding these virtues within the fire service's established ethos and signaling their importance with clear definitions, leaders can safeguard identity while advancing resilience, inclusivity, and operational effectiveness.*

Psychology, defined by the Oxford English Dictionary (2022) as "the scientific study of the human mind and behavior," offers critical frameworks for tackling both institutional and interpersonal resistance within the fire service. Firefighters, often perceived as infallible heroes, experience high rates of occupational injury (National Fire Protection Association [NFPA], 2023), posttraumatic stress disorder (Gershon et al., 2008), and elevated suicide rates (Stanley et al., 2016). Addressing resistance effectively means moving upstream: targeting the root causes rather than merely managing downstream crises (Heath, 2020). Embedding evidence-based psychological education and integrating licensed psychologists into department structures may catalyze lasting culture change, strengthen individual resilience, and improve long-term health, safety, and career longevity.

Resistance to change within the fire service is not merely an administrative or cultural inconvenience but also a psychological phenomenon rooted in social identity processes, systemic loyalty, and existential meaning-making. Firefighters, as a professional group, adopt highly salient identities centered on heroism, bravery, control, and stoic self-sacrifice. Identities are reinforced by societal mythologies, internal hierarchies, and generational norms (Moore & Gillette, 1990). These identities become fused with personal narratives; therefore, challenging the culture is

K. Wheldon, *Fire Service Psychology*,
https://doi.org/10.1007/978-3-032-02126-7_5

also challenging the self. Social identity theory explains that individuals derive self-worth from group membership, and any perceived threat to the group's values or norms can lead to psychological discomfort and resistance (Tajfel & Turner, 1979). This experience is particularly relevant in fire departments, where group cohesion and loyalty influence effective functioning and survival.

System justification theory adds another layer of complexity by explaining that people often defend the status quo, even when it is personally or collectively harmful, because existing systems provide a sense of order, predictability, and symbolic meaning (Jost & Banaji, 1994; Jost et al., 2004). Within fire and emergency services, traditional practices such as critical incident stress debriefing, rigid command structures, or emotional suppression are often preserved not because they are effective but because they are familiar and affirm group norms. Efforts to introduce practices focusing on genuineness, emotional expression, or psychological safety may be met with resistance because they clash with the established mythos of the "infallible hero." This resistance is further amplified when external sources perceive change as imposed, particularly those who do not share the firefighter identity, such as civilians or mental health professionals. Therefore, understanding the psychological mechanisms behind group resistance is important for designing interventions that do not alienate the individuals they seek to support.

Extensive research on social psychology and organizational behavior supports the idea that successful change should be aligned with the values and identities of the target group rather than being in opposition to them (Haslam et al., 2011, 2018). Therefore, reframing new practices in ways that reinforce, rather than dismantle, the group's sense of mission and pride is important. For example, positioning psychological resilience training as a form of elite performance, akin to physical conditioning, can help reframe help-seeking as a sign of strength rather than weakness. Framing psychological services as mission critical rather than ancillary allows them to be interpreted through the lens of duty and responsibility, values that are already central to the firefighter identity. Moreover, research has shown that change is more likely to be embraced when it is championed by respected in-group members rather than being imposed through top-down mandates (Haslam et al., 2011). This peer-led model of change is supported by programs such as Stamp Out Stigma, which has reduced internalized stigma among firefighters by utilizing testimonial videos from fellow firefighters and department-specific workshops (Gulliver et al., 2023). This way, cultural change becomes an internal evolution rather than an external imposition.

Leadership also plays a critical role in navigating resistance and embedding change. According to Edmondson (1999), organizations that foster psychological safety, where individuals feel secure in expressing concerns, admitting mistakes, and questioning norms without fear of retribution, are significantly more adaptive and resilient. In contrast, passive leadership models, which fail to actively promote a safe culture or provide emotional support, have been shown to increase stress and anxiety and diminish compliance with safety behaviors (Smith et al., 2023). Within the fire service, which operates under high-pressure and unpredictable conditions, proactive leadership encourages open dialog, and emotional intelligence is important for safety outcomes and the successful implementation of new practices. Similarly, Barton and Sutcliffe (2009) argue that change in high-reliability organizations often hinges not on sweeping policy shifts but rather on micro-level social processes, i.e., the day-to-day interactions in which team members voice concerns, question assumptions, and interpret shifting environmental cues. Over time, these seemingly small acts of cognitive and social flexibility can dismantle dysfunctional momentum and create space for innovation and reflection.

Ultimately, the fire service cannot afford to treat resistance as a barrier to work around; it should be viewed as a signal of an identity threat that can be transformed through inclusive, psychologically grounded strategies. Psychologists embedded within the service can offer critical insights into this process by helping cocreate language, rituals, and training frameworks that align with firefighter values while promoting growth, safety, and well-being. When change efforts honor the cultural bedrock of the fire service while creating new pathways for support and development, resistance can be softened, not through force but through understanding.

Overcoming resistance to change in fire and emergency services requires an integrative understanding of cultural dynamics, psychological theory, and evidence-based strategies rooted in social and clinical science. Psychology, as defined by the Oxford English Dictionary, is the scientific study of the human mind and its functions, especially those affecting behavior in a given context. Historically, in line with the medical model, psychology was once limited to diagnosing and treating illness. However, in the last two decades, the field has expanded to encompass human potential, performance, and adaptability. Advances in psychological science now allow us to examine genetic and neurobiological markers that predispose individuals to mental health challenges, enabling proactive and preventive approaches to behavioral health within high-risk professions such as firefighting. This shift reflects a broader transformation in psychology from a deficit-based model to a strengths-based model, which considers human potential, resilience, and the conditions under which individuals thrive.

Understanding the psychological foundations of change is critical. Psychology offers a rigorous framework for examining individual and collective behaviors that emerge in complex, hierarchical systems, such as fire and emergency services. Resistance to change, whether institutional or interpersonal, is rarely irrational; rather, it reflects deeply held values, fears of identity loss, and the perceived risks of adopting unfamiliar norms. Social identity theory suggests that individuals derive meaning and self-esteem from group membership and respond defensively when changes threaten the group's coherence or values (Tajfel & Turner, 1979). In the fire service, group identity is intimately tied to ideals of bravery, stoicism, and technical competence. New policies or practices emphasizing emotional openness, vulnerability, or psychological intervention may inadvertently trigger resistance because they may be perceived as contradicting these core values.

Moreover, system justification theory posits that people tend to defend existing institutional structures, even if flawed or harmful, because these systems offer predictability, order, and a shared reality (Jost & Banaji, 1994; Jost et al., 2004). With respect to fire and emergency services, long-standing traditions such as the command structure, rites of passage, and cultural norms serve both practical and symbolic purposes. They reinforce a shared sense of purpose and belonging. Consequently, reform efforts perceived as undermining these traditions may be interpreted as operational changes and existential threats. To address this dynamic, psychological principles should be employed not to force change but rather to frame it as an extension of existing values, an evolution rather than a revolution. This framing is important in reconciling the psychological conflict between idealism (the heroic self-concept) and fallibility (recognizing human limits and mental health needs).

Cognitive dissonance theory (Festinger, 1957) offers another valuable lens. When individuals encounter information or directives that contradict their beliefs or behaviors, they experience discomfort and seek ways to resolve this tension. In fire and emergency services, initiatives aimed at mental health awareness, trauma support, or emotional regulation may provoke dissonance for personnel who have internalized messages equating emotional vulnerability with weakness. To reduce this dissonance, these interventions should be presented in a way that affirms, rather than challenges, the individual's self-concept as capable, strong, and mission-oriented. For example, programs can frame psychological resilience as an elite skill akin to physical readiness rather than a remedial response to dysfunction. When framed appropriately, change becomes a means of enhancing operational performance and personal mastery.

The cultural dynamics of fire and emergency services are closely intertwined with public perception and internal identity. Society has long viewed firefighters as saviors who run into danger when others flee. This archetype is cemented in popular culture, public ceremonies, and children's education. It contributes to adopting symbolic roles within the fire service beyond functional job duties. In these interpretations, firefighters are not merely viewed as employees but as guardians, protectors, heroes, and members of a special group. Such roles shape how firefighters perceive themselves and how they interact with others. Role formation can lead to psychological rigidity, where any deviation from the traditional script feels like a betrayal of identity. As Jungian psychology and narrative identity theory suggest, people are motivated to maintain coherent life stories. Changing the narrative of what it means to be a firefighter, especially when it involves acknowledging emotional complexity or psychological struggle, requires careful attention to meaning-making processes (Jung, 1959a, 1959b).

These symbolic frameworks influence more than just individual identity. They shape crew dynamics, organizational behavior, and interagency relationships. Fire crews function as cohesive units, often developing high levels of interdependence and mutual accountability. However, this can also result in insularity and resistance to outside influence, particularly from civilian professionals such as psychologists or researchers. The belief that only individuals with firsthand firefighting experience can fully understand the profession fosters an exclusionary mindset that limits interdisciplinary collaboration. However, this alliance is needed to address complex issues such as trauma, suicide, and organizational stress. Bridging this gap requires cultural humility, sustained engagement, and leadership support. Psychologists should be embedded within the fire service, not as outsiders delivering abstract theories but as partners co-developing solutions grounded in lived experience.

The barriers to change associated with fire and emergency services are multifaceted. Mental health stigma is a primary concern. Despite growing awareness, many firefighters still fear judgment, career repercussions, or loss of status if they seek psychological support. Internalized stigma can be particularly damaging, leading individuals to view their struggles as personal failures rather than predictable responses to chronic stress exposure. Programs such as "Stamp Out Stigma" have demonstrated that peer-led interventions can reduce these harmful beliefs (Gulliver et al., 2023). However, stigma is only one layer of it. Entrenched systems, such as critical incident stress management (CISM), persist despite limited evidence of their efficacy. The reluctance to abandon familiar models, even in the face of contrary evidence, reflects the psychological inertia of institutional norms. Therefore, change efforts should address both individual attitudes and systemic reinforcements.

Another critical barrier is leadership. Studies have shown that passive leadership is correlated with higher stress levels, increased anxiety, and reduced compliance with safety protocols (Smith et al., 2023). Firefighters working under disengaged leaders may feel unsupported, unvalued, and reluctant to speak up. Conversely, proactive leadership fosters psychological safety, where individuals feel safe in taking interpersonal risks, admit mistakes, and express concerns (Edmondson, 1999). Psychological safety is not merely a "soft" concept; it can have a direct impact on operational outcomes. Teams with high levels of psychological safety respond more adaptively to emergencies, communicate more effectively, and recover quickly from setbacks. Therefore, leadership development programs within fire and emergency services should prioritize emotional intelligence, trauma-informed supervision, and inclusive communication.

Upstream thinking represents a shift from reactive problem-solving to proactive system design. Instead of responding to crises after they occur, upstream approaches seek to identify and address the conditions that give rise to them (Heath, 2020). In the context of firefighter mental health, this includes implementing psychological screening during the hiring process, providing resilience training during the academy, and offering ongoing mental health education throughout one's career. It also includes conducting psychological autopsies following suicides or critical incidents, not to assign blame but to extract lessons and identify prevention opportunities (Pennington et al., 2018). Accountability frameworks could be reframed from punitive to restorative and designed to foster growth, learning, and system improvement (Fixsen et al., 2005).

Empowering the workforce through education is a cornerstone of sustainable change. Psychological education demystifies mental health, reduces stigma, and equips individuals with tools to manage stress, build resilience, and support peers (Corrigan, 2004). These messages carry greater weight when delivered by credible messengers, such as experienced firefighters or embedded psychologists. Programs such as Trauma Risk Management (TRiM) and Mental Health First Aid (MHFA) offer structured, evidence-based approaches that can be tailored to the fire service context (Jones et al., 2017). Moreover, integrating psychological principles into technical training reinforces that mental readiness is as critical as physical readiness (Luthar & Cicchetti, 2000). This alignment enhances buy-in and makes psychological training an integral part of professional development rather than an optional add-on.

Psychologists play a unique and necessary role in the cultural transformation of fire and emergency services. Their expertise in behavior change, trauma recovery, organizational dynamics, and leadership development positions them as key change agents (Haslam et al., 2018). However, their effectiveness depends on integration and trust. To collaborate effectively, psychologists should understand the culture, language, and rhythm of fire and emergency services. This developmental process should involve engaging in specialized training for psychologists working specifically with the fire service. Additionally, interdisciplinary teams include psychologists, fire service leaders, medical professionals, and policy experts who can co-create strategies that are both culturally congruent and scientifically grounded (Fixsen et al., 2005).

Research continues to shed light on the complexities of behavioral health in fire and emergency services. For example, the SOS initiative revealed statistically significant reductions in internalized and self-stigma after peer-led interventions (Gulliver et al., 2023). Longitudinal studies have also shown that pre-employment trauma exposure is predictive of depression among recruits, underscoring the importance of early identification and intervention (Pennington et al., 2018). Moreover, the presence of both posttraumatic stress disorder (PTSD) and posttraumatic growth (PTG) among firefighters highlights the dual nature of trauma responses and the potential for psychological growth even after adverse events (Kehl et al., 2014). Understanding these nuances enables the development of more sophisticated and individualized support systems.

Studies by Barton and Sutcliffe (2009) emphasize the importance of micro-level social processes in safety and performance. Organizational safety is achieved not only through rigid protocols but also through dynamic communication, reevaluation, and adaptability. Wildland firefighting, in particular, offers lessons in decision-making under uncertainty. Recognizing early warning signs, seeking diverse perspectives, and adjusting tactics in real time are social achievements that hinge on trust, humility, and vigilance. These represent psychological attributes that manifest within operational contexts.

Finally, fire and emergency services should address the moral complexities of suicide. We should honor lives without normalizing or mythologizing suicide; prevention hinges on accurate risk framing, access to care, and safe messaging. Suicide is often the result of distorted cognitions and overwhelming psychological pain and is not an inevitable consequence of occupational stress (Joiner, 2005). Labeling suicide as a line-of-duty death may offer symbolic closure, but it also risks normalizing behavior and diminishing the sense of agency for those still struggling. As mental health professionals, we should walk the line between compassion and prevention, ensuring that our responses support healing without reinforcing harmful narratives (Jobes, 2006).

In conclusion, resistance to change in fire and emergency services is not a singular obstacle but rather a complex interplay of identity, tradition, psychology, and leadership. Addressing this resistance requires more than policy changes; it requires a cultural shift rooted in psychological insight and sustained by collaborative effort. Integrating psychological science across the full continuum, from proactive prevention to post-incident recovery, supports the development of a fire service that is resilient, ethically grounded, and sustainably well.The evolution of leadership begins with understanding psychology, specifically the human mind.

In addition to these foundational concepts, the psychology of resistance to change within the fire service deeply intersects with theories of organizational identity and role conflict. When individuals internalize their professional roles to such a degree that they become indistinguishable from their identity, as is often the case in high-intensity, mission-driven fields such as firefighting, any critique or modification of institutional norms can be interpreted as a personal attack. This results in a psychological phenomenon known as "identity fusion," where the boundaries between self and group dissolve, heightening loyalty and increasing defensiveness (Swann Jr. et al., 2012). When firefighters are asked to adapt to cultural shifts prioritizing psychological safety, emotional expression, or trauma responsiveness, some may experience an existential disorientation. They may ask: If I am not the version of a firefighter tradition glorifies, stoic, untouchable, always in control, then who am I? Addressing this conflict requires psychological interventions to do more than offer new tools; they should also support identity reformation in ways that preserve core values while allowing for evolution.

One effective strategy for navigating this terrain is the use of narrative reframing. Narrative therapy and narrative psychology underscore the importance of the stories people tell about themselves, their purpose, and their place in the world (White & Epston, 1990). By helping firefighters reauthor their internal narratives to include psychological resilience, emotional intelligence, and posttraumatic growth as integral components of the heroic ideal, not contradictions to it, leaders and psychologists can reduce internal resistance to change. This process also opens the door to incorporating alternative leadership models, which value empathy, adaptability, and distributed decision-making alongside traditional traits such as bravery and decisiveness (Fletcher, 2004).

Moreover, there is growing support for psychological practices that focus on meaning-making and existential psychology in high-risk professions. Viktor Frankl's logotherapy, for instance, emphasizes the human capacity to derive meaning from suffering and adversity (Frankl, 1984). Within the fire service, this approach can be used to reframe occupational stress, loss, and trauma not as evidence of weakness but as pathways to deeper purpose. In practice, this could involve guided reflection groups facilitated by trained psychologists, where firefighters discuss critical incidents in ways that foster meaning, growth, and moral clarity. Such interventions can serve as individual therapy and collective rituals, strengthening personal resolve and reinforcing group cohesion.

These psychosocial dynamics are further compounded by institutional systems that may inadvertently reinforce harmful norms. For example, promotional processes in fire departments often reward tenure, technical skill, and command conformity over emotional intelligence or leadership development (Bass & Riggio, 2006). These choices perpetuate a cycle in which individuals ascending into positions of influence often lack the interpersonal skills necessary to create a psychologically safe environment (Edmondson, 1999). They also marginalize those with leadership strengths in terms of relational intelligence, mentoring, or culture building. As a result, progressive change is slowed not by a lack of awareness but by a misalignment between what the system rewards and what it needs.

Organizational development research offers valuable insights here. The concept of "learning organizations," popularized by Peter Senge (1990), highlights the importance of continuous growth, reflection, and systems thinking. Fire departments can adopt these principles by fostering environments where learning from error is institutionalized, not punished; where feedback is sought, not suppressed; and where adaptive thinking is considered a strength, not a liability. This process can be operationalized through after-action reviews, including tactical analysis and emotional processing; leadership retreats that focus on personal growth; and cross-functional collaborations with behavioral health experts to design interventions grounded in science and culture.

Finally, the conversation about resistance to change should account for intersectionality, as factors such as gender, race, and sexuality intersect with fire service culture to create additional layers of exclusion or resistance (Crenshaw, 1991). Female firefighters, LGBTQ+ personnel, and people of color may face unique stressors and barriers, not only in accessing mental health services but also in being fully accepted as members within the fire service culture. These identities can be seen as "disruptive" to the normative script of who a firefighter is, adding another layer of complexity to resistance. Diversity, equity, and inclusion (DEI) initiatives are often met with resistance in fire and emergency services, not because their goals are rejected outright but because they challenge the institution's implicit identity norms (Mor Barak, 2016). A psychologically informed approach to DEI should move beyond training modules and focus on sustained cultural mentoring, inclusive storytelling, and structural policy change.

To move forward meaningfully, we should confront one of the fire service's most deeply embedded protective mechanisms: emotional suppression. Firefighters are trained and socialized to remain calm under pressure, to compartmentalize their fears, and to act decisively in life-threatening scenarios. These attributes are important in operational contexts. However, these traits can become maladaptive in interpersonal relationships, family life, and quiet moments following traumatic calls. The inability or unwillingness to process emotion is not just a personal issue but a cultural one. Left unaddressed, emotional suppression leads to a buildup of unresolved grief, anger, and moral injury, which often manifests as anxiety, depression, substance misuse, or suicidal ideation (Litz et al., 2009). These concerns are not merely isolated clinical issues; they are indicative of a broader systemic culture that prioritizes performance over psychological processing and reinforces silence rather than support.

What psychology teaches us is that culture and behavior are mutually reinforcing. When a behavior such as help-seeking is culturally coded as weak, belief is perpetuated not only by leadership attitudes or policy gaps but also by the stories told in kitchens, locker rooms, and after calls (Corrigan, 2004). Therefore, any effort to reshape behavior should also reshape culture, and culture shifts through repeated, consistent experiences contradicting old narratives and offering new possibilities. When a respected captain speaks openly about seeking therapy, a department normalizes post-incident decompression rather than brushing it off. When rookies are told from day one that strength includes self-awareness, that is, how the culture begins to change.

In this sense, we should stop treating cultural resistance as a wall to push through and start understanding it as a language to translate. When firefighters reject wellness programs, it is not always because they deny their utility. More often, they do not see themselves in the message, or worse, accepting the message means abandoning an identity they have worked their entire career to embody (Tajfel & Turner, 1979). We must offer them an identity-expanding rather than identity-eroding message, saying, "You are not less of a firefighter for doing this; you're more equipped to do the job, to lead, and to survive it in the long term." This kind of shift is not theoretical. It is actionable. As a result, programs, outreach materials, and even our tone of conversation may need to be intentionally reviewed to ensure that they reflect clinical accuracy and cultural fluency (Haslam et al., 2011).

At the same time, there is a need for honest reckoning with what systems have allowed to persist under the guise of tradition. Leadership often avoids accountability, mental health support lacks confidentiality, and peer support programs are often performative rather than relational; these are not benign shortcomings. They reinforce distrust and the belief that change is cosmetic, not substantive. To support firefighters in embracing evolving roles, as mentors, emotionally intelligent leaders, and integrated individuals, organizational change must be modeled both from the top down and from within the culture itself (Bass & Riggio, 2006).

Examining how the brain and body encode and retain traumatic experiences is also necessary. Firefighters are subjected to cumulative stress throughout their careers, a phenomenon known in the literature as the allostatic load (McEwen, 1998). This concept extends beyond conventional definitions of stress, referring instead to the physiological wear and tear that results from chronic hypervigilance, sleep disruption, exposure to secondary trauma, and the emotional burden of routinely witnessing human suffering. Over time, such demands can lead to nervous system dysregulation, manifesting as emotional numbing, heightened reactivity, and interpersonal strain. These consequences are not merely abstract; they are profoundly embodied and impactful. Advances in neurobiological research now offer evidence-based strategies to mitigate these effects. Interventions such as mindfulness-based stress reduction (MBSR), eye movement desensitization and reprocessing (EMDR), and trauma-informed somatic therapies have demonstrated promise in helping first responders recalibrate their physiological arousal and restore emotional regulation (Van der Kolk, 2014). However, while EMDR is widely recognized as effective for posttraumatic stress disorder (PTSD), recent evidence highlights that its safety profile has been underexamined. A review of 51 randomized controlled trials found that adverse effects were rarely monitored systematically, with only nine studies even mentioning them and just one employing structured protocols. Reported effects were typically mild and temporary, but their anecdotal documentation limits clear conclusions about EMDR's risk–benefit balance, especially as the intervention expands beyond PTSD into populations with complex comorbidities (van Schie et al., 2025).

Alongside evolving operational demands, the need for clear role definition within the fire service has become increasingly critical. In recent years, firefighters have assumed a wide array of responsibilities, including emergency medical response, public education, and community outreach, that, while reflective of shifting societal needs, have also blurred the traditional boundaries of the firefighter role. Although this specific dynamic has not been extensively studied within the fire service, research in broader occupational contexts indicates that such role ambiguity can contribute to role conflict and identity strain, particularly among individuals who entered the profession with a well-defined operational identity (Burke, 2006). Today, firefighters are expected to function as dispatchers, paramedics, crisis counselors, arson investigators, behavioral health responders, and SWAT medics, all under a single professional identity. While adaptability is a vital skill, this continuous shifting between roles, without sufficient psychological support, can foster burnout, disengagement, and cynicism. Role clarity, anchored in comprehensive training, mentorship, and realistic expectations, is not an optional benefit but a foundational requirement for the long-term sustainability of the workforce.

There is a need for a systemic cultural realignment that honors tradition while guiding its evolution. Fire service culture is deeply rooted in rich rituals, enduring symbols, and shared values. Rather than posing obstacles to reform, these cultural elements can serve as effective conduits for change. By integrating new cognitive and emotional frameworks into established practices, such as embedding moments of mindfulness into shift transitions or incorporating structured emotional check-ins into after-action reviews, reform efforts can align with, rather than oppose, existing cultural norms. The fire service preserves its foundational strengths while intentionally expanding its resilience, inclusivity, and capacity for psychological well-being. This integrative approach is not a rejection of legacy but a continuation of it, adapted to meet contemporary needs.

Central to the cultural evolution of fire and emergency services is a reevaluation of what constitutes strength itself. Strength has often been conflated with emotional detachment, stoicism, and invulnerability. However, emerging psychological research and organizational behavior literature suggest that true resilience encompasses broader competencies, including self-awareness, emotional regulation, and the capacity to seek support when needed (Luthar & Cicchetti, 2000). These qualities do not compromise operational effectiveness; instead, they enhance it. The evidence suggests that teams with high emotional intelligence exhibit improved performance under pressure, as well as greater cohesion and adaptability during crises (Jordan & Troth, 2004). As fire service responsibilities grow increasingly complex and community expectations evolve, cultivating these strength dimensions becomes relevant and an integral component of organizational success.

The challenge lies in creating environments where these traits are encouraged and modeled. Leadership, once again, becomes a critical lever. Leaders set the emotional tone of an organization. Those values begin to cascade if officers model emotional intelligence, transparency, and humility. However, when leaders reinforce stoicism, dismiss mental health needs, or punish emotional expression, they create an environment of psychological rigidity. Transformational leadership, characterized by vision, inspiration, intellectual stimulation, and individualized consideration, has been shown to predict higher levels of engagement, satisfaction, and well-being across various emergency service professions (Bass & Riggio, 2006). Fire service leaders need to be developed with this model in mind.

However, the transformation of fire service culture requires more than the development of emotional competencies; it also necessitates cultivating moral courage. This form of courage extends beyond physical bravery; it involves the willingness to act ethically and responsibly in situations where doing so may affect personal or professional risk (Kidder, 2005). In the context of fire service, moral courage may be expressed through actions such as intervening when a colleague exhibits signs of psychological distress, advocating for enhanced behavioral health support, or challenging entrenched cultural norms that undermine individual or organizational well-being. These behaviors must be consistently supported, modeled, and institutionally recognized to become an integral part of everyday practice. Without such reinforcement, acts of moral courage risk becoming isolated exceptions rather than embedded in cultural expectations.

An additional consideration in the cultural evolution of fire and emergency services is the imperative of system alignment. Psychological and organizational research consistently demonstrates that individual behavior is shaped by personal beliefs and attitudes, as well as the broader systemic context in which individuals function (Bronfenbrenner, 1979). For example, if a firefighter is inclined to seek therapeutic support but encounters prohibitive insurance barriers or fears punitive consequences for disclosing psychological distress, the organizational environment implicitly discourages help-seeking behavior. Sustainable change, therefore, necessitates structural reform. By implementing clear policies that protect confidentiality, provide nonpunitive pathways for addressing psychological health, support mental health leave, and ensure that wellness efforts do not jeopardize opportunities for career progression, culture can evolve to meet the needs of fire service members. Organizational health is not an ancillary but rather a critical determinant of operational effectiveness. High functioning teams are the product of well designed, equitable, and accessible systems. When these systems are misaligned, fragmented, or punitive, they fail to promote resilience and become active sources of harm.

Effective organizational change requires the intentional application of implementation science principles. Evidence-based interventions often fall short not because of flaws in their design or efficacy but because of poorly executed or contextually misaligned implementation strategies (Fixsen et al., 2005). The success of any initiative depends not only on the content of the intervention but also on how it is introduced and sustained within the organization. As such, the "how" of implementation is as critical as "what." Research emphasizes that successful implementation necessitates visible leadership commitment, adequate resource allocation, continuous capacity building, and mechanisms for ongoing feedback and adaptation to local contexts (Aarons et al., 2011; Fixsen et al., 2005).

In the context of fire and emergency services, where organizational culture is shaped by trust, experiential learning, and interpersonal credibility, implementation strategies must be culturally congruent. Programs are more likely to be accepted and internalized when they are facilitated by individuals who possess technical expertise and a deep understanding of the operational environment and cultural norms (Aarons et al., 2014). Cultural competence should not be viewed as a peripheral consideration but rather as a central pillar of practical implementation. When cultural alignment is prioritized, interventions have a greater chance of achieving sustained behavioral change and long-term organizational impact.

Equally important is the concept of recovery, not only in the context of trauma but also with respect to operational fatigue. Accumulated stress, disrupted sleep patterns, and insufficient recovery time have implications that extend beyond individual well-being, influencing team safety, cognitive performance, and public trust. Empirical research on shift work and circadian misalignment has established strong associations with cardiovascular disease, mood dysregulation, and cognitive impairment (Wagstaff & Sigstad Lie, 2011). Despite this evidence, many fire departments utilize traditional shift schedules that do not adequately support physiological or psychological recovery. Integrating scientifically supported recovery protocols, such as revisiting duty cycles, incorporating structured opportunities for psychological decompression, and promoting sleep hygiene, should be prioritized within operational planning and policy development. These adjustments are not ancillary but critical to sustaining a healthy, high-performing workforce.

Ultimately, efforts to transform fire service culture must be grounded in understanding relational dynamics. Organizational transformation does not occur solely through policy mandates; it is facilitated through interpersonal interactions that communicate values, foster psychological safety, and establish new behavioral norms. It is important to cultivate peer support programs, mentorship structures, and informal leadership networks. Social connectedness has been found to protect against occupational stress, trauma exposure, and burnout (Pines & Maslach, 1978). However, adequate support extends beyond availability; it requires preparation. Peer supporters should receive training in empathetic communication and active listening, maintaining boundaries, navigating referral pathways, and serving as cultural intermediaries. While firefighters do not need to assume the role of clinicians, they can serve as accessible conduits to critical resources, including behavioral health services, medical care, and financial assistance. In this way, the relational infrastructure becomes a cornerstone of individual resilience and systemic reform.

In conclusion, fostering meaningful change within the fire service extends beyond implementing new policies or procedures. This necessitates a foundational reexamination of the constructs that define strength, the development of emotionally attuned leadership, the alignment of supportive organizational systems, and the intentional cultivation of psychological safety and mutual regard. Empirical research and practical tools are increasingly available to guide this process; however, the pivotal challenge lies in undertaking the cultural and emotional labor required for genuine transformation. Ultimately, systemic change is rooted in structural shifts and the evolution of narratives. Through the deliberate reinterpretation and reintegration of shared stories, fire and emergency services can cultivate a resilient, inclusive, and adaptive culture that is equipped to endure and progress.

Safeguarding Firefighters' and EMS Providers' Mental Health

Over the past decade, fire and emergency services have made notable progress in addressing the behavioral health needs of firefighters and emergency medical service personnel. At the national level, the National Fallen Firefighters Foundation formally recognized the importance of integrating psychological support across the career span of fire service members. The International Association of Fire Chiefs (IAFC) has committed resources to its Safety, Health, and Survival Section. At the same time, the International Association of Fire Fighters (IAFF), in partnership with Advanced Recovery Systems, has established the IAFF Center of Excellence, a dedicated facility for treating behavioral health and substance use issues among firefighters. In parallel, numerous initiatives have emerged to identify and respond to mental health challenges within the profession. At the local level, many departments have implemented peer support programs and partnered with licensed mental health clinicians to deliver targeted services. In some cases, departments have expanded their commitment by hiring in-house psychologists to oversee and coordinate comprehensive behavioral health strategies.

Given that firefighters frequently rely on their peers for initial emotional support, many departments have invested in strengthening the capacity of peer support teams to address behavioral health concerns. While peer responders play a critical role in early identification and intervention, distinguishing their function from that of licensed mental health professionals is important. Most firefighters are not formally trained clinicians, although some pursue dual roles through additional education and licensure. Mental health providers typically complete graduate-level degree programs, undergo supervised clinical training, and pass national and state licensing examinations before being authorized to deliver therapeutic services. In contrast, peer support certification, while valuable, is not equivalent to licensure and does not permit the provision of clinical treatment under legal or ethical standards.

Peer support programs, which have roots in military contexts, are designed to foster early risk recognition, provide empathetic listening, and facilitate referrals to appropriate services. Their effectiveness lies in the ability of peer responders to offer culturally congruent support, normalize emotional responses, and serve as trusted conduits for further care. These programs can reduce stigma and increase help-seeking behaviors by providing individuals with a nonjudgmental, familiar context in which to process their experiences.

However, a critical gap remains: the shortage of culturally competent mental health clinicians with specific knowledge of fire and emergency services and EMS environments. This deficit continues to undermine access to appropriate care, as firefighters may struggle to establish rapport or feel misunderstood by providers unfamiliar with the nuances of their occupational experiences. To bridge this gap, some organizations have begun offering rapid-response clinical interventions following critical incidents, often incorporating modalities such as eye movement desensitization and reprocessing (EMDR). While early EMDR interventions may provide benefits in managing acute distress, there are valid concerns regarding the timing and implementation of such protocols. These interventions may yield unintended psychological consequences if delivered prematurely or without proper contextual assessment. As such, careful consideration is required to ensure that these clinical tools are applied within evidence-based, trauma-informed frameworks that prioritize safety and efficacy.

In addressing posttraumatic stress within the fire and emergency medical services (EMS) community, safeguarding mental health begins with a structured, evidence-informed approach:

1. **Promotion of natural recovery**: Empirical research indicates that approximately 80% of individuals exposed to traumatic events will recover without clinical intervention within the first 30 days (Bonanno, 2004). Therefore, immediate postexposure responses should prioritize supportive environments for natural psychological processing.
2. **Implement trauma risk management (TRiM) protocols**: To support those who may not experience spontaneous recovery, a structured assessment system such as Trauma Risk Management (TRiM) can help identify individuals at greater risk for prolonged or complicated psychological responses and refer them to appropriate care.
3. **Premature pathologization:** Premature pathologization is important not to prematurely label individuals as clinically impaired during the natural recovery phase, as doing so can inadvertently stigmatize normal responses to trauma and disrupt the recovery process.
4. **Define the scope of peer support**: Peer support team members must not engage in activities that constitute clinical mental health treatment unless appropriately licensed. Providing therapy without proper credentials violates both legal and ethical standards, posing risks to both the provider and the recipient of care.
5. **Protect peer support providers**: When peer responders overstep their role, there is a potential for significant emotional burden if an adverse outcome occurs. Through clear role definition and training, peer support personnel should be shielded from undue psychological liability.
6. **Prevent role overload**: Firefighters and EMS providers already bear considerable professional and emotional responsibilities. Asking peer support members

to assume the additional role of therapist may contribute to burnout and role strain, undermining both peer support efforts and operational readiness.

7. **Strengthening collaboration with licensed clinicians**: Long-term resilience requires partnership with the professional mental health community. Peer support should serve as a bridge, not a substitute, for clinical care. Encouraging licensed providers to engage with the unique culture and needs of the fire service enhances both the access to and relevance of support services.

Together, these strategies ensure a continuum of care that respects natural recovery, safeguards peer responders, and reinforces the critical role of professional mental health services in the fire and EMS environment.

As mental health professionals seek to integrate more effectively into fire and emergency services, it is important to center the ethical imperative of nonmaleficence, "first, do no harm." This foundational principle, rooted in the Hippocratic tradition, remains central to the ethical codes of contemporary clinical practice. The American Psychological Association (APA) outlines guiding principles, including beneficence, nonmaleficence, respect for autonomy, and justice, which are directly relevant when high-risk occupational groups such as firefighters and EMS personnel are supported.

In this context, the development and implementation of peer support programs must align with these ethical standards, ensuring that such interventions complement, rather than replace, qualified clinical care. While the fire service continues to face a shortage of culturally competent clinicians and stigma around help-seeking behavior, these structural barriers should be addressed through sustainable, systemic strategies rather than ad hoc or provisional measures that may inadvertently compound existing challenges. Upholding ethical integrity and professional standards is vital to fostering trust, enhancing care, and preventing unintended harm within fire service mental health initiatives.

Character-Based Leadership: A Developmental and Cultural Framework for Ethical Performance

Character-based leadership is an evolving model in leadership theory that focuses on the moral and ethical dimensions of leadership rather than solely on competencies or personality traits. It posits that leadership effectiveness is determined by what a leader does and who the leader is, particularly in moments of uncertainty, pressure, or moral ambiguity (Crossan et al., 2017). This framework prioritizes cultivating virtues such as integrity, humility, courage, and justice as core capacities for sound judgment and ethical influence.

Unlike traditional personality theories such as the five-factor model, which view traits such as extraversion or conscientiousness as biologically rooted and relatively stable over time (McCrae & Costa Jr., 1999), character-based leadership emphasizes that character is malleable. It can be developed through intentional practice, reflective learning, and social engagement (Crossan et al., 2017; Seijts et al., 2015). The concept repositions leadership development from a static model based on inherited traits to a dynamic process grounded in experience, culture, and moral reasoning.

At the heart of this model is the multidimensional structure of leader character. Crossan et al. (2017) identify eleven interrelated dimensions (accountability, judgment, humanity, and transcendence), each contributing to leadership efficacy and resilience. Among these, judgment is regarded as a central integrative virtue, enabling the application of other traits in contextually appropriate and ethically sound ways.

Character-based leadership also recognizes the social environment as an ideal determinant of behavior. Rather than viewing leadership performance as an outcome of individual disposition alone, this model reflects ecological systems theory (Bronfenbrenner, 1979) in asserting that organizational norms, peer influence, and institutional values shape the expression of leadership. This distinction is especially critical in high-stakes professions such as fire and emergency services.

Scarborough (2017) reported that firefighters' decisions during rescue operations are often shaped more by shared cultural values within the firehouse than by individual ethical reasoning. Similarly, the National Safety Culture Change Initiative (USFA, 2014) emphasizes that institutional culture, characterized by recurring assumptions, behaviors, and traditions, is a decisive factor in determining safety outcomes, ethical consistency, and team integrity.

Consequently, character-based leadership invites a shift in focus from individual correction to systemic cultivation. The development of character in leaders requires not only personal effort but also supportive environments and organizations that model, reward, and reinforce ethical behavior. Research shows that leaders who embody strong moral character are associated with greater trust, psychological safety, team performance, and adaptive problem solving in crisis conditions (Hannah & Avolio, 2011; Jordan & Troth, 2004).

In the context of fire and emergency services, where risk, tradition, and camaraderie profoundly shape behavior, character-based leadership offers a culturally congruent yet reformative path forward. It aligns psychological insight with operational demands, emphasizing that true strength includes empathy, reflective judgment, and a commitment to the collective good. Leadership, therefore, becomes not only an individual capacity but also a shared cultural achievement shaped by the systems we build and the values we uphold.

From Resistance to Resilience: Leading Cultural Change in the Fire Service

The evolution of fire and emergency services requires more than procedural updates or isolated mental health initiatives; it necessitates a comprehensive reevaluation of the psychological, cultural, and organizational frameworks that influence how firefighters think, feel, and lead. Resistance to change in this context is not simply obstinacy but rather a psychologically complex response to perceived threats against identity, belonging, and purpose. Drawing from psychological science, particularly theories of social identity, system justification, and cognitive dissonance, we recognize the importance of aligning reform with the enduring strengths of the fire service rather than challenging them outright.

Real and lasting transformation will depend on cultivating leadership that is not only operationally effective but also ethically grounded, emotionally attuned, and culturally competent. This means embedding mental wellness into the profession's identity, redefining strength to include vulnerability, and building systems that protect, rather than punish, psychological honesty. It involves re-authoring the firefighter narrative to reflect heroism and humanity, enabling individuals to find coherence between their roles and realities. Above all, interventions must be relational, contextual, and built in partnership with those they serve.

The fire service stands at a pivotal moment. With the right tools, language, and leadership, it can become a model of integrated, psychologically informed practice in high-risk professions. Change will not happen overnight, but with a collective commitment, cultural humility, and sustained investment in mental and organizational health, the fire service can emerge as stronger, more resilient, inclusive, and better prepared for the complex demands of the future.

Chapter Review

Assignment: Academic Exercise: Translating Resistance—A Strategic Cultural Change Plan for the Fire Service

Learning Objectives: By completing this assignment, students will be able to:

- Apply psychological theories such as social identity theory, system justification theory, and cognitive dissonance to interpret resistance to change within the fire service.
- Analyze the interplay between fire service culture, leadership, and behavioral health initiatives.
- Design a multitiered change strategy that balances cultural fidelity with evidence-based psychological practice.
- Integrate implementation science and ethical considerations to address structural and interpersonal barriers to reform.
- Demonstrate cultural competence by developing reforms that resonate with firefighters' values and traditions while advancing psychological resilience and operational effectiveness.

Assignment Instructions—Scenario:

You are a behavioral health and organizational consultant brought in by a metropolitan fire department to help lead a cultural transformation. Despite administrative support for new behavioral health programs, training on emotional intelligence, and leadership development initiatives, internal surveys reveal widespread skepticism, low participation, and informal resistance among rank-and-file firefighters.

Your task is to develop a Strategic Cultural Change Plan that explains this resistance and outlines a practical, psychologically grounded path forward.

Final Product: Strategic Cultural Change Plan (2000–2500 Words).

Your paper should include the following six sections:

1. Psychological Foundations of Resistance (Approx. 400–500 Words)
   - Explain how resistance in the fire service reflects adaptive psychological processes, not simply noncompliance.
   - Apply at least two psychological theories (e.g., social identity theory, system justification theory, and cognitive dissonance theory) to explain common responses to behavioral health reform, emotional expression, or leadership restructuring.
   - Use relevant examples from the chapter to support your analysis.
2. Cultural and Structural Analysis (Approx. 400–500 Words)
   - Identify at least three cultural or systemic contributors to resistance (e.g., stoicism, identity fusion, command structure, and stigma).
   - Explain how these factors function as both protective and limiting influences in the fire service context.
   - Address intersectional challenges that affect underrepresented members (e.g., gender, race, and sexual orientation).
3. Identity-Aligned Reframing Strategy (Approx. 400–500 Words)
   - Propose a reframing approach that aligns new practices with firefighters' core values (e.g., duty, bravery, and team loyalty).
   - Incorporate narrative psychology or existential theory to support re-authoring firefighter identity to include psychological resilience.
   - Provide example messaging or metaphors that demonstrate cultural fluency.
4. Leadership and Character Development (Approx. 300–400 Words)
   - Propose a leadership development model informed by character-based leadership theory.
   - Discuss how emotional intelligence, moral courage, and reflective judgment can be cultivated in officers and senior personnel.
   - Identify leadership practices that promote psychological safety and trust.
5. Implementation Strategy (Approx. 300–400 Words)
   - Outline a staged plan based on implementation science (e.g., stakeholder engagement, pilot testing, and feedback mechanisms).
   - Address ethical boundaries for peer support programs and the integration of licensed mental health professionals.
   - Recommend systems to support confidentiality, role clarity, and trauma-informed supervision.

6. Evaluation and Long-Term Sustainability (Approx. 200–300 Words)
    - Identify metrics to evaluate success (e.g., utilization rates, cultural readiness assessments, and peer support participation).
    - Propose structural supports (e.g., ongoing training, embedded psychology roles, and policy revision) to maintain momentum.
    - Reflect briefly on how cultural transformation should be measured not only in compliance but also in identity integration and lived experience.

Formatting and Submission Guidelines
Word Count: 2,000–2,500 words (excluding references)
APA format required.

Chapter 6
Implementing Upstream Solutions for Firefighter Safety and Well-Being

Firefighters face unique occupational hazards that place them at elevated risk for a range of behavioral health challenges, including posttraumatic stress disorder (PTSD), depression, substance use, and burnout. Addressing these concerns requires a comprehensive, multilevel prevention framework that engages the individual firefighter and the workplace, broader organizational systems, and the evidence base guiding interventions. The application of primary, secondary, tertiary, and quaternary prevention models in fire and emergency services emphasizes the importance of fostering psychological resilience, promoting early identification and intervention, providing specialized treatment and recovery support, and safeguarding against overmedicalization. Locus of control, organizational culture, and specialized peer support systems influence behavioral health outcomes. Furthermore, there are limitations in the use of generalized mental health programs with fire service populations, such as Employee Assistance Programs (EAPs), due to the lack of cultural competence among providers. Integrating evidence-based strategies tailored to the fire service enables a proactive, holistic approach to strengthening mental wellness and operational readiness across all levels of prevention.

Identifying Upstream Solutions in the Fire Service: A Multilevel Prevention Framework

Effectively addressing behavioral health outcomes within fire and emergency services requires a comprehensive, multilevel approach that considers the individual, social, and organizational factors influencing firefighter well-being. Firefighters routinely operate in high-stress environments and are frequently exposed to potentially traumatic events, placing them at elevated risk for a range of behavioral health challenges, including posttraumatic stress disorder (PTSD), depression, anxiety, substance use disorders, burnout, and elevated suicide risk (Carleton et al., 2019;

K. Wheldon, *Fire Service Psychology*,
https://doi.org/10.1007/978-3-032-02126-7_6

Haddock et al., 2012; Stanley et al., 2015). Additionally, while research is limited, emerging concerns suggest that problematic behaviors, such as unhealthy risk-taking, interpersonal conflict, and intrateam aggression, may negatively affect both individual well-being and overall team performance within the fire service. Fire service organizations should adopt a comprehensive prevention framework encompassing primary, secondary, tertiary, and quaternary prevention strategies to mitigate these risks and promote psychological well-being. Each level serves a distinct function: fostering resilience and healthy coping, early detection of emerging issues, providing evidence-based treatment, and safeguarding against overmedicalization. An integrated, systemic approach is important for sustaining the behavioral health of firefighters throughout their careers.

Substance abuse is a notably prevalent concern within fire and emergency services. Research suggests that a significant proportion of firefighters engage in binge drinking, potentially as a coping mechanism for occupational stressors (National Volunteer Fire Council [NVFC], 2015). The incidence of PTSD among firefighters is also substantially higher than that in the general population, with estimates suggesting that nearly 20% of firefighters experience PTSD symptoms (Kim et al., 2018). These mental health challenges are further complicated by organizational factors such as shift work, sleep disruption, and a culture that may stigmatize seeking psychological help (Regehr & Hill, 2001).

To address these behavioral health issues, prevention strategies are implemented across multiple levels:

> *Primary* Prevention: This method focuses on preventing the onset of behavioral health problems by promoting resilience and healthy coping mechanisms. This concept includes mental health education, stress management training, and fostering a supportive organizational culture (Institute for Work & Health, 2015).
>
> *Secondary Prevention:* Targets early detection and intervention for individuals exhibiting signs of behavioral health issues. Regular mental health screenings and peer support programs are examples of secondary prevention strategies (Greenberg et al., 2008).
>
> *Tertiary Prevention:* Provides treatment and support to individuals already affected by behavioral health problems, aiming to reduce the impact and facilitate recovery. Access to counseling services, therapy, and rehabilitation programs are key components in prevention (StatPearls, 2023).
>
> *Quaternary Prevention:* Aims to prevent overmedicalization and protect individuals from interventions that may cause more harm than benefit. This includes ensuring that mental health treatments are evidence-based and tailored to the unique needs of firefighters (StatPearls, 2023).

A comprehensive, multilevel prevention approach provides a structured pathway to address the complex behavioral health challenges faced by firefighters. By understanding and addressing the underlying factors that contribute to these outcomes, fire service organizations can better support the well-being and performance of their personnel.

Primary Prevention: Building Resilience and Promoting Mental Wellness

In the context of fire and emergency services, primary prevention has traditionally referred to Community Risk Reduction (CRR) strategies, which focus on proactively identifying and mitigating risks before they result in emergencies. CRR activities, such as fire safety inspections, public education, building code enforcement, and hazard mitigation, aim to prevent incidents from occurring, thereby reducing the need for emergency responses (National Fire Protection Association [NFPA], 2023; United States Fire Administration [USFA], 2022). By minimizing the frequency and severity of fire-related emergencies, the CRR serves as the frontline defense for safeguarding not only the public but also the health and safety of firefighters, effectively reducing the need for hazardous deployments and associated risks of injury, trauma, or fatality (USFA, 2022).

From a behavioral and public health standpoint, primary prevention focuses on reducing the risk of developing mental and behavioral health disorders among firefighters by minimizing harmful exposure. However, given the inherent nature of emergency response work, eliminating exposure to traumatic events, an exposure that is a core criterion in the development of posttraumatic stress disorder (PTSD), is not feasible (Institute for Work & Health, 2015). Therefore, within this framework, primary prevention focuses on developing psychological resilience, enhancing healthy coping skills, providing access to preventive psychoeducation, and cultivating an organizational culture that destigmatizes behavioral health support (Wild et al., 2020). These interventions aim to strengthen individual and team capacity to anticipate and manage occupational exposures and stressors, thereby reducing the likelihood of developing mental health conditions (Carleton et al., 2019).

Both primary prevention strategies are fundamentally aligned in their ultimate goal of risk reduction, albeit targeting different domains. While the CRR addresses environmental and situational risk factors external to the firefighter, the other primary prevention strategies focus on internal psychological preparedness and resilience. A comprehensive primary prevention strategy within the fire service should therefore integrate CRR initiatives to reduce exposure risks alongside psychological preparedness to mitigate the impact of inevitable exposures. This dual-pronged approach acknowledges the reality of firefighters' emergency response role while promoting a holistic model of occupational health and safety (Wild et al., 2020).

To support the development of psychological resilience among firefighters, training can incorporate foundational concepts such as emotional regulation, cognitive appraisal, and the psychological dimensions of moral injury. When firefighters become emotionally activated, they benefit from having accessible, healthy coping strategies to manage their responses to stress. For many, these strategies are not consciously examined or deliberately practiced. Moving coping mechanisms from unconscious habits to intentional actions can enhance personal effectiveness and emotional control. Preventive psychoeducation, when integrated at the organizational level, allows leaders and personnel to better understand the psychological effects of trauma and prepare for the demands inherent in emergency response work. Efforts to reduce stigma around behavioral health support may be more impactful when they not only encourage care seeking but also highlight those who have experienced tangible improvements in quality of life and professional performance as a result (Wild et al., 2020).

Resilience training programs have demonstrated effectiveness in enhancing firefighters' capacity to cope with occupational stressors. For example, a study by Wild et al. (2020) revealed that resilience-building interventions targeting first responders improved emotional regulation, reduced perceived stress, and enhanced overall psychological well-being. Such programs often incorporate components such as mindfulness, cognitive reappraisal, and peer support integration, equipping firefighters with practical skills to navigate the cumulative stressors of their profession (Leppin et al., 2014).

Organizational culture can play a significant role in primary prevention. Leadership endorsement of mental health initiatives and the promotion of psychological safety within teams are associated with greater willingness to seek help and lower stigma (Armstrong et al., 2016). Proactive efforts, such as mental health literacy campaigns and routine wellness checks, can create a work environment that prioritizes well-being and fosters resilience at the organizational level (Haddock et al., 2012).

Secondary Prevention: Early Identification and Intervention

Secondary prevention in fire and emergency services involves the early detection of behavioral health issues and timely intervention to prevent them from escalating into chronic or severe conditions. Given the occupational stressors faced by firefighters, strategies such as routine mental health screenings, early identification of stress injuries, and structured peer support programs are recommended to support this detection (Carleton et al., 2019; Wild et al., 2020).

One secondary prevention strategy used to address occupational exposure to potentially traumatic events (PTEs) is the integration of trauma risk management (TRiM) systems, which serve as the screening component of a psychological first aid model. TRiM is a peer-led, evidence-informed framework designed to support personnel following exposure to PTEs by promoting psychological monitoring, education, and referral pathways (Greenberg et al., 2008). TRiM-trained peer support teams are equipped to distinguish between normal acute stress reactions and patterns of distress that may necessitate professional intervention. This strategy helps to avoid unnecessary clinical referrals for individuals undergoing natural recovery processes (Bryant, 2019).

Following trauma exposure, individuals may experience one of several psychological trajectories: (1) resilient, no symptoms at baseline or thirty days after exposure; (2) natural recovery, where symptoms resolve without formal intervention; (3) persistent symptomatology; or (4) delayed onset, where symptoms emerge after an initial period without impairment (Bonanno, 2004; Bryant, 2019). Recognizing these potential outcomes informs decisions regarding the timing and necessity of clinical referrals. A "watchful waiting" approach, where individuals are monitored over time, allows peer supporters to track recovery and initiate further intervention only when appropriate (National Institute for Health and Care Excellence [NICE], 2018). This approach aligns with efforts to avoid overmedicalization and respects the natural course of recovery.

Another method within secondary prevention is the use of annual behavioral health checks. These methods are comparable to medical methods but focus on psychological well-being rather than fitness-for-duty evaluations. Behavioral health checks offer firefighters the opportunity to meet with a mental health professional who assesses current stressors, coping resources, and work–life balance, thereby facilitating the development of personalized coping strategies and mental health approaches. Unlike reactive assessments, these proactive check-ins encourage self-reflection and help identify areas for maintenance or improvement before clinical problems arise Annual behavioral health checks (e.g., universal depression screening once per year) have been shown to be cost-effective compared to less frequent or no screening in adolescent primary care settings (Doan et al., 2025). Although annual behavioral health checks show promise in general and clinical populations, dedicated research is still needed to determine their utility among firefighters, who face unique occupational stressors.

The incorporation of validated tools such as the Holmes-Rahe Life Stress Inventory enhances the value of these assessments. This instrument quantifies cumulative life stress from recent events, offering a structured means to evaluate an individual's overall stress load and potential vulnerability to stress-related health outcomes (Holmes & Rahe, 1967). In the firefighting context, where professional demands often intersect with personal life challenges, the Holmes-Rahe scale provides valuable insights to guide early proactive coping strategies.

Peer support programs remain a primary mechanism for identifying and addressing emerging stress responses. Research shows that peer-led interventions within fire departments contribute to early symptom recognition and increase the likelihood of referral to professional services (Creamer et al., 2012a). These programs facilitate access to support, particularly in environments where stigma may inhibit formal help-seeking behaviors (Wild et al., 2020).

In summary, secondary prevention in fire and emergency services involves a coordinated system of peer-led support, structured monitoring (e.g., TRiM), proactive behavioral health assessments, and validated screening tools. These strategies promote early identification and intervention while avoiding the premature medicalization of normal stress responses, thereby contributing to a comprehensive model for firefighter behavioral health care.

Tertiary Prevention: Treatment and Recovery Support

Tertiary prevention focuses on supporting firefighters who are already experiencing behavioral health challenges to reduce symptom severity, facilitate recovery, and prevent further functional decline. This level of intervention typically involves access to evidence-based treatment modalities such as cognitive–behavioral therapy

(CBT), trauma-focused therapies, substance use treatment, and rehabilitation programs tailored to the individual's clinical presentation (Haugen et al., 2012).

However, it is essential to acknowledge that interventions are considered evidence-based only if they are grounded in validated research. Such validation requires clinical language that reflects the actual diagnostic criteria for a condition, ensuring that researchers and clinicians discuss and treat the same presentation. The use of terms such as posttraumatic stress disorder (PTSD), posttraumatic stress symptoms (PTSS), and posttraumatic stress injury (PTSI) interchangeably can create ambiguity in research and clinical practice, potentially leading to misclassification, inappropriate treatment approaches, and confusion in outcome measurement (Bryant, 2019). A formal diagnosis of PTSD, as defined by standardized criteria (e.g., DSM-5-TR), serves as a benchmark for clinical trials and treatment protocols, ensuring the reliability and generalizability of findings (American Psychiatric Association, 2022). Addressing stigma needs to focus on the meaning attributed to the terminology rather than changing the words, which can complicate the process of establishing best-practice standards.

Although there is a robust evidence base for PTSD treatments within the general population, the unique occupational context of firefighters introduces nuances that may not be fully captured by generalized research. Factors such as cumulative trauma exposure, fire service culture, moral injuries, childhood trauma, and the intersection of operational and organizational stressors can influence both symptom presentation and treatment responsiveness (Carleton et al., 2019). Therefore, while interventions such as cognitive processing therapy (CPT) and prolonged exposure therapy (PE) have demonstrated efficacy in first responder populations (Haugen et al., 2012), the absence of firefighter-specific research necessitates cautious adaptation and ongoing evaluation of these methods within this occupational group.

Comprehensive Employee Assistance Programs (EAPs) remain a critical component of tertiary prevention, offering confidential access to counseling, crisis intervention, and referral services. Notably, effective Employee Assistance Programs (EAPs) should encompass culturally competent care, with mental health provider lists that reflect specialized training so that providers understand the unique dynamics of fire service work.

Additionally, workplace-based tertiary interventions often incorporate return-to-work programs and ongoing peer support mechanisms to help firefighters reintegrate into their roles after treatment (Carleton et al., 2019). These interventions may not only support functional recovery but also reduce the risk of relapse by addressing work-related exposures in a gradual, supportive manner.

Research by Paul Bartone (2006, 2022) further highlights the critical role of peer support programs in tertiary prevention. Bartone identified three primary functions of peer support in high-risk occupations: (1) facilitating the processing of grief and loss, which is common after traumatic incidents; (2) strengthening group cohesion, thereby enhancing collective resilience and team functioning; and (3) early identification of suicide risk, enabling timely intervention and referral to professional mental health services (Bartone, 2006). These peer-led initiatives complement formal clinical interventions by providing a trusted and stigma-reducing avenue for support, which is particularly relevant in the culture of the fire service.

In summary, tertiary prevention in fire and emergency services requires evidence-based, diagnosis-driven interventions that are adapted to the specific needs of firefighters. While best practices from the general population provide a foundational guide, the fire service context demands nuanced application and rigorous evaluation. Integrating clinical treatments with peer support, EAP resources, and occupationally informed strategies enhances recovery outcomes and promotes sustained mental health among firefighters.

Unique Dynamics of EAPs

While Employee Assistance Programs (EAPs) are often positioned as a primary resource for tertiary prevention in fire and emergency services, it is essential to critically examine their structure and limitations. EAPs typically consist of contracted provider networks where clinicians agree to offer services at predetermined reimbursement rates set by the employer or insurance carrier. These contracted rates are often significantly lower than market rates, which can deter specialized providers, such as those with advanced training in complex PTSD, moral injury, or occupational trauma specific to first responders (Merrick et al., 2022).

As a result, many EAP panels are populated by generalist clinicians, who may lack the cultural competence and specialized knowledge required to address the unique behavioral health needs of firefighters. Unlike mandated certifications for treating substance use disorders or trauma-specific therapies, there is no uniform requirement for EAP providers to be trained in the complexities of chronic occupational trauma, cumulative stress, or the moral injuries often encountered in fire service work (Litz et al., 2009).

Moreover, opportunities for EAP-affiliated providers to gain meaningful exposure to the fire service culture are limited. Few EAP organizations offer targeted continuing education or immersion experiences that help providers understand the operational demands, organizational stressors, and peer dynamics inherent in firefighting (Carleton et al., 2019). Consequently, EAP networks sometimes include providers who are spouses or family members of firefighters. While these individuals may be familiar with their lifestyle, they may also bring personal biases or emotional entanglements that compromise the objectivity and efficacy of care delivered to other firefighters.

The misalignment between firefighter-specific behavioral health needs and EAP provider expertise raises concerns about the quality and appropriateness of care. This gap can lead to misdiagnosis, inadequate treatment planning, and even disengagement from care, especially if firefighters perceive that their unique experiences are misunderstood or minimized.

Furthermore, the reliance on low reimbursement models creates economic disincentives for highly qualified providers to participate in EAP networks, thereby reducing the availability of clinically competent and culturally informed practitioners (Merrick et al., 2022. Without addressing these structural barriers, EAPs risk perpetuating a cycle in which firefighters are referred to providers who are ill-equipped to meet their complex needs, thereby undermining the intent of tertiary prevention efforts.

In this context, enhancing the clinical quality and cultural competence of EAP providers is important. This may involve advocating for higher reimbursement rates, specialty training mandates, and fostering fire service-specific provider development programs to ensure that EAPs truly function as adequate tertiary prevention resources within firefighter behavioral health frameworks.

Quaternary Prevention: Preventing Overmedicalization and Ensuring Evidence-Based Care

Quaternary prevention in fire and emergency services focuses on protecting individuals from overmedicalization or overdiagnosis and ensuring that behavioral health interventions are both evidence-based and culturally appropriate. Given the high-stress and trauma-laden nature of firefighting, there is a natural inclination toward immediate intervention following critical incidents. However, quaternary prevention emphasizes the importance of avoiding unnecessary or premature clinical interventions, particularly when common psychological responses are misinterpreted as pathological.

Historically, interventions such as critical incident stress debriefing (CISD) have been widely employed post-incident in emergency services. However, empirical evidence has questioned their efficacy, with systematic reviews suggesting that indiscriminate, mandatory debriefings may be ineffective and disrupt natural recovery processes (McNally et al., 2003; Rose et al., 2002). This has prompted a shift away from universal, immediate debriefing models toward more flexible and individualized approaches that respect the diversity of trauma responses (Hobfoll et al., 2007).

A similar concern pertains to the early application of intensive trauma-focused interventions such as eye movement desensitization and reprocessing (EMDR) shortly after trauma exposure. While EMDR has robust evidence for treating chronic PTSD, its premature use before a diagnosis is warranted may interfere with the natural recovery trajectory of acute stress reactions (Shalev et al., 2012). Notably, Bryant (2019) emphasized in his work Acute Stress Disorder: A Handbook of Theory, Assessment, and Treatment that acute stress disorder (ASD) represents a cluster of psychological and physiological responses occurring within the first

30 days following a traumatic event. These symptoms, while distressing, often resolve without formal clinical intervention as part of a natural recovery process (Bryant, 2019).

Overmedicalizing these ASD symptoms by introducing aggressive clinical treatments prematurely risks pathologizing adaptive stress responses and may inadvertently prolong or complicate recovery (Bryant, 2019; Ruzek et al., 2017). Hence, quaternary prevention advocates for stepped-care models, where initial support emphasizes psychological first aid, peer support, and monitoring, with escalation to formal interventions only for those whose symptoms persist beyond the acute phase (Hobfoll et al., 2007; Ruzek et al., 2017).

Furthermore, quaternary prevention in fire and emergency services may emphasize the importance of patient-centered care, informed consent, and continuous evaluation of intervention outcomes. A balanced approach integrates psychotherapy, peer support, and lifestyle interventions where clinically indicated while cautioning against reflexive reliance on pharmacological treatments that fail to address underlying psychosocial factors (Sussman & Sussman, 2011).

In summary, quaternary prevention ensures that firefighters receive behavioral health interventions in a timely, appropriate, and evidence-based manner, preventing harm from overmedicalization while promoting natural recovery and long-term psychological resilience.

Engaging the Individual: Locus of Control across Prevention Levels

Locus of control is a well-established psychological concept that refers to an individual's general expectations about the extent to which they can influence events in their life (Rotter, 1966). Those with an internal locus of control believe that their actions and decisions directly shape outcomes. In contrast, individuals with an external locus of control tend to attribute outcomes to outside forces such as luck, fate, or the influence of others (Rotter, 1966; Lefcourt, 2014).

This belief system plays a critical role in how individuals interpret and respond to stress and trauma, making it especially relevant to behavioral health outcomes in fire and emergency services. Supporting firefighters in adopting a more internal or balanced locus of control can help them manage stress more effectively. Empowering individuals to actively engage in their mental health by using preventive strategies and seeking professional support when needed can strengthen their resilience. Conversely, those with a predominantly external locus of control may be more susceptible to maladaptive responses. Therefore, fostering a more balanced sense of control holds significant promise for improving mental health and operating performance in high-stress environments.

To assess locus of control, Rotter's Internal-External Locus of Control Scale (I-E Scale) remains one of the most widely used instruments (Rotter, 1966). Over time, domain-specific measures have been developed, such as the Work Locus of Control Scale (WLCS), which explicitly evaluates perceptions of control within occupational contexts (Spector, 1988). The WLCS has strong psychometric properties and is frequently used in high-risk occupational populations, including firefighters (Spector, 1988; Onyedire et al., 2017). These tools allow for the identification of individuals who may be more vulnerable to maladaptive stress responses owing to an external locus of control orientation.

In firefighting, locus of control has been identified as a critical psychological factor influencing susceptibility to posttraumatic stress disorder (PTSD) symptoms following trauma exposure. Individuals with an external locus of control often experience a diminished sense of agency, making them more vulnerable to feelings of helplessness, maladaptive coping, and, ultimately, greater PTSD symptomatology (Benight & Bandura, 2004). Conversely, firefighters with a strong internal locus of control are more likely to engage in adaptive coping strategies and exhibit greater psychological resilience posttrauma (Benight & Bandura, 2004).

Additional empirical evidence supports the association between psychological factors and PTSD outcomes in firefighters. A study by Onyedire et al. (2017) examining PTSD symptoms, resilience, and work locus of control among Nigerian career firefighters revealed that higher resilience scores significantly predict lower levels of PTSD symptoms. Conversely, firefighters with a stronger external locus of control reported more severe PTSD symptoms. The study also identified demographic variables, such as longer service duration, greater tenure, and higher educational attainment, as being associated with reduced PTSD symptom severity. On the basis of these findings, the authors recommended that interventions to mitigate PTSD risk should incorporate both resilience-building strategies and efforts to shift the external locus of control beliefs toward a more internal orientation.

Primary Prevention: Building an Internal Locus of Control Before Exposure

Within primary prevention, fostering an internal locus of control is foundational for building psychological resilience and preparing firefighters to manage stress before it escalates. Preexposure interventions enhance self-efficacy, cognitive appraisal, and coping mechanisms, empowering individuals to perceive greater control over their stress responses (Benight & Bandura, 2004; Meichenbaum, 2017). These programs reduce feelings of helplessness and are associated with lower PTSD risk posttrauma (Wild et al., 2020).

Secondary Prevention: Early Identification and Self-Efficacy in Help-Seeking

In secondary prevention, locus of control significantly affects whether firefighters recognize emerging stress symptoms and engage with support services. Individuals with an internal locus (internally motivated) are more likely to seek help proactively and respond positively to peer support interventions, such as trauma risk management (TRiM). In contrast, an external locus may contribute to avoidance and passivity (Greenberg et al., 2008). Screening tools such as the WLCS can help identify individuals at greater risk due to external control beliefs, informing targeted secondary interventions (Onyedire et al., 2017).

Tertiary Prevention: Engagement and Recovery in Treatment

For firefighters requiring tertiary-level interventions, the locus of control continues to shape treatment engagement and recovery trajectories. Individuals with an internal locus are more likely to perceive therapy as beneficial and engage actively. In contrast, those with an external locus may attribute recovery to external forces, which can potentially hinder treatment adherence (Lefcourt, 2014). The incorporation of self-efficacy-enhancing components, such as skill-building and personalized coping strategies, into treatment can mitigate these barriers and improve outcomes (Benight & Bandura, 2004).

Quaternary Prevention: Empowering Self-Regulation and Avoiding Overmedicalization

In quaternary prevention, fostering an internal locus of control aligns with principles of avoiding overmedicalization. Educating firefighters on the natural course of acute stress reactions and equipping them with self-monitoring tools promotes empowerment and reduces reliance on unnecessary clinical interventions. This approach supports watchful waiting, ensuring that interventions are reserved for those who require them while reinforcing individual agency in mental health maintenance.

Summary

Locus of control represents a pivotal cognitive variable influencing how firefighters perceive and respond to trauma across all levels of prevention. While it is important to identify at-risk individuals early, it is also imperative that individuals are empowered to take a proactive role in their mental health. Interventions designed to increase the internal locus of control have shown promise in reducing PTSD symptom severity and improving overall mental health outcomes in high-risk occupational groups (Wild et al., 2020; Kinman et al., 2020). Integrating locus of control-focused strategies into firefighter behavioral health programs not only empowers individuals but also enhances the overall effectiveness of prevention efforts.

Engaging the Workplace: Organizational Role in Firefighter Behavioral Health Prevention

The workplace represents a critical context for implementing behavioral health prevention strategies in fire and emergency services. Engaging the organizational environment, encompassing leadership, culture, policies, and peer networks, is important for the practical application of primary, secondary, tertiary, and quaternary prevention models. The unique stressors of firefighting, including repeated trauma exposure, high operational demands, and strong team dynamics, necessitate workplace-level interventions that extend beyond individual responsibility (Carleton et al., 2019).

Primary Prevention: Cultivating a Resilient and Supportive Organizational Culture

At the primary prevention level, workplace engagement focuses on cultivating an organizational culture that promotes psychological resilience, mental health literacy, and proactive wellness initiatives. Fire departments can implement programs to normalize conversations about mental health, reduce stigma, and provide psychoeducation on stress management and coping strategies. Leadership plays a pivotal role in shaping workplace norms; leaders who model healthy coping behaviors and prioritize mental health signals to employees that their psychological well-being is valued (Armstrong et al., 2016).

Organizational policies support work–life balance, adequate rest periods, and access to preventive resources (e.g., wellness workshops, mindfulness training), further reinforcing a proactive approach to mental health. These efforts align with the Community Risk Reduction (CRR) model by reducing the likelihood of behavioral health crises through systemic, environmental modifications (National Fire Protection Association [NFPA], 2023).

Secondary Prevention: Early Detection through Workplace-Embedded Systems

Secondary prevention in the workplace emphasizes the establishment of systems for the early detection and intervention of behavioral health concerns. Initiatives such as regular behavioral health screenings, peer support programs, and trauma risk management (TRiM) are most effective when they are embedded within the organizational fabric of the agency (Greenberg et al., 2008). These programs rely on the workplace to provide infrastructure, training, and administrative support, ensuring that at-risk individuals are identified and referred to appropriate resources when appropriate.

Workplace engagement in secondary prevention also involves fostering a climate where seeking help is normalized and psychological safety is maintained. When peer supporters are formally recognized and supported by the organization, they are better positioned to assist colleagues without fear of stigma or reprisal (Creamer et al., 2012a). Additionally, annual behavioral health check-ins, supported by employers, provide structured opportunities for early identification of stress-related issues, akin to routine medical physicals.

Tertiary Prevention: Supporting Recovery and Reintegration

In the context of tertiary prevention, engaging the workplace involves developing systems that support firefighters in recovery and facilitate reintegration into their roles after treatment. This includes return-to-work programs, modified duty options, and ongoing peer support networks that address the challenges of transitioning back to operational duties following behavioral health treatment (Haddock et al., 2012).

Moreover, the effectiveness of employee assistance programs (EAPs) is largely contingent upon the organization's commitment to ensuring culturally competent, specialized care tailored to firefighters' unique needs (Merrick et al., 2022). Organizations that actively vet EAP providers, advocate for fair reimbursement rates, and provide training on firefighter-specific variables are more likely to deliver meaningful tertiary interventions. Workplace engagement ensures that recovery is not solely the individual's responsibility but is supported through coordinated, organizationally endorsed efforts.

Quaternary Prevention: Organizational Responsibility in Avoiding Overmedicalization

Quaternary prevention requires the workplace to actively prevent overmedicalization and promote evidence-based, individualized care. This involves developing policies and protocols that emphasize "watchful waiting" strategies post-incident, ensuring that clinical interventions are pursued only when indicated by evidence and diagnosis (NICE, 2018). Fire service organizations should also guard against knee-jerk implementations of interventions (e.g., mandatory debriefings) that have not been demonstrated to be effective and may inadvertently cause harm (McNally et al., 2003).

Through ongoing education, data-driven decision-making, and partnerships with behavioral health professionals, organizations can ensure that care pathways reflect current best practices while respecting their personnel's natural recovery trajectories. This organizational vigilance helps strike a balance between providing needed support and avoiding unnecessary clinical interventions.

Four Levels of Prevention

Engaging the workplace across all levels of prevention transforms the fire service from a passive strategy to a proactive force in supporting firefighter behavioral health. By embedding prevention strategies within the organizational culture, leadership, policies, and support systems, fire departments can create environments that foster resilience, facilitate early intervention, support recovery, and ensure the delivery of ethical, evidence-based care. Therefore, workplace engagement is not ancillary but rather integral to the successful implementation of behavioral health prevention frameworks in fire and emergency services.

Prevention Related to Substance Abuse

Substance use, particularly alcohol misuse, represents another prevalent concern among firefighter populations. Paulus et al. (2017) examined the associations between posttraumatic stress, depression, and alcohol use among firefighters. Their findings revealed that depression was directly related to alcohol dependence. Posttraumatic stress is significantly associated with multiple alcohol-related outcomes, including symptoms of alcohol dependence, positive alcohol dependence screenings, and increased alcohol consumption per occasion (Paulus et al., 2017). Furthermore, the interaction between posttraumatic stress and depression had a significant effect on alcohol use outcomes, with this interaction persisting even after controlling for demographic variables and covariates. Interestingly, higher depression levels are more strongly associated with adverse alcohol outcomes among individuals with lower levels of posttraumatic stress (Paulus et al., 2017).

Prevention Programs for High-Risk Occupational Groups

High-risk occupational groups, such as firefighters, police officers, military personnel, and healthcare workers, face elevated risks of substance misuse because repeated exposure to trauma, high occupational stress, irregular work schedules, and workplace cultures may normalize substance use (Carleton et al., 2019; Haddock et al., 2017; Substance Abuse and Mental Health Services Administration [SAMHSA], 2015). Among firefighters, studies indicate a high prevalence of alcohol misuse, with approximately 50% of career firefighters engaging in binge drinking (Haddock et al., 2017). Similar trends are observed among police officers and military personnel, with approximately 30% of police officers reporting monthly binge drinking and high levels of alcohol use among service members postdeployment (Ballenger et al., 2011; Schumm & Chard, 2012). Co-occurring conditions, including PTSD, depression, and anxiety, further compound the risk of substance misuse in these populations (Carleton et al., 2019).

Key Components of Effective Prevention Programs

Effective substance abuse prevention programs share several core components:

Organizational Support and Leadership Buy-In: Programs are most effective when endorsed by organizational leaders, fostering a culture that prioritizes wellness and substance use prevention (SAMHSA, 2022).

Confidentiality and Trust: Ensuring confidentiality encourages participation, especially in professions where stigma and fear of job loss deter help-seeking behaviors (Hoge et al., 2004).

Evidence-Based Interventions: Programs grounded in cognitive–behavioral therapy (CBT), motivational interviewing (MI), and psychoeducation are consistently shown to be effective in reducing substance use (Benight & Bandura, 2004; Carey et al., 2006).

Multilevel Approach: Combining individual-level interventions (e.g., resilience training, coping skills) with organizational policies (e.g., wellness initiatives, employee assistance program [EAP] access) yields better long-term outcomes (Wild et al., 2020).

Peer Support Integration: Peer-led initiatives reduce stigma and facilitate early intervention, particularly in first responder and military populations (Creamer et al., 2012a).

Effective Program Types and Evidence

Cognitive-Behavioral and Skills Training Programs: Cognitive–behavioral interventions (CBIs) have been shown to be effective in reducing alcohol misuse among military personnel and police officers by enhancing coping skills and modifying maladaptive thought patterns (Carey et al., 2006). The "Team Awareness" program, a team-focused CBT-based intervention, has demonstrated success in reducing workplace substance use in high-risk industries (Bennett & Lehman, 2001).

Resilience and Stress-Inoculation Training: Building psychological resilience through structured training helps individuals develop healthier coping mechanisms, thereby reducing the likelihood of substance misuse following trauma (Meichenbaum, 2017). Resilience-focused interventions in firefighters and police officers have been associated with improved stress management and reduced maladaptive behaviors (Wild et al., 2020).

Peer Support Programs: Peer support models have become integral in substance use prevention for first responders. Programs such as "peer support teams" in fire departments and "Battle Buddy" systems in the military have been effective in promoting help-seeking and reducing substance-related stigma (Creamer et al., 2012a).

Organizational Policies and Health Promotion: Comprehensive wellness initiatives, including substance use education, fitness programs, and mental health resources, have been shown to improve overall employee well-being and reduce substance misuse (Kinman et al., 2020). Random drug testing and alcohol-free workplace policies further reinforce a culture of safety and accountability, although evidence suggests that they are most effective when combined with supportive interventions (Frone, 2013).

Outcomes and Effectiveness

Effective prevention programs have led to reductions in substance use frequency and severity, improved coping skills, and enhanced mental health outcomes among high-risk occupational groups (Carey et al., 2006; Wild et al., 2020). For example, brief interventions in military populations have led to short-term decreases in alcohol use (Carey et al., 2006), whereas peer support programs have increased early help-seeking behaviors in first responders. Comprehensive programs that address both individual and organizational factors are associated with sustained improvements in workplace culture and a reduction in stigma surrounding substance use.

Conclusion: Advancing a Multilevel Prevention Model for Firefighter Behavioral Health

Addressing the complex behavioral health needs of firefighters requires a shift from reactive, crisis-driven responses toward a proactive, systemic, and culturally attuned prevention framework. It is essential to employ a comprehensive model that encompasses primary, secondary, tertiary, and quaternary prevention strategies, each of which is informed by psychological science, occupational health literature, and research specific to fire and emergency services. Rather than focusing solely on individual pathology, this approach emphasizes resilience-building, early identification, evidence-based treatment, and protection against the harm of overmedicalization. Central to this framework is the recognition that behavioral health outcomes are shaped not only by individual traits but also by organizational culture, leadership practices, peer dynamics, and systemic access to competent care.

The inclusion of psychological constructs such as locus of control adds nuance to prevention efforts across all levels, providing actionable insights into how firefighters perceive stress, engage with services, and recover from trauma. Moreover, organizational engagement emerges as an important force multiplier; when departments cultivate environments of psychological safety, embed prevention strategies into their policies, and equip leaders to model mental health literacy, the entire system becomes more resilient. Similarly, critical examination of employee assistance programs (EAPs), along with the integration of peer-led initiatives and trauma-informed care, reveals the importance of aligning interventions with the unique realities of fire service work.

Substance abuse prevention, a particularly pressing concern, underscores the need for a multifaceted, evidence-based approach that integrates individual skill development with peer support and organizational commitment. Research from other high-risk occupations reinforces the value of combining cognitive-behavioral interventions, resilience training, and peer mentoring to reduce risk behaviors and promote well-being.

Ultimately, the implementation of upstream solutions in fire and emergency services is not a singular intervention but a cultural transformation. It requires investment in workforce education, leadership development, structural reform, and the integration of mental health expertise tailored to the occupational context. By committing to this holistic, multilevel prevention model, fire service organizations can safeguard not only the operational readiness of their personnel but also their long-term psychological health, dignity, and humanity.

Chapter Review

Assignment: Designing a Multilevel Behavioral Health Prevention Framework for Fire Service Populations

Learning Objectives

- By the end of this assignment, students will be able to:
- Differentiate and critically evaluate the four levels of behavioral health prevention (primary, secondary, tertiary, and quaternary) within the context of fire and emergency services.
- Analyze the psychological, organizational, and cultural determinants that influence behavioral health outcomes in firefighters.

- Apply principles of psychological theory (e.g., locus of control, trauma trajectories, resilience science) to inform prevention strategies.
- Identify limitations in existing systems (e.g., EAPs) and propose culturally competent, evidence-based reforms.
- Design an integrated, upstream-focused behavioral health strategy for a fire service agency, addressing both individual and systemic factors.

Assignment Prompt

You have been retained by a state fire marshal's office to develop a comprehensive, multilevel behavioral health prevention framework for adoption across regional fire departments. The goal is to reduce rates of psychological injury, improve resilience, support early intervention, and ensure ethical, evidence-based care.

The office is particularly interested in a strategy that:

- Differentiates among primary, secondary, tertiary, and quaternary prevention levels.
- Applies psychological constructs (e.g., locus of control) to prevention design.
- Improves or replaces underperforming systems such as EAPs.
- Integrates individual, organizational, and policy-level recommendations.

You are tasked with developing a written strategic prevention proposal for review and implementation.

Deliverable: Strategic Prevention Proposal.

Length: 2000–2500 words.

Format: APA seventh edition, with headings corresponding to the sections below.

Required Sections

1. Conceptual Foundations (Approx. 500 Words)
    - Briefly define the four levels of prevention (primary, secondary, tertiary, quaternary) as applied to firefighter behavioral health.
    - Explain the rationale for a multilevel prevention approach in this occupational context.
    - Introduce one or more psychological constructs (e.g., locus of control, trauma recovery trajectories) that will guide your proposal design.
2. Strategic Prevention Design (Approx. 1200–1400 Words Total)

    Break this section into four subsections, each addressing a level of prevention:

    - Primary Prevention: Resilience and Preparedness
        - Explore community risk reduction strategies.
        - Outline prevention strategies targeting psychological readiness before exposure.
        - Propose organizational culture and leadership interventions to promote resilience and normalize mental wellness.
        - Include strategies for building an internal locus of control.

- Secondary Prevention: Early Identification and Peer Intervention
  - Recommend methods for early detection, including peer support, TRiM, or behavioral health screenings.
  - Address how to avoid overdiagnosis while ensuring timely care.
  - Discuss use of tools like the Holmes-Rahe Scale or Work Locus of Control Scale.
- Tertiary Prevention: Clinical Treatment and Return-to-Work Support
  - Identify evidence-based treatments suitable for firefighters (e.g., CPT, EMDR) and discuss how to adapt them culturally.
  - Recommend improvements to existing EAP structures or alternatives.
  - Discuss reintegration supports such as modified duty, peer bridging, or clinician-peer collaboration.
- Quaternary Prevention: Ethical Safeguards Against Overmedicalization
  - Propose strategies to prevent premature clinical intervention (e.g., watchful waiting, stepped-care models).
  - Include a critique of past interventions (e.g., CISD) and how new systems can avoid similar pitfalls.
  - Recommend education strategies to distinguish natural recovery from pathology.

3. Organizational and Policy Recommendations (Approx. 400–500 Words)
   - Provide specific organizational changes (e.g., policy revisions, leadership training, structural supports) to embed prevention across all levels.
   - Include a proposal for improving provider access and competence, including EAP reform or the development of fire-service-specific clinician networks.
   - Identify key metrics for program evaluation (e.g., stigma reduction, symptom tracking, utilization trends).

   Submission Requirements
   Word Count: 2000–2500 (excluding references)
   Citation Style: APA seventh edition

Chapter 7
The Role of Psychologists in the Fire Service

As the psychological demands of emergency response work gain national attention, the role of psychologists in public safety settings has expanded significantly, particularly in law enforcement. However, within the fire service, this integration remains nascent, fragmented, and often overshadowed by models developed for police populations. Despite overlapping stressors across first responder roles, firefighters face a distinct constellation of psychological challenges shaped by operational tempo, cultural expectations, trauma exposure, and team dynamics that differ in nature, not just degree, from their law enforcement counterparts. Current frameworks within police and public safety psychology (PPSP), while foundational, often lack specificity and relevance for fire service applications. There should be a critical examination of the divergence between these two fields, which may lead to the formal development of a specialized field of fire service psychology. It explores the historical trajectory of psychological support in emergency services, legal and operational considerations unique to fire and emergency services, and the emerging need for culturally competent, evidence-based psychological practices tailored to firefighters. In doing so, it highlights the opportunities and ethical imperatives for psychologists to serve not only as adjunct providers but also as embedded, strategic partners in promoting resilience, performance, and systemic health within fire departments.

Fire Service Psychology: Parallel Paths and the Need for Divergence

Over the past fifteen years, police and public safety psychology have developed significantly. In 2011, the American Board of Police and Public Safety Psychology was formally established, followed shortly by the recognition of the police and public safety psychology (PPSP) specialty by the American Psychological Association

K. Wheldon, *Fire Service Psychology*,
https://doi.org/10.1007/978-3-032-02126-7_7

in 2013 (Corey et al., 2011; American Psychological Association, 2014; Kitaeff, 2019). These developments were key to legitimizing psychological work in law enforcement settings and laid the foundation for a growing body of research, clinical tools, and operational practices.

However, while fire and emergency services are now occasionally mentioned within PPSP reference materials, the foundational research used to inform these guidelines remains rooted almost entirely in law enforcement populations. As a result, professionals and policymakers tend to treat police officers, firefighters, and emergency medical services personnel as a single, homogeneous group of "first responders." This assumption has led to the widespread belief that their psychological needs and service strategies should be the same.

However, those working with or exclusively connected to fire service psychology consider another perspective. The difference is not merely in degree but in kind. Firefighters encounter a unique set of stressors, team dynamics, and cultural expectations that warrant their own study, standards, and voice within public safety psychology. While there are distinctions between fire and emergency services and other first responder populations, there are shared experiences that can be identified and honored. Nonetheless, there is a need for fire service-specific research to support truly effective and sustainable psychological practices to support the health, safety, and longevity of our firefighters.

The American Psychological Association's PPSP specialty outlines four domains in which psychology is applied: assessment, intervention, operations, and consultation (American Board of Professional Psychology [ABPP], n.d.). These domains encompass pre-employment psychological evaluations, fitness-for-duty assessments, workers' compensation evaluations, and psychological autopsies. They also include prevention and treatment efforts, operational support in high-risk environments, and guidance to leadership for improving system functioning. These areas are well suited to the law enforcement environment but do not yet reflect the full scope of what is needed within fire service settings. For example, although not included in current PPSP guidelines, fire and emergency services would greatly benefit from incorporating human factor analysis following injuries or line-of-duty fatalities, an area where psychological consultation could meaningfully improve outcomes and safety culture.

What complicates matters further is that both psychology and fire and emergency services are developing standards for behavioral health simultaneously yet independently. Psychology does so through clinical science, ethics, and legal precedent, including the Frye and Daubert standards, which govern the admissibility of expert psychological testimony in court (Daubert v. Merrell Dow Pharmaceuticals, Inc., 1993; Frye v. United States, 1923). These legal frameworks require expert opinions to be based on methods that are empirically tested, peer reviewed, widely accepted within the scientific community, and held to known standards of error and reliability.

In contrast, the fire service develops its behavioral health framework through organizations such as the National Fire Protection Association (NFPA), with a focus on occupational safety rather than psychological treatment. The NFPA has issued two major standards addressing mental health in fire and emergency services: NFPA

1500 and NFPA 1582. NFPA 1500: The Standard on Fire Department Occupational Safety, Health, and Wellness Program provides a high-level view of what behavioral health programs could include access to licensed clinicians, peer support programs, critical incident stress management (CISM), and basic training in mental health awareness for department personnel (National Fire Protection Association [NFPA], 2021a). The intent is to reduce stigma and encourage early help-seeking behaviors.

NFPA 1582: Standard on Comprehensive Occupational Medical Program for Fire Departments complements 1500 by incorporating mental health screenings into regular medical evaluations (NFPA, 2021b). While primarily medical in scope, this standard acknowledges the link between mental and physical readiness and recommends that departments assess posttraumatic stress disorder (PTSD), depression, anxiety, and substance use disorders. These standards represent a significant step in recognizing behavioral health as an integral part of operational readiness.

However, it is important to understand that the NFPA is not a psychological authority. It does not establish clinical standards, and its guidelines are not developed through psychological research or subjected to legal scrutiny under the Frye or Daubert standards. Its behavioral health directives are written from a safety and risk management standpoint, not a therapeutic one. While this approach is valuable in setting a minimum threshold for behavioral health programming, it cannot substitute for the ethical and evidence-based standards that guide clinical care.

These dynamics create real and often problematic tension for clinicians operating in fire service environments. A psychologist may be asked to implement or consult programs that meet NFPA requirements. However, those requirements may not align with the clinical standards dictated by the psychologist's license, training, or legal obligations. For example, the NFPA may emphasize peer support and CISM without addressing the limitations or controversies around their efficacy in the scientific literature (Everly & Mitchell, 2000; McNally et al., 2003). Meanwhile, the psychologist is expected to uphold scientific integrity, use validated interventions, and stay within the bounds of their ethical code. These competing standards generate confusion over priorities, intervention structure, and even liability, especially when the organizational culture is unfamiliar with or resistant to clinical nuance.

From the perspective of the fire service, this misalignment is not only confusing but also potentially harmful. Programs may be created to check compliance boxes, but they often lack clinical grounding. Peer support teams may be deployed without adequate training, boundaries, or supervision. Outdated practices may be maintained simply because they are written into policy. In the absence of true collaboration with the psychological community, departments risk perpetuating models that do little to move the needle on firefighter mental health and, in some cases, may even reinforce stigma or contribute to delayed care.

Ultimately, we observe the results of two parallel systems, psychology and fire service, each of which aims to address firefighter mental health strategies but does so in isolation. Without coordination, a gap forms between what is operationally recommended and what is clinically sound. Bridging the gap will require better communication between disciplines and recognition that firefighters deserve more than generalized solutions pulled from adjacent professions. They need, and have earned, behavioral health programs built from the ground up, on the basis of the realities of the job and grounded in data specific to their lived experience. It cannot happen without sustained research, meaningful partnerships between clinicians and departments, and a willingness to rethink how behavioral health is delivered in the fire service. Firefighters are not just another branch of "first responders." They are a unique and deeply specialized community; our standards, practices, and research should reflect reality.

Fire Service Psychology: Historical Context

Military Psychology

The origins of psychology in the military date back to the early 1900s, when initial studies on the mental and emotional aspects of warfare were conducted (Yerkes, 1921). During World War I, the introduction of the Army Alpha and Beta tests marked a significant step in screening soldiers for service, representing one of the earliest systematic applications of psychology in the military (Jones & Wessely, 2007). In 1921, the first formal publication of military psychology research appeared in the Journal of Applied Psychology. World War II saw a significant expansion of military psychology into personnel selection, combat stress, and morale studies (Jones & Wessely, 2007). After the war, the focus shifted to the psychological rehabilitation of veterans, and the growing recognition of posttraumatic stress disorder (PTSD), which was later formally recognized in the Diagnostic and Statistical Manual of Mental Disorders. Research during the Korean War explored the psychological impact of captivity and the experiences of prisoners of war (Jones & Wessely, 2007). At the same time, the Vietnam War era furthered the study of combat stress, morale, and PTSD, leading to long-term clinical recognition and treatment advancements. In the 1970s, the American Psychological Association (APA) established Division 19, the Society for Military Psychology, and in 1979, PTSD was formally included in the DSM-III (American Psychiatric Association, 2022). The Gulf War highlighted the importance of psychological preparation and post-deployment mental health. The post-9/11 period focused on PTSD, traumatic brain injury (TBI), and psychological resilience during the wars in Iraq and Afghanistan (Adler et al., 2011). Today, military psychology research continues to evolve, addressing emerging challenges such as cyber warfare, the mental health of drone operators, and the long-term care of veterans (Adams et al., 2004).

Psychology in Other First-Respondent Agencies

Psychologists were first hired by police departments in the 1960s. During the same period, the Federal Bureau of Investigation hired a psychologist to expand its Behavioral Sciences Unit. These law enforcement agencies sought to understand the underlying factors that contributed to criminal behavior. The New York Police Department (NYPD) acquired its first psychologist, Dr. Sloussenburg, in 1964. His primary job duty was to assist with the department's hostage negotiation tactics. During this time, the NYPD developed the "East Coast Model," in which a negotiation team was initially deployed, and if the crisis was not resolved, the tactical team responded. Similarly, the Los Angeles Police Department (LAPD) hired its first psychologist in the 1960s. This psychologist helped create the "West Coast Model" of crisis negotiations, where the Special Weapons and Tactics Team trained members in tactical and negotiation strategies but deployed them together (American Board of Police and Public Safety Psychology, n.d.; American Psychological Association, 2022).

Police departments seek psychologists to train them in negotiation tactics and strategies for addressing challenging community members. Since fire departments do not hire psychologists at the same rates as their police counterparts do, many have been unable to see the practical application of professional psychology. Police departments began using psychologists for management consultation, ongoing training, and direct psychological services after specific incidents (American Psychological Association, 2022). The presence of psychology in law enforcement has increased. Currently, police psychologists are assigned to many departments across the United States, and the research pool is growing substantially (American Psychological Association, 2014). Unfortunately, the growth of fire psychology has fallen behind (Addis & Mahalik, 2003).

The origins of psychology in law enforcement can be traced back to 1916, when Lewis Terman adapted the Stanford-Binet test for screening police applicants in California. Following World War II, the 1940s and 1950s saw an increased focus on psychological assessments and officer selection. In the 1960s, the civil rights movement prompted a shift toward improving officer training and managing stress. The 1970s marked significant development as the American Psychological Association (APA) integrated psychologists into law enforcement, focusing on crisis intervention and handling critical incidents. During the 1980s, the scope of concern widened to address officers' mental health, stress management, and trauma response. In 1991, the APA formally recognized police and public safety psychology as a specialty, underscoring the growing importance of psychology in law enforcement (American Psychological Association, 2014, 2022). Post-9/11, there was increased emphasis on trauma, counterterrorism, and disaster response. In 2013, the APA granted specialty recognition to police and public safety psychology (American Psychological Association, 2014). Recent trends in the field have focused on improving community–police relations, enhancing officers' mental health, training diverse populations, and advocating for law enforcement reform (American Board of Professional Psychology, n.d.).

The integration of psychology into law enforcement took a significant step forward with the involvement of the first police psychologists in the Los Angeles Police Department (LAPD) and the New York Police Department (NYPD). In the 1960s, Dr. Martin Reiser became the first full-time police psychologist for the Los Angeles Police Department (LAPD), pioneering the use of psychological techniques in law enforcement, particularly in hostage negotiation and crisis intervention. His work laid the foundation for developing crisis negotiation models, which focused on understanding the psychological dynamics of perpetrators and victims during high-stress situations (American Board of Police and Public Safety Psychology, n.d.).

Similarly, in the NYPD, psychologist Harvey Schlossberg, who was also a police officer, played a critical role in developing the department's crisis negotiation team in the 1970s. Schlossberg's expertise in psychology, combined with his experience in law enforcement, helped create the first formal hostage negotiation model. This model emphasizes the importance of communication, active listening, and de-escalation techniques in resolving high-stakes situations without violence. The contributions of these early police psychologists not only revolutionized how hostage and crisis negotiations were handled but also shaped the broader role of psychology in law enforcement, particularly in handling critical incidents and managing officer stress (American Psychological Association, 2022). These developments also contributed to the APA's increased involvement in law enforcement psychology in the following decades (American Psychological Association, 2014).

Fire Service Psychology

In the early 1900s, firefighters faced significant mental and emotional challenges with little to no psychological support. Following World War II, there was a growing acknowledgment that trauma and stress in firefighters mirrored the experiences of soldiers and law enforcement personnel (Berger et al., 2012). By the 1980s and 1990s, critical incident stress management (CISM) had been adopted by fire departments to help manage stress following critical incidents (Bledsoe, 2003). Moreover, peer support programs began to be implemented to address the stress and trauma that firefighters experienced (Bartone et al., 2019; Creamer et al., 2012). In the 1990s and post-9/11 eras, research on PTSD, depression, and stress in firefighters increased significantly (Berger et al., 2012; Bartlett et al., 2018).

The late 2010s marked a turning point for fire service mental health, with a Ruderman Foundation report revealing that firefighters were more likely to die by suicide than in line with their duties, leading to widespread acknowledgment of mental health concerns. In 2013, the American Psychological Association (APA) included emergency responder psychology in its guidelines for occupational health psychology, emphasizing the importance of addressing the mental health needs of firefighters (American Psychological Association, 2022). By the late 2010s, fire departments nationwide began adopting behavioral health programs, including wellness initiatives, counseling, and resilience-building programs (Bartone, 2006). The formation of the Fire Service Psychology Association in 2018 further advocated for the evolution of fire service psychology as a distinct discipline. Today, fire departments focus on crisis intervention, peer support training, PTSD, and suicide prevention to support the mental health of firefighters nationwide (Bartlett & Schmitz, 2023; Arbona et al., 2016).

Fire Service Psychology: Legal Considerations of Frye and Daubert

In the legal system, the admissibility of psychological expert testimony is guided primarily by Frye and Daubert's standards. Although both serve to regulate the use of expert evidence in court, they differ significantly in how they evaluate scientific validity, particularly within the context of psychological practice. The Frye standard, originating from Frye v. United States (1923), holds that expert testimony should be based on scientific techniques or principles that are "generally accepted" within the relevant professional community. For psychologists, methods such as diagnostic assessments, risk evaluations, or therapeutic models should be widely endorsed by the field to be considered admissible. While this standard offers clarity through consensus, it can also exclude newer, empirically supported methods that have not yet achieved widespread recognition, potentially slowing innovation in psychological practice (American Board of Police and Public Safety Psychology, n.d.).

In contrast, the Daubert standard, established in Daubert v. Merrell Dow Pharmaceuticals, Inc. (1993), takes a more rigorous and nuanced approach. It designates judges as "gatekeepers" responsible for evaluating whether expert testimony is scientifically valid and relevant to the case. Under Daubert, psychological evidence should satisfy several criteria: it should be testable, subjected to peer review, have a known error rate, and be grounded in standards of scientific rigor. While general acceptance in the field is still considered, it is no longer the sole determining factor for success. For psychologists, this means that any tools or opinions introduced in legal contexts, such as fitness-for-duty evaluations, psychological autopsies, or trauma assessments, should withstand scrutiny not only from a clinical standpoint but also from a scientific and methodological standpoint (American Board of Police and Public Safety Psychology, n.d.).

In practical terms, the Daubert standard requires psychologists to rely on evidence-based, validated instruments and be able to clearly articulate the scientific underpinnings of their work in court. This expectation is particularly relevant in forensic and public safety settings, where psychological conclusions can have a profound impact on employment, criminal justice outcomes, and civil liability. As such, Daubert has elevated the standard for psychological testimony, encouraging greater methodological transparency and ensuring that mental health assessments presented in court are both reliable and relevant. Psychologists working in environments such as law enforcement or fire and emergency services should be especially mindful of these standards, as the tools they use and their opinions may one day be subject to legal challenges (American Board of Police and Public Safety Psychology, n.d.).

Fire Service Psychology: Options for Employment

Psychologists are professional minorities in fire and emergency services. Since there are no national standards for applying psychological services within fire and emergency services, they are not required to have a role within a fire department. Unlike law enforcement agencies, which have legal requirements for pre-employment psychological screenings or fitness-for-duty evaluations, many professional applications are tied to clinical services or the management of behavioral health programs. As such, many clinical providers are fulfilling roles within the fire service.

The Embedded Psychologist: Lessons from Military Integration

One model of psychological service delivery that has gained considerable traction in recent years, particularly within military settings, is the embedded psychologist. This role represents a departure from the traditional clinic-based model, in which mental health services are accessed reactively and often removed from the operational environment. Instead, embedded psychologists are physically and operationally integrated within their unit. In the military context, the psychologist trains, eats, and sometimes deploys with the unit, becoming a familiar and trusted presence rather than an outside consultant brought in during a crisis (Kennedy, 2019).

The value of proximity cannot be overstated. By living and working alongside service members, embedded psychologists are positioned to observe stress reactions in real time, provide early interventions, and respond to emerging needs before they escalate. Their presence reduces the stigma often associated with seeking mental health care because they are seen not as clinical authorities who diagnose and refer but as team members who understand the unique stressors and tempo of the unit (Martinez et al., 2023). This model has proven especially effective in high-intensity environments, where quick access to mental health expertise can mitigate acute stress reactions, improve performance, and prevent long-term psychological harm.

Embedded psychologists also play an important consultative role. They advise leadership on matters ranging from morale and cohesion to fatigue management, operational stress, and personnel readiness. They can offer insights that align clinical concerns with operational goals because they understand the psychological landscape and the demands of the mission. In this way, they serve both the individual service member and the unit, functioning as a bridge between behavioral health science and the command structure (Kitaeff, 2019).

One of the most powerful aspects of the embedded model is its ability to normalize help-seeking. Mental health becomes part of everyday conversation rather than a separate and stigmatized domain. When the psychologist is part of the team, visible, and accessible, personnel are far more likely to engage in brief check-ins, stress management strategies, or even formal therapy if needed. The embedded model shifts care from reactive to preventive and from external to internal (Kennedy, 2019).

While this model has been developed and tested primarily in military settings, it has important implications for fire and emergency services and other public safety professions. Like military personnel, firefighters operate in close-knit teams, face repeated exposure to trauma, and often work in environments where help-seeking is perceived as weak. Embedding a psychologist within a fire department, or at least integrating them more directly into station life and shift structure, could replicate the success seen in the military. It would enable clinicians to gain cultural competence, build rapport over time, and provide targeted support that aligns with the values and rhythms of the profession.

As fire service psychology evolves, the embedded model presents a promising framework for delivering practical, accessible, and mission-aligned care. It calls for reimagining the clinician's role not as a distant authority but as a proactive, integrated presence that can support individuals and systems alike from the inside out.

Contracted Psychological Services in Government Settings

Another prevalent model for delivering psychological care within public safety and governmental systems involves individual psychologists or group practices contracting directly with local, state, or federal agencies. These contracts enable agencies to access specialized mental health services without having to hire full-time, in-house providers. Instead, psychologists serve as external consultants or providers under formal agreements, offering assessments, treatments, training, or consultations tailored to the agency's specific needs.

At the local level, municipal fire departments, police agencies, or emergency medical services may contract with private psychologists or practice groups to deliver fitness-for-duty evaluations, pre-employment psychological screenings, trauma-informed counseling, or peer support training. These arrangements are particularly valuable for smaller departments lacking the resources to sustain an internal behavioral health unit. Contracted providers often become trusted partners, offering continuity and expertise while maintaining professional independence.

At the federal level, psychologists can secure contracts through systems such as the General Services Administration (GSA) or SAM.gov, where agencies such as the Department of Defense (DoD), the Department of Veterans Affairs (VA), the U.S. Forest Service, and the Federal Bureau of Prisons solicit behavioral health services. These contracts may be awarded to individual licensed psychologists, group practices, or behavioral health companies through a competitive bidding process. Services can range from direct clinical services, leadership consultation, psychological evaluations, crisis response, or resiliency training for disaster response teams.

The structure of these contracts varies. Some are fee-for-service agreements on the basis of hourly rates or per-assessment or therapy hour costs, whereas others are retainer-based or built into broader consulting contracts. Regardless of the format, contracted psychologists should adhere to high standards of licensure, scope of practice, documentation, confidentiality, and, when appropriate, forensic defensibility, particularly when the services include evaluations that could influence employment status or legal decisions.

Contracted providers often balance maintaining clinical independence with responding to the agency's organizational needs. This balance requires an understanding of organizational psychology, public sector dynamics, and the ethical challenges that arise when working with individual clients (e.g., firefighters, officers, or service members) and system-level stakeholders (e.g., department leadership, human resources, and legal counsel).

In recent years, group practices have increasingly specialized in providing psychological services to public safety sectors, offering integrated models that combine clinical care, assessments, training, and program development under one umbrella. This approach has proven especially useful for agencies seeking comprehensive behavioral health solutions without having to build internal infrastructure.

Overall, contracted psychological services offer a flexible and scalable means for government entities to meet the mental health needs of their personnel. For psychologists, these contracts provide opportunities to make a meaningful impact at the systems level, supporting both individual well-being and organizational resilience.

Regional Behavioral Health Support: A Shared Services Model for Rural Agencies

The regional or mutual aid psychological services model can effectively address the behavioral health needs of small and rural public safety agencies. In this framework, multiple departments, often across several towns or counties, form a shared-services agreement to jointly fund and utilize a single licensed psychologist or group practice. This collaborative approach enables agencies to access specialized mental health services without hiring full-time, in-house providers, which is particularly beneficial for smaller departments with limited resources (North & Pfefferbaum, 2013).

Rural and volunteer departments often lack the call volume, staffing, or budget to justify dedicated behavioral health staff. However, the psychological demands of the job—exposure to trauma, operational stress, burnout, and suicide risk—are significant in these communities. A regional model enables agencies to pool their limited resources to provide a level of care that none can afford independently (North & Pfefferbaum, 2013).

In this model, a memorandum of understanding (MOU) or interagency agreement outlines the financial contribution of each participating agency, the services included, and access protocols. Services may include pre-incident training, critical incident response, posttraumatic debriefing, individual therapy, and family support. The psychologist may rotate between agencies on a set schedule or remain based in a central location with travel options as needed. Some models also incorporate telehealth to increase access across broad geographic areas.

Regional psychologists embedded in these systems are trained to understand public safety culture, ensure confidentiality, and work across different organizational climates. They serve as a consistent behavioral health presence across multiple agencies, allowing for rapport-building, ongoing education, and timely interventions. Because no single department employs these psychologists, they often maintain greater clinical neutrality, which enhances trust and reduces concerns about stigma or professional consequences (North & Pfefferbaum, 2013).

This shared model mirrors what has been effective in other regionalized care systems, particularly in emergency medicine and disaster response, where limited resources are stretched across broad service areas. It also reflects the growing consensus in public safety psychology that access to care should be scalable and culturally informed, particularly for rural responders, who face greater service barriers (North & Pfefferbaum, 2013).

By emphasizing collaboration over competition, the regional model ensures that behavioral health care is treated as a collective responsibility. It levels the playing field between large urban departments and smaller, underserved communities, allowing all responders, regardless of geography, to access competent, confidential, and effective psychological support.

Employee Assistance Programs (EAPs): Accessibility, Limitations, and Cultural Gaps in Fire Service Care

Employee assistance programs (EAPs) are among the most widely used models for delivering mental health services to employees across both the public and private sectors. Designed as short-term, confidential counseling and support services, Employee Assistance Programs (EAPs) are intended to help employees manage personal and work-related problems that may impact job performance, health, or overall well-being (Attridge, 2009). While the model is well established and commonly used within public safety organizations, it has notable limitations, particularly in its application to specialized populations, such as firefighters.

EAPs are typically funded by employers, who contract with external vendors, such as national EAP companies or regional behavioral health firms, or establish internal EAP programs staffed by licensed mental health professionals. External models are more common, especially in municipal or county-based fire departments. Employers pay a per-employee-per-month (PEPM) rate or a flat annual fee to the EAP provider, which grants employees access to a defined number of counseling sessions per year, typically ranging from three to six (Masi, 2005). The cost to the employer is relatively low compared with traditional insurance coverage, making EAPs an attractive option from a budgeting perspective.

Psychologists and clinicians who wish to become EAP providers should apply through the EAP vendor's credentialing process. The process typically involves submitting documentation of licensures, malpractice insurance, and possibly experience in brief, solution-focused therapy. Once accepted, clinicians are placed on a referral panel and may receive clients through Employee Assistance Program (EAP) referrals.

However, providers should agree that contracted reimbursement rates are often significantly lower than standard private pay or insurance-based rates, sometimes as low as \$35–\$75 per session (Masi, 2005). This economic model can make EAP work financially unsustainable for many clinicians, particularly those in solo or specialty practices. As a result, many EAP panels are populated by generalist providers and clinicians who are trained and competent but who may lack direct experience with trauma, shift work, or high-stakes occupational stress environments such as fire and emergency services.

One of the most significant critiques of EAPs in fire and emergency services is their lack of cultural competency. Firefighters operate within a unique professional culture defined by strong peer bonds, repeated trauma exposure, hierarchical structure, and a tendency to underreport psychological distress due to stigma (Haugen et al., 2012). However, EAP clinicians are rarely trained to navigate these dynamics.

Because EAPs function primarily as volume-driven, fee-for-service models, their primary focus is on accessibility and short-term resolution rather than deep clinical specialization. Providers are expected to see clients for limited sessions and refer them for long-term care if necessary. While this structure may serve the general workforce adequately, it often falls short for firefighters, who may be experiencing complex trauma, burnout, or cumulative stress and require more nuanced, sustained care.

Moreover, a lack of familiarity with the realities of fire service culture, such as sleeping at the station, exposure to death and injury, or the emotional toll of being the "strong one" in family and community, can create a disconnect between client and clinician. This disconnect may result in poor engagement, early dropout, or harm if providers unintentionally minimize or misinterpret occupational stressors.

While EAPs offer a convenient and cost-effective pathway for care, they are not always aligned with the specific needs of high-risk occupational groups, such as firefighters. Their generalist structure, brief treatment model, and economic pressures often prevent specialized, culturally attuned care that fire and emergency services require. Departments that rely solely on employee assistance programs (EAPs) for behavioral health support may inadvertently underserve their personnel, missing an opportunity to provide more meaningful, effective, and trusted interventions.

In light of these limitations, many departments are exploring supplemental behavioral health models, such as embedded clinicians, fire-specific referral networks, or regional collaborators, to address the gap left by traditional Employee Assistance Program (EAP) coverage. A culturally competent mental health response is not just a clinical concern but also an operational imperative that supports safety, performance, and long-term organizational health.

Fire Service Psychology: Four Domains Including Assessment, Intervention, Operational Support and Organizational Consultation

First Domain: Psychological Assessment in the Fire Service: Tools, Applications, and Legal Considerations

Psychological assessment is pivotal in ensuring individual readiness and organizational integrity within fire and emergency services. Traditionally, these assessments have centered around pre-employment psychological screenings and fitness-for-duty evaluations. However, the field has since expanded to include various tools for evaluating psychological wellness, trauma exposure, resilience, and risk throughout a firefighter's career. As these tools become more specialized and empirically supported, departments are better equipped to assess, monitor, and support their personnel in ways that are not only clinically valid but also legally and operationally defensible. Note that there is an important distinction between the tools or assessments themselves and the standards against which those assessments are evaluated.

Tools of Psychological Assessment in the Fire Service

One of the most frequently used instruments in public safety settings is the Minnesota Multiphasic Personality Inventory-3 (MMPI-3). It has demonstrated strong validity in identifying psychological risk factors, particularly externalizing behaviors, impulse control issues, and interpersonal difficulties, which are important factors to assess when individuals are selected for high-risk occupations such as firefighting. The MMPI-3 has shown applicability across public safety roles and demographic categories, making it useful in diverse applicant pools (Whitman et al., 2023).

These standardized inventories are more dynamic and context-specific tools, such as biographical data inventories and statistical prediction rules, which are rooted in military psychology. Garb et al. (2018) reported that structured background data can reliably predict attrition and disciplinary issues. With respect to fire and emergency services, this predictive screening could reduce turnover and improve team cohesion by identifying red flags before hiring decisions are finalized.

In the context of fitness-for-duty evaluations, particularly following incidents of concern or extended leave, fire service psychologists increasingly rely on tools designed specifically for this population. The Firefighter Coping Self-Efficacy (FFCSE) Scale assesses a firefighter's perceived ability to manage occupational stress and trauma. It has been found to correlate positively with psychological well-being and negatively with stress-related symptoms, providing helpful insight into an individual's readiness to return to duty (Lambert et al., 2012).

Another emerging tool, the Firefighter Assessment of Stress Test (FAST), offers a brief but psychometrically sound method for identifying stress across three domains: operational challenges, administrative burdens, and workload intensity. It is particularly valuable for identifying stress before it escalates into clinical conditions such as burnout or PTSD (Schuhmann et al., 2022). Tools such as the FAST may assist with annual wellness checks, enabling departments to track the health of their workforce proactively.

Population-specific instruments are gaining traction as professional psychology and academic communities become more attuned to the psychological nuances of fire service members. The Emergency Services Moral Injury Scale–Firefighter Version (EMIS-F) helps differentiate between PTSD and moral injury, two overlapping but distinct constructs with different treatment implications (DeMoulin et al., 2023). Similarly, Steinberg and Vujanovic (2024) validated the PTSD Checklist for DSM-5 (PCL-5) in a firefighter sample, confirming that it can be used reliably as a unidimensional scale, which simplifies interpretation without compromising clinical accuracy.

Not all tools have been effectively translated to the context of fire and emergency services. Studies evaluating instruments such as the Sports Mental Toughness Questionnaire (SMTQ) and the Military Training Mental Toughness Inventory (MTMTI) have shown that their psychometric reliability does not hold up in firefighter samples, highlighting the limitations of transferring tools from other high-performance professions (Stamatis et al., 2024).

In contrast, broad psychological constructs such as sense of coherence (SOC), trait resilience, and internal locus of control have shown promise in predicting lower distress and greater well-being in firefighters. Schäfer et al. (2020) reported that these traits were associated with reduced symptoms of PTSD, burnout, and general psychopathology, suggesting that they may be helpful both for assessment and for guiding departmental wellness initiatives.

Historical Legal Precedents Supporting Psychological Assessment

The legal system has consistently upheld the use of psychological assessments in public safety settings, affirming the rights of fire departments to require such evaluations under conditions of reasonable concern. In Rogers v. City of San Antonio, the court upheld the city's decision to require a fitness-for-duty evaluation for a firefighter with a known history of mental health issues, emphasizing the employer's duty to ensure public and crew safety.

Similarly, Fisher v. City of San Jose addressed the termination of a firefighter deemed psychologically unfit for duty. The court ruled the city within its rights, noting that psychological fitness is an important requirement in high-risk occupations. These rulings underscore that departments are not only permitted but also obligated to ensure that their members are psychologically capable of performing their duties.

In Harris v. City of New York, a firefighter claimed discrimination after being required to undergo a fitness-for-duty evaluation. However, the court found that the city's actions were justified, given the need to assess fitness in roles where impaired functioning can lead to catastrophic outcomes. Garcia v. City of New York reinforced this stance, emphasizing that employers should balance their duty to maintain safety with respect to employee rights, a balance best achieved through valid and well-documented psychological evaluations. These cases clarify that psychological assessments are not only clinical tools but also risk management strategies designed to protect the public, departments, and firefighters. The key to their defensibility lies in their validity, consistency, and connection to job-relevant criteria.

2025: The Sintos Case and the Need for a Fire-Specific Psychological Standard

The case of Nicholas Sintos v. City of Chicago highlights the legal and ethical pitfalls of applying generalized or misaligned psychological screening tools to fire service applicants. In this 2025 ruling, a federal district court determined that the City of Chicago violated the Americans with Disabilities Act (ADA) and the Illinois Human Rights Act (IHRA) when it rescinded Sintos' job offer due to a psychological screening that failed to properly assess whether his mental health history actually affected his ability to perform the essential duties of a firefighter/EMT. The city relied on a "suitability screening" designed for broad "risk of poor outcome" prediction rather than a true, validated fitness-for-duty evaluation tied to fire service job demands (Varone, 2025; *Sintos v. City of Chicago*, 2025).

The court found this practice discriminatory and unlawful, particularly because the screening was only imposed on candidates with disclosed mental health histories—despite its admitted irrelevance to determining whether the candidate could safely and effectively carry out firefighting or emergency medical tasks. Notably, the psychologist who performed the screening testified that her tool did not determine fitness for duty. The city's own medical director misunderstood or misapplied the tool's purpose, resulting in an illegal denial of employment (Varone, 2025; *Sintos v. City of Chicago*, 2025).

This case illustrates a critical issue: in the absence of a fire-service-specific psychological standard, agencies may improperly import general forensic or law enforcement psychological tools or frameworks that do not align with the unique realities of firefighting and emergency medical services. Law enforcement pre-employment psychological evaluations, for example, are designed to assess risks and job competencies specific to policing: use of force, authority dynamics, and continual high-conflict interactions with the public. Firefighters and EMTs, by contrast, operate in environments with team-based, trust-heavy, and often physically hazardous conditions requiring endurance, cooperative risk-taking, and split-second life-or-death decisions under extreme physical and emotional stress. Fire service members are also embedded in tight-knit subcultures with unique stressors like exposure to mass casualties, pediatric deaths, and moral injury stemming from perceived failed rescues.

The fire service has evolved dramatically beyond suppression to include high-level emergency medical services, community risk reduction, and even complex public health interventions. These layered responsibilities differentiate the cognitive, emotional, and ethical burdens of fire service work from those of police officers or other public safety personnel. Therefore, the profession deserves a purpose-built, empirically validated psychological evaluation standard, one rooted in rigorous job analysis, scientific research, and ongoing oversight by licensed subject matter experts (American Psychological Association, 2023).

Without this, fire departments risk repeating the missteps of the Sintos case: deploying tools that unfairly screen out qualified applicants, misalign with actual essential job functions, and fail to comply with federal civil rights protections. As this ruling confirms, psychological evaluations must be directly linked to actual job performance, risk, and functional demands, not generic "suitability" constructs that cannot withstand legal or scientific scrutiny.

Conclusion

Modern psychological assessment in fire and emergency services reflects a convergence of clinical science, operational necessity, and legal precedent. Whether screening applicants, determining fitness for duty, or monitoring wellness throughout a firefighter's career, these tools support individual health, organizational performance, and public trust. As more population-specific instruments emerge and departments deepen their understanding of psychological resilience and risk, assessment practices will continue to evolve, becoming a form of risk management, legally defensible hiring standards, and a cornerstone of sustainable fire service leadership.

Second Domain: Intervention

Firefighters face a unique constellation of psychological stressors, cumulative trauma, operational fatigue, exposure to death and injury, and cultural expectations of stoicism, which increase their risk for PTSD, anxiety, depression, substance misuse, and suicide. While awareness of these issues is increasing, access to mental health care remains inconsistent, and stigma continues to inhibit help-seeking behaviors. Emerging research highlights the need for more services, as well as clinically effective, culturally informed, and logistically feasible interventions within the fire service context.

Paraprofessional-Delivered Narrative Exposure Therapy (eNET)

One promising approach involves expanding the traditional clinical workforce by training paraprofessionals to deliver structured, evidence-based interventions. In a recent study, virtual narrative exposure therapy (eNET) was delivered to firefighters by trained paraprofessionals via video conferences. The intervention targeted individuals with clinical or subclinical PTSD and consisted of 10–12 sessions of trauma-focused, exposure-based therapy. The results revealed significant reductions in PTSD, anxiety, depression, and functional impairment from baseline to posttreatment, with improvements being sustained at the two- and six-month follow-ups (Olthuis et al., 2023). The participants emphasized the approachability and support of paraprofessionals, and no adverse events were reported, suggesting that, with appropriate training and supervision, paraprofessional-led care may help scale access to treatment in underserved or rural fire departments.

Brief Intensive Counseling (BIC) for Complex Needs

In Korea, a mental health promotion program for firefighters resulted in significant reductions in PTSD, anxiety, suicidal ideation, insomnia, and alcohol use. Among participants who received brief intensive counseling (BIC), a targeted, short-duration intervention, improvements were even more pronounced, particularly in the domains of depression, anxiety, and substance use (Won et al., 2020). These findings suggest that the BIC can function either as a stepping stone to longer-term treatment or as focused standalone support for firefighters experiencing acute psychological distress.

Peer-Led Referral Training: The Reach Out Program

Another impactful intervention focuses not on direct clinical care but on empowering firefighters to act as early identifiers and connectors to behavioral health resources. The Reach Out program trains firefighters in motivational interviewing, community reinforcement techniques, and mental health education. A randomized controlled trial comparing two program formats, group-based and video-based formats, revealed that the video format significantly increased the number of successful peer referrals. It was rated as more credible than a behavioral health video control (Gulliver et al., 2016). These findings support the use of structured, peer-delivered training as a powerful tool for reducing stigma and improving engagement in care.

Public Health and Social Work Integration

In addition to individual-level interventions, systemic solutions are emerging. O'Dare et al. (2024) described a public health model of behavioral wellness that integrates clinical intervention with social work, policy reform, leadership development, and community partnerships. This collaborative approach recognizes that mental health care does not exist in a vacuum; it requires the coordinated involvement of researchers, clinicians, fire service leaders, families, and public health infrastructure to create sustainable change. Their model emphasizes trauma-informed assessment, culturally competent care, and upstream prevention, which are all important components of a comprehensive fire service behavioral health strategy.

Complementary and Physiological Interventions

Complementary techniques also show promise. A recent study investigated cranial osteopathy, a manual therapy designed to modulate autonomic nervous system activity, as a means to reduce cardiovascular stress, as measured by heart rate variability (HRV). Firefighter cadets who received five weeks of cranial techniques experienced statistically significant improvements in HRV markers of stress regulation, suggesting a potential physiological benefit from integrating body-based interventions into mental health support for firefighters (Wójcik & Siatkowski, 2023).

These diverse interventions reflect a growing recognition that psychological care for firefighters should be accessible, population specific, and flexible. The most effective programs, whether delivered by licensed clinicians, trained peers, or paraprofessionals, share several key characteristics:

- Grounding in evidence-based protocols.
- Accessibility across shifts and geographic regions.
- Cultural competency specific to fire service norms.
- Integration with both preventive and responsive strategies.

As the behavioral health response of fire and emergency services evolves, the field should move toward multitiered preventive, inclusive, and clinically sound care models. This strategy ensures that psychological support is available, trusted, normalized, and embedded in the firehouse's culture.

Third Domain: Consultation

According to the American Board of Police and Public Safety Psychology (ABPPSP), psychological consultation is one of four foundational domains in public safety psychology, alongside assessment, intervention, and operational support (ABPPSP, n.d.). Within the fire service, consultation refers to the strategic, systems-level role psychologists play in advising leaders, union representatives, policy developers, and frontline personnel on matters affecting the mental health, organizational climate, and cultural functioning of the department. Unlike individual therapy or crisis intervention, consultation focuses on the broader operational environment, emphasizing prevention, systemic improvement, and evidence-informed policy guidance.

Psychological consultants often assist fire departments in evaluating and shaping organizational culture. Consultation addresses morale, burnout, peer relationships, trust in leadership, and cultural attitudes toward mental health. For example, a consulting psychologist might help identify how stigma, traditional masculine cultural norms, or communication breakdowns within or between shifts contribute to emotional suppression or reluctance to seek help. In addition, psychologists are frequently called upon to contribute to policy development, especially in the context of fitness-for-duty evaluations, substance use policies, peer support team implementation, or critical incident response protocols. They ensure that these policies are both legally and ethically sound and sensitive to the fire service's operational and cultural realities (Kitaeff, 2019).

Leadership consultation is another critical function. Psychologists may coach fire officers or chiefs in managing personnel distress, navigating interpersonal conflict, or practicing trauma-informed leadership. These consultations help leaders avoid pathologizing normal stress reactions and create psychologically safe environments that foster accountability and resilience. In the context of critical incidents, such as line-of-duty deaths, mass casualty events, or particularly traumatic calls, psychologists may guide departments in designing or refining response protocols, advising when to activate peer support, how to structure after-action reviews, and what to consider when planning return-to-duty for impacted personnel.

Consultation also plays a key role in education and training. Psychologists help departments design and evaluate their mental health training curricula, ensuring that content is evidence-based, delivered by credible voices, and reinforced over time. In many cases, psychologists also evaluate the broader impact of wellness programs. A department may have peer support teams, embedded clinicians, or mental toughness training in place, but without a feedback loop, it becomes difficult to know what is working. Psychological consultants can design evaluation metrics, collect data, and offer recommendations grounded in outcomes rather than assumptions (Kitaeff, 2019).

Additionally, when conflict emerges between labor and management, within crews, or involving individuals with behavioral difficulties, psychologists may serve as neutral, trusted facilitators. Using systems theory, organizational behavior principles, and cultural awareness, consultants help fire departments address conflict without escalation or punitive fallout. Ultimately, psychological consultants operate not as command staff or clinicians in these moments but as strategic advisors, shaping decisions with insight, ethics, and a deep understanding of fire service culture and psychological science. Their influence often extends beyond individual care, driving meaningful, lasting change at the organizational level (Kitaeff, 2019).

Fourth Domain: Operations

Firefighting is more than a physically demanding job; it is rooted in rapid decision-making, emotional containment, team interdependence, and exposure to high-stakes environments. As fire departments advance in their understanding of behavioral health, there is increasing recognition that psychological operations should extend beyond individual clinical care to include interdisciplinary collaboration, team-level psychological functioning, and integrated operational support. The fire service should provide access to treatment and foster a culture and infrastructure that actively promotes mental resilience, psychological safety, and trauma-informed practices (Gonzalez et al., 2024).

Embedded Clinical Care in Complex Medical Contexts

Research suggests that incorporating mental health providers into complex medical cases involving firefighters may be beneficial (Heyda et al., 2023). A powerful example of integrated psychological operations can be found in the case of a firefighter undergoing oncology treatment while simultaneously managing comorbid mental health conditions, including PTSD, OCD, and substance use. In this instance, a psychotherapist was embedded within the oncology team and delivered daily clinical intervention via trauma-informed modalities such as mindfulness and breathwork to regulate arousal, enhance distress tolerance, and support emotional containment (Heyda et al., 2023). The collaborative care team, comprising physicians, nurses, dietitians, and mental health professionals, coordinated to ensure that physical treatment was not derailed by escalating psychological symptoms. This case illustrates how interdisciplinary, context-sensitive clinical work can be life-saving, particularly when tailored to the complex psychological profiles common among first responders.

Mental Health Integration into Fire Service Operations

While individual therapy remains critical, fire and emergency services are increasingly recognizing the operational dimension of psychological functioning, including how team communication, leadership behavior, and organizational culture affect mental wellness and safety outcomes. For example, the REST-Q fire questionnaire was developed to assess team-related psychological stressors and resources. The findings revealed that team reliability and skill familiarity were perceived as major psychological support, whereas leadership behavior and interpersonal conflict were seen as stressors (Heinemann et al., 2024). These insights provide a foundation for targeting operational interventions, such as leader training, team debriefings, and trust-building practices, as key levers for enhancing psychological safety on firegrounds.

Further supporting this idea, research by Jouanne, E. et al. (2017) revealed that closed-loop communication, positive emotional interactions, and adaptive teamwork behaviors were associated with greater effectiveness during real emergency operations. Conversely, communication breakdowns and emotional disengagement reduce team functionality. These findings affirm the importance of "nontechnical" skills, such as emotional intelligence, self-awareness, and real-time interpersonal feedback, as central to operational psychology in firefighting contexts.

Clinical and Community Collaboration: The TAPP-C Model

In prevention and youth intervention, the TAPP-C program offers a model of interdisciplinary collaboration between fire service professionals and mental health clinicians to address juvenile firesetting behaviors. This program is not only a clinical tool; it represents a knowledge translation model in which mental health and operational fire service teams cocreate and codeliver interventions (Henderson et al., 2010). The success of the TAPP-C highlights the importance of protocol-driven, cross-disciplinary partnerships, particularly when complex behaviors that emerge at the intersection of safety, trauma, and community well-being are addressed.

Occupational Health Culture as a Psychological Barrier

Ultimately, psychological operations should consider organizational culture as a key risk or resilience factor. A UK study revealed that firefighters who internalized contaminated PPE as a "badge of honor" were significantly more likely to engage in risky post-incident behaviors, including neglecting PPE cleaning and wearing sooty gear (Wolffe et al., 2023). These behaviors are not simply hygiene concerns; they reflect deeper cultural norms of invulnerability, which are known to suppress mental health help-seeking and reinforce stigma. Changing this narrative requires psychological operations at the cultural level, reframing health-preserving behaviors (e.g., decontamination, therapy, emotional expression) as acts of professionalism and strength, not weakness.

The studies reviewed here suggest a maturing perspective on psychological operations in fire and emergency services, one that integrates individual clinical care, team dynamics, leadership behavior, and organizational culture. The key themes include the following:

- Clinicians are embedded within medical and operational teams to support trauma-exposed or medically vulnerable firefighters (Heyda et al., 2023).
- To develop tools such as REST-Q Fire to assess and intervene in teamwork-related psychological stressors (Wolffe et al., 2023).
- Community-based clinical programs, such as the TAPP-C, can be utilized to address juvenile fires through interdisciplinary care models (Henderson et al., 2010).
- Leaders are trained in communication, motivation, and interpersonal safety to increase team performance (Jouanne et al., 2017).
- Addressing cultural attitudes normalizes risk and suppresses emotional expression (Addis & Mahalik, 2003; Wong et al., 2017).

This integrated perspective does not focus only on "treating" firefighters once symptoms emerge; it represents a shift toward designing fire service systems that promote psychological health from the inside out.

The Expanding Role of Psychologists in the Fire Service: From Assessment to Operational Support

Psychologists are increasingly important in promoting individual well-being and organizational effectiveness within fire and emergency services. Their contributions span four interrelated domains: assessment, clinical intervention, organizational and industrial psychology, and operational support (American Board of Police and Public Safety Psychology [ABPPSP], n.d.). As the mental health needs of firefighters gain attention, psychologists are becoming indispensable advisors, clinicians, and consultants in building a psychologically resilient and high-performing workforce.

Psychological Assessment: Screening, Monitoring, and Risk Mitigation

Psychological assessment remains a foundational function in fire service psychology. Many career firefighters first encounter a psychologist during pre-employment psychological evaluations, which are designed to assess emotional stability, impulse control, and interpersonal functioning. In addition to traditional personality assessments, biographical data inventories and statistical prediction rules have also proven useful. In a large-scale military study, Garb et al. (2018) demonstrated that structured background screening could predict early attrition and disciplinary incidents. These findings can directly impact fire service recruitment, as early risk identification can enhance long-term retention and cohesion.

While potentially valuable tools for promoting occupational health and safety, psychological assessments are often misunderstood or stigmatized within the fire service. This stigma may stem from a perception among fire service leaders that such assessments pathologize individuals rather than support their capacity to meet professional demands. There is often an implicit belief that the firehouse environment can shape individuals to adapt and conform, minimizing the perceived need to identify psychological vulnerabilities early. However, unrecognized or untreated psychological disorders can pose significant risks to team cohesion and operational safety, making early detection essential for informed risk management and organizational accountability (Sterud et al., 2006).

Fitness-for-duty evaluations, in particular, are frequently associated with fear, suspicion, and potential career consequences. Many firefighters equate these evaluations with punitive disciplinary measures, in part owing to the limited integration of mental health professionals into routine, non-evaluative aspects of fire service culture (Johnson, 1983). The limited visibility of psychological services outside of high-stakes assessments reinforces this apprehension. Moreover, research specific to fitness-for-duty evaluations within fire and emergency services is limited. As a result, most clinicians draw upon assessment tools and protocols developed initially and validated for law enforcement populations, raising concerns about contextual relevance and diagnostic validity (Johnson, 1983). Without occupation-specific standards (even with assessment tool norms) or culturally attuned guidelines, the credibility and perceived fairness of these evaluations may be undermined, potentially decreasing their effectiveness and acceptance within the fire service.

Behavioral Health Intervention: From Peer Support to Treatment

Firefighters are disproportionately affected by health conditions, including PTSD, depression, substance abuse, and suicide (Stanley, Hom, Hagan, & Joiner, 2015). Psychologists address these issues through direct clinical care and training of paraprofessionals and peer supporters. Innovative interventions, such as virtual narrative exposure therapy delivered by paraprofessionals, have shown promising results. In a recent study, firefighters receiving online narrative exposure therapy experienced significant reductions in PTSD symptoms, anxiety, depression, and functional impairment, with gains sustained over six months (Olthuis et al., 2023).

Psychologists also support the evolution of peer support programs and psychological first aid models, which are important early intervention strategies. By training peer supporters in active listening, psychological first aid, and referral protocols, psychologists extend the reach of mental health support into informal networks that firefighters already trust.

Organizational and Industrial Psychology: Shaping Culture and Leadership

The influence of psychologists goes well beyond individual treatment. Through the lens of organizational psychology, they work to improve fire department culture, communication, and leadership. Psychological safety, the belief that one can express concerns or admit struggles without fear of reprisal, is crucial in high-risk, high-accountability environments, such as firefighting (Edmondson & Lei, 2014). Psychologists help departments build this safety through leadership coaching, policy development, and trust-building strategies.

Recent research has also highlighted that organizational stressors contribute to mental health challenges. For example, the REST-Q Fire, developed by Heinemann et al. (2024b), noted that firefighters often perceive interpersonal reliability and shared team knowledge as psychological resources, whereas inconsistent leadership behavior and team conflict are experienced as stressors. These findings suggest that systemic interventions, such as improved supervision, crew continuity, and transparent communication, can serve as behavioral health strategies.

By supporting decision-making under stress, team coordination, and human factor analysis following incidents in the operational domain (Jouanne, E. et al., 2017), psychologists have observed that communication breakdowns, poor emotional regulation, and ineffective leadership adaptation directly undermine team performance during emergency operations. Conversely, emotionally intelligent leadership and closed-loop communication were associated with better outcomes.

Psychologists are also involved in cancer care support, especially as increasing numbers of firefighters face occupationally linked cancers. Heyda et al. (2023)

described a case in which an embedded psychotherapist supported a firefighter undergoing cancer treatment. This approach, which combines mindfulness, trauma-focused therapy, and interdisciplinary care, has proven critical in stabilizing firefighters' mental health during intensive treatment. As occupational health risks such as cancer and toxic exposure gain attention, psychologists will be integral in addressing not only the physiological impact but also the psychological toll of long-term medical treatment and reintegration.

Effective engagement in these roles demands advanced cultural competence to maintain professional objectivity and appropriately manage transference and countertransference dynamics (Sue et al., 1992). Fire service culture is characterized by shared trauma exposure, strong intraunit loyalty, the use of gallows humor, and a pronounced aversion to displays of vulnerability (Henderson et al., 2010). Interventions that fail to account for these cultural dimensions are unlikely to achieve lasting impact (Henderson et al., 2010). Accordingly, psychologists embedded within fire departments must have a deep understanding of this ethos and tailor their language, methods, and interpersonal stance to align with its established norms and values (Sue et al., 1992; Henderson et al., 2010).

Insights from military and law enforcement psychology suggest that trauma-informed care, resilience training, and decision-making support, proven in high-stress occupations, may be adapted to the fireground (Adler et al., 2011). However, whereas police psychology benefits from formalized national practice guidelines and specialty certification pathways (American Psychological Association, 2013), fire service psychology remains largely unstandardized, lacking dedicated credentialing, specialized training curricula, and a robust empirical base. Consequently, psychologists in fire departments often operate in a state of professional isolation, lacking tailored tools and peer networks

There may be value in adopting an embedded psychological services model in firefighting, encompassing defined psychologist roles, the development of firefighter-specific assessment instruments, and longitudinal research into mental health trajectories. The leadership development literature further emphasizes the integration of psychological safety and wellness competencies into training programs, alongside continuous professional education, to address stigma and clarify practitioner functions (Bass & Riggio, 2006; Haslam et al. 2011). As the discipline evolves, building culturally competent training, evidence-based interventions, and collaborative partnerships that reflect the operational realities of firefighting is essential for embedding psychological services as foundational elements of safety, resilience, and performance (McEwen, 1998; Van der Kolk, 2014).

Conclusion

The integration of psychology into fire and emergency services reflects a broader shift toward recognizing the behavioral health needs of high-risk occupational groups. Psychologists now serve across four core domains, assessment, intervention, consultation, and operations, supporting both individual well-being and organizational effectiveness. Drawing on developments in military and police psychology, fire service psychology has begun to establish itself as a distinct field shaped by the unique demands of firehouse culture, trauma exposure, and team dynamics. While progress is evident through emerging tools, care models, and interdisciplinary practices, key gaps remain in standardization, empirical research, and field-specific guidance. Ongoing collaboration among mental health professionals, fire leaders, and national organizations will be crucial to advancing the field in an evidence-based and operationally relevant manner.

Chapter Review

Assignment: Building Behavioral Health in the Fire Service: A Comparative Program Proposal

Assignment Context: You are a psychologist applying for a consulting role with a mid-sized metropolitan fire department. The department has no current behavioral health program and is evaluating how best to integrate psychological support into their operations. Leadership is aware of options such as embedded clinicians, peer support teams, EAPs, and regional partnerships but is unclear on which approach is most appropriate for their culture and needs.

Your task is to create a proposal that compares and contrasts at least two models of service delivery described in Chap. 7, culminating in a recommendation tailored to this department's context.

Learning Objectives

By completing this assignment, students will be able to:

- Differentiate between behavioral health delivery models used in the fire service (e.g., embedded psychologist, contracted services, shared regional models, and EAPs).
- Critically evaluate the cultural, logistical, and clinical implications of each model.
- Apply psychological and organizational principles to propose an ethically sound and operationally viable program.
- Integrate legal, historical, and evidence-based perspectives to support a culturally competent approach.

Assignment Instructions

Prepare a 2000–2500-word proposal (excluding references) structured as follows:

Section I—Introduction and Department Context (Approx. 300–400 Words).

Describe the hypothetical fire department, including its size, call volume, and any known issues related to stress, morale, or behavioral health. Identify what leadership is looking for in a behavioral health program and what constraints (budget, staffing, geography, etc.) they may face.

Section II—Compare and Contrast: Program Models (Approx. 1000–1200 Words).

Using at least two distinct models from Chapter 7, such as:

- Embedded Psychologist.
- Contracted Psychological Services.
- Regional Shared Services Model.
- Employee Assistance Programs (EAPs).

For each model:

- Describe how the model operates in a fire service context.
- Highlight clinical, logistical, and cultural benefits and limitations.
- Reference relevant APA guidelines, NFPA standards, and legal/ethical considerations.
- Draw upon historical or empirical foundations (e.g., military or police parallels).
- Use side-by-side comparison where appropriate.

Note: Role of Paraprofessional and Peer Support Integration.

Section III—Recommendation and Justification (Approx. 500–700 Words).

Recommend the most appropriate model—or a hybrid approach—for the department you described. Your justification should be:

- Grounded in fire service-specific needs and organizational culture.
- Aware of resource and implementation constraints.
- Sensitive to stigma and help-seeking behaviors.
- Supported by course readings and outside literature (APA 7 citation required).

Submission Requirements

- Word Count: 2000–2500 words.
- Citation Style: APA 7th edition.
- Format: APA format, typed, double-spaced, 12-pt font, with clear section headings.

Evaluation Criteria

- Clarity and accuracy of model comparison—30%.
- Depth of analysis and cultural application—25%.
- Strength of recommendation and justification—20%.
- Use of evidence and APA citations—15%.
- Organization, writing, and formatting—10%.

Chapter 8
Advancing Fire Service Safety Through Human Factors and Behavioral Insights

Analysis of the Effects of Human Factors on Firefighter Safety

Human factor analysis is critical in accident investigations across various industries, such as aviation, nuclear power, and transportation. The National Transportation Safety Board (NTSB) investigates accidents to prevent future occurrences. Initially, focused on mechanical failure, aviation accident investigations emphasized human factors, recognizing that systemic variables influence human behavior, which can lead to accidents involving injury or death. This shift exemplifies how data analysis and safety recommendations can improve safety. The fire service has not yet adopted human factor analysis within the National Institute for Occupational Safety and Health (NIOSH)'s Fire Fighter Fatality Investigation and Prevention Program, which was meant to reduce occupational injuries and fatalities. The Human Factors Analysis and Classification System (HFACS) provides a framework for identifying both systemic and individual errors, thereby enhancing safety. Expert teams with diverse skill sets are crucial for conducting reliable investigations.

Human factors are an interdisciplinary field concerned with understanding human interactions, behaviors, and the complex systems in which they operate. By examining how people interact with tools, technologies, environments, and organizational structures, human factors seek to enhance human well-being and optimize overall system performance.

Early human factor approaches were informed by behaviorism, particularly the work of B.F. Skinner (1953, 1974), who proposed that a framework of antecedents and consequences shapes behavior. According to Skinner, reinforcement, either positive (the introduction of a stimulus) or negative (the removal of a stimulus), increases the likelihood of a recurring behavior. Conversely, punishment reduces the likelihood of a behavior, either by introducing an aversive stimulus (positive punishment) or by removing a reinforcing stimulus (negative punishment).

K. Wheldon, *Fire Service Psychology*,
https://doi.org/10.1007/978-3-032-02126-7_8

While behaviorism provides foundational insights into how behavior can be modified through external stimuli, it does not encompass the full scope of human factors. Modern human factor analysis has evolved beyond behaviorist principles, integrating cognitive psychology, systems engineering, ergonomics, and sociotechnical systems theory (Wickens et al., 2013). This broader perspective acknowledges observable behaviors and internal cognitive processes such as attention, perception, memory, and decision-making (Norman, 1988).

Human factors now consider how individual actions are influenced by organizational culture, environmental design, interface usability, and social dynamics. This systems-oriented approach is especially critical in high-risk domains such as healthcare, aviation, and emergency services, where human performance and safety outcomes are closely interlinked.

While early safety systems and training models drew heavily from behaviorist theories, contemporary human factor practices adopted a more comprehensive view. It integrates behavioral, cognitive, and systemic insights to better understand and support human performance in complex environments (Salas & Maurino, 2010).

In occupational contexts such as fire and emergency services, this behavioral lens can clarify how cultural norms, perceived accountability, and identity influence decision-making and risk-taking. Unsafe practices often stem from normalized behaviors reinforced by perceived rewards, such as peer approval or a heroic image, rather than formal consequences. Despite the technical focus of fatality investigations by agencies such as NIOSH, human factors, particularly cultural and psychological dynamics, remain insufficiently studied. Even as OSHA standards provide behavioral benchmarks, there is limited application of consequence-based strategies, as outlined in Skinner's behavioral framework, that are designed to reduce the recurrence of unsafe behaviors.

Human factors analysis constitutes an interdisciplinary field dedicated to understanding how humans interact with their environments, technologies, and organizational systems. Its primary aim is to enhance both human well-being and system performance by addressing the interface between people and the complex settings in which they operate—initially influenced by behavioral psychology, particularly the work of B.F. Skinner (1953, 1974), who noted that early human factor approaches focused on observable behavior shaped by external stimuli. Skinner proposed that behavior operates within a framework of antecedents and consequences, wherein reinforcement, positive (the introduction of a stimulus) or negative (the removal of a stimulus), increases the likelihood of a behavior recurring. In contrast, punishment decreases behavior either through the addition of an aversive stimulus (positive punishment) or the removal of a reinforcing stimulus (negative punishment) (Skinner, 1953, 1974).

Although behaviorism provides foundational insights into behavior modification, it does not fully capture the complexity of human behavior in modern systems. Contemporary human factors have since evolved to incorporate cognitive psychology, ergonomics, systems engineering, and sociotechnical systems theory (Wickens et al., 2013). This evolution has expanded the scope of human factors beyond observable behaviors to encompass internal processes, including attention, memory, perception, and decision-making (Norman, 1988). The field now recognizes that behavior emerges not only from external contingencies but also from the interplay between individuals' cognitive functions and their broader sociotechnical environments.

Currently, human factor analysis considers how organizational culture, interface design, environmental constraints, and social norms influence decision-making and behavioral norms. This systems-oriented approach is particularly vital in high-risk industries such as aviation, healthcare, and emergency services, where the consequences of human error can be severe. Human factors play a crucial role in these settings, as they enable the identification and mitigation of risks, enhance system resilience, and improve safety outcomes (Salas & Maurino, 2010).

In occupational domains such as fire and emergency services, the behavioral lens remains relevant for understanding how norms, accountability, and professional identity influence risk-taking. Unsafe practices often normalize through social reinforcement, such as peer validation or alignment with heroic imagery, rather than being mitigated by formal corrective consequences. Despite the technical emphasis in post-incident investigations, particularly by agencies such as the National Institute for Occupational Safety and Health (NIOSH), human factors, primarily cultural and psychological dynamics, are often underexplored. While the Occupational Safety and Health Administration (OSHA) standards provide behavioral guidelines, the systematic use of consequence-based strategies, which are consistent with Skinner's framework, to deter unsafe behaviors remains limited (Skinner, 1953, 1974).

Furthermore, within the sociocultural context of the fire service, there is a tendency to honor all line-of-duty deaths equally, regardless of whether the incident arose from a commendable action or a preventable error. This uniform reverence can hinder critical inquiry into the behavior and culture of contributors to fatal outcomes. Investigations that attempt to address underlying psychological or systemic factors often face resistance, which is perceived as attributing blame or tarnishing the legacy of the deceased. This resistance is compounded by the presence of multiple stakeholders (colleagues, families, unions, and institutions), each with vested interests in preserving a specific legacy or collective identity of the profession (Bartone, 2006; Barton & Sutcliffe, 2009). As a result, the meaningful exploration of the human factors behind occupational failure remains largely absent from standard investigative protocols, limiting opportunities for organizational learning and safety improvement (Barton & Sutcliffe, 2009).

When mechanical and technological systems function as intended, human factors often emerge as critical contributors to accidents. It is well understood within psychology that individual behavior is shaped by various variables, many of which may operate beyond conscious awareness. To understand behavior fully, we must move beyond moral attributions and examine the broader system within which behavior occurs. Reducing investigations to a "blame and train" approach does little to create safer work environments, as it oversimplifies the complex conditions under which decisions are made (Reason, 1997).

Historically, accident investigations have relied on root cause analysis (RCA) to identify underlying contributors to adverse events. This method includes techniques such as fault tree analysis, causal-effect diagrams, and the "5 Whys" approach. These tools encourage investigators to trace chains of events by continuously asking "why" a failure occurred to identify the primary cause and disrupt the chain of causation, thereby improving system safety (Anderson & Fagerhaug, 2006). While effective for mechanical or procedural failure, traditional root cause analysis (RCA) has shown limitations when applied to human behavior. Its linear structure does not accommodate the dynamic nature of human decision-making or the influence of organizational culture, environmental stressors, and psychological pressures (Dekker, 2011).

Investigative models must evolve beyond traditional approaches that focus solely on equipment or procedural lapses to reduce firefighter injuries and fatalities effectively. A systems-oriented, psychologically informed approach is crucial for addressing the complexity of behavior in high-risk environments. Human error rarely stems from a single misstep; rather, it arises from a convergence of individual characteristics, team dynamics, environmental factors, task demands, supervision quality, and organizational climate (Omodei et al., 2005).

When applied to human performance, traditional RCAs oversimplify the multifactorial nature of accidents. In high-stakes fields such as firefighting, linear causal models cannot adequately account for the layered psychological, cultural, and systemic influences that shape behavior (Wiegmann & Shappell, 2003). In response, experts have advocated redesigning RCA by integrating principles from human factor science and psychological theories of error. Notably, the Swiss Cheese Model illustrates how accidents occur when multiple system-level vulnerabilities align, each represented as a "hole" in a layer of defense, allowing failure to pass through unimpeded (Reason, 1990). As Socrates once stated, "No one errs willingly." This philosophical insight aligns with contemporary human factors theory, reminding us that behavior is contextually driven and influenced by latent variables, risk perception, and cultural norms.

Modern investigative frameworks, such as the Human Factors Analysis and Classification System (HFACS) and the Human Factors Intervention Matrix (HFIM), provide structured tools for analyzing not only what happened but also why it happened and how it can be prevented (Wiegmann & Shappell, 2003; Ma et al., 2022). HFACS enables investigators to examine latent organizational factors that contribute to unsafe acts, such as poor supervision or a compromised safety culture. The HFIX complements this by offering actionable recommendations for systemic reform, such as targeted policy changes, improved training, or procedural revisions.

These models are already standard in high-reliability industries, such as aviation, nuclear energy, and transportation, where organizations such as the National Transportation Safety Board (NTSB) prioritize human error as a primary investigative focus rather than solely identifying mechanical failure (Zhang et al., 2018; Zarei, 2023). The adoption of human factor frameworks in fire and emergency services reflects the shift in these industries toward proactive prevention and systems thinking.

This transition also aligns with a nuanced psychological understanding of fire service culture. Firefighters often engage with risk guided by deeply internalized ideologies of duty, sacrifice, and valor, motivated by reinforcement histories, cultural expectations, and shared identity (Bartone, 2006; Dangermond et al., 2022). Unlike fires, which have no agency or intent, firefighter engagement strategies are driven by value-based decision-making shaped by perceived obligations and rewards (Bartone, 2004; Benight & Bandura, 2004). From a research perspective, analyzing such behavior requires a balance between objective observation and contextual sensitivity. To uncover the strategies that drive action, we must withhold moral judgment and instead focus on the conditions and frameworks that shape behavior. Moreover, it is important to recognize that individuals make choices on the basis of their internal value judgments about how to behave in specific situations. These two principles—nonjudgmental analysis and recognition of value-driven decision-making—are not in conflict. Instead, they are complementary approaches that support a comprehensive understanding of human behavior (Benight & Bandura, 2004; Bartone, 2006).

Within the broader context of societal norms, fire, and emergency services tend to respond to line-of-duty fatalities with equal reverence, regardless of whether the death resulted from a heroic act or behavior deemed operationally irresponsible. Efforts to explore the psychological and cultural.

The dynamics underlying these incidents often involve resistance, as such inquiries are perceived as assigning blame or diminishing the honor of the deceased (Dangermond et al., 2022). Consequently, the human factors contributing to these events remain largely unexamined. This reluctance is further complicated by multiple stakeholders—colleagues, families, unions, leadership, and the broader community—each invested in different aspects of a firefighter's life and legacy, who may interpret investigative scrutiny as undermining the profession's collective values or identity (Bartone, 2006; Barton & Sutcliffe, 2009).

Advancing safety within fire and emergency services requires a multidisciplinary approach that combines psychology, engineering, and fire science. Investigative models should be reimagined to reflect the full scope of human behavior, enabling a deeper understanding of past failures and the prevention of future tragedies. Behavioral analysis, leadership assessment, and cultural audits offer practical strategies to foster safety-oriented organizational change. By adopting modern tools such as HFACS and a psychologically grounded RCA, fire departments can transition from reactive investigations to proactive prevention strategies that honor lessons learned and protect future generations.

From a broader systems view, psychology intersects every level of the fire service. Humans influence land use, policy, and development patterns, which are key factors shaping wildfire exposure and structural fire risk. Governments determine building codes and land management strategies that impact incident frequency and severity. When fatalities occur, societal narratives often emphasize bravery and sacrifice, framing the event through a lens of valor. However, alongside honoring service, there must be a commitment to reducing fatalities through a deeper understanding of behavioral motivation and operational strategy. Recognizing that firefighters intentionally engage in fire, driven by perceived reinforcement, duty, and cultural identity, offers critical insight for designing safer systems. To change behavior, we must understand why that behavior occurred first.

Historical Review of Human Factor Analysis in Fire-Related Incidents

Human factors play a central role in the cause and prevention of fireground accidents and safety-compromising events. Human error has consistently emerged as the leading contributor to incident occurrence across diverse settings, from wildland fires to ship engine rooms and laboratory environments. Estimates suggest that 70–80% of accidents are rooted in human factors, underscoring the urgent need for systematic approaches to their identification and analysis (Omodei et al., 2005).

In wildland firefighting, investigations often overlook the human elements that lead to operational failure. Ryerson and Whitlock reported that accident reviews within the U.S. Federal Wildland fire program frequently lack a structured analysis of human factors, even though such factors are often the root causes of decision-making breakdowns and procedural oversight. To address this gap, the Human Factors Analysis and Classification System (HFACS), initially developed for aviation, has been adapted to improve the reliability and depth of fire service accident investigations. HFACS provides a hierarchical framework that enables investigators to examine underlying influences, such as unsafe supervision, the organizational climate, and individual decision-making errors, thereby moving beyond surface-level attributions to deeper, system-wide contributors.

Similarly, research in Australian bushfire settings has emphasized the cognitive and organizational dimensions of human error. Omodei et al. (2005) introduced a post-incident interview protocol that enhances the accuracy of recollections following incidents by taking into account memory limitations and self-preservation biases. The protocol is specifically designed to identify cognitive traits (e.g., risk propensity) and the perceived influence of safety culture on decision-making on firegrounds. Importantly, this approach is not limited to formal investigations; it can also be applied during training debriefs and no-fault reporting, enabling organizations to create safer environments through proactive learning (Omodei et al. 2005).

Beyond wildland fire contexts, large-scale industrial and maritime investigations have underscored the importance of integrating HFACS with other analytical tools to capture human–system interactions. For example, in laboratory fire and explosion events, organizational factors, such as lapses in safety oversight and inconsistent training protocols, were identified as root causes when analyzed via hybrid models such as HFACS integrated with fuzzy set theory and Bayesian networks (Ma et al., 2022). These findings parallel observations in fire and emergency services, where cultural, managerial, and procedural deficiencies often create conditions that lead to individual human errors.

Recent advancements have also proposed the use of machine learning to automate human factor analysis. Ensemble learning techniques, for example, can parse complex accident data to extract patterns and causal chains more efficiently than manual reviews can (Zarei, 2023). This evolution holds promise for fire service agencies seeking to implement predictive analytics in their risk mitigation efforts, especially in high-temperature environments where near misses and minor errors can rapidly escalate into critical incidents.

Ultimately, integrating human factor analysis into routine fire service operations, from training debriefings to accident investigations, offers a powerful mechanism for improving safety. By acknowledging the multifactorial nature of human error and using structured frameworks such as the HFACS, fire departments can move beyond individual blame toward systemic prevention, thereby fostering a culture of learning and resilience across the organization.

Applications of HFACS Across Contexts

The Human Factors Analysis and Classification System (HFACS) has been effectively applied across various high-risk industries to better understand systemic and human contributors to accidents. In the maritime sector, the adapted HFACS-MA model, when used in conjunction with gray relational analysis (GRA), has proven effective in identifying recurring organizational and human factors that contribute to accidents. Similarly, in aviation and rail transport, HFACS has been validated as a reliable framework for identifying causal factors ranging from unsafe acts to latent systemic conditions (Daramola, 2014; Reinach & Viale, 2006). Comparative research highlights HFACS's strengths when used in conjunction with broader system-based models, such as AcciMap and STAMP, particularly in its ability to provide a granular classification of human errors within complex accident trajectories (Underwood & Waterson, 2013). These applications demonstrate the flexibility and depth of HFACS in diagnosing failures across various safety-critical domains, thereby supporting a systematic approach to risk mitigation and accident prevention.

Training and Development

In addition to incident analysis, HFACS has informed the evolution of training programs designed to enhance nontechnical skills, which are critical for safety in dynamic, high-pressure environments. Research on organizational psychology and emergency response underscores the importance of competencies such as communication, emotional regulation, decision-making, and teamwork in shaping safe and effective field operations (Salas et al., 2005). In the fire service, this recognition has prompted efforts to integrate psychosocial and behavioral dimensions into firefighter training, with a focus on developing resilience, clarifying roles, and fostering interdependence. Moreover, recent initiatives have begun to apply HFACS insights to identify key stressors and support mechanisms across different experience levels, helping tailor interventions for both recruits and seasoned personnel. This integration of human factors into training reflects a proactive shift from reactive post-incident analysis to preventive, culturally informed skill development aimed at long-term operational safety.

Human Factors Analysis and Classification System (HFACS)

Unsafe Acts: Errors and Violations

In the Human Factors Analysis and Classification System (HFACS), *unsafe acts* are divided into two broad categories: errors and violations. Errors are unintentional actions, such as lapses in memory, judgment, or attention, that can compromise safety during high-stakes operations. These behaviors are not rooted in negligence but occur when cognitive, perceptual, or situational demands exceed the responder's capacity at a given moment. Fire service environments, characterized by dynamic risk, time pressure, and limited information, are fertile ground for such errors.

Understanding and mitigating these errors requires more than disciplinary measures; proactive systems thinking supported by data-informed decision-making is also needed. Recent research highlights the role of predictive analytics in reducing the likelihood of error by anticipating operational demands. For example, Guyeux et al. (2023) analyzed over 200,000 fire service interventions in France, using machine learning algorithms to forecast incident volume and type within 3-h windows. Although not explicitly framed through HFACS, the implications of this study are clear: by predicting operational tempo and call volume, departments can better allocate resources, reduce fatigue-related errors, and increase readiness. These findings underscore the potential of integrating technological tools into fireground psychology, shifting from reactive error correction to anticipatory risk management. From a human factor perspective, such data-driven approaches help shape conditions that reduce cognitive strain and enhance decision-making under pressure (Guyeux et al., 2023).

Decision Errors

Within the HFACS framework, poor choices are categorized under decision errors, a subtype of unsafe acts. These errors involve selecting an inappropriate course of action, even when all necessary information is available. In fire service psychology, understanding the cognitive processes behind such decisions is crucial for enhancing on-scene performance and minimizing adverse outcomes. Okoli et al. (2022)

expand upon the naturalistic decision-making (NDM) framework to examine how experienced fireground commanders manage complex, non-routine incidents. Their study, which included commanders from both the UK and Nigeria, utilized the critical decision method (CDM) to elicit detailed accounts of challenging fireground scenarios. The findings emphasize that expert decision-making is not merely about pattern recognition; it also involves nuanced *information filtering*, the ability to detect, prioritize, and act on subtle but critical environmental cues.

This capacity to discriminate between relevant and irrelevant information emerged as a core determinant of fireground competence. The researchers identified 42 specific cues that informed tactical decisions and developed a classification model to aid in future training and assessment. From a human factor perspective, poor choices often reflect cognitive overload or impaired cue discrimination under stress rather than incompetence. As such, enhancing decision quality requires more than procedural drills; it involves training firefighters to process uncertainty, manage attentional resources, and develop intuition through experience-rich learning environments. Okoli et al.'s (2022) work supports the integration of psychological insights into fireground command training, reinforcing the HFACS principle that unsafe acts, particularly decision errors, must be understood within the broader cognitive and environmental context in which they occur.

Skill-Based Errors

Within the Human Factors Analysis and Classification System (HFACS), skill-based errors are defined as unintentional execution failures during routine, well-practiced tasks. These include lapses in memory, attention, or perception that lead to actions such as forgetting a step in a procedure, mishandling controls, or misjudging familiar conditions (Shappell & Wiegmann, 2003). Unlike decision errors, which involve flawed judgment or problem solving, skill-based errors often occur without conscious thought, typically when an individual is operating under stress, fatigue, or distraction.

In fire and emergency services, such errors are particularly consequential. High-pressure environments, such as firegrounds, increase cognitive load, making firefighters more susceptible to lapses in attention or motor performance. These errors may present as task fixations, missed procedural steps, or failures in basic safety protocols, despite adequate training and experience. Gough (2022) reported that the majority of firefighter injuries documented during emergency response operations were associated with either decision errors or skill-based execution failures, which are often linked to degraded attention or skill fading in real-time operational contexts. These findings underscore the reality that even seasoned professionals can falter during routine tasks when operating under high stress.

Apparatus operation is another domain where skill-based errors frequently emerge. Firefighters may fail to engage a pump correctly, skip a step in aerial ladder deployment, or forget to apply wheel chocks, all of which have been identified in accidents and near-miss reports (National Fire Fighter Near-Miss Reporting System

[NFFNMRS], 2006). Such errors are often the result of momentary lapses in procedural memory or attentional slips. NFFNMRS data indicate that more than 90% of analyzed near misses are attributed to human error, with a significant proportion involving failures in attention, perception, or basic operational skill.

Skill-based errors are also present in routine, nonemergency tasks such as equipment checks or SCBA maintenance. These errors, although less dramatic, can create latent conditions for future incidents. For example, neglecting to refill an air cylinder after training or improperly storing hose couplings may lead to critical failures during deployment. Gough (2022) emphasized the importance of frequent, high-fidelity training to combat skill fading, particularly for low-frequency, high-consequence tasks.

Line-of-duty death investigations by the National Institute for Occupational Safety and Health (NIOSH) have repeatedly highlighted skill-based lapses in fatal incidents. For example, in a 2011 high-rise fire, a captain attempting to share air during a Mayday incident failed to control the air release, resulting in the rapid depletion of the partner's SCBA cylinder (NIOSH, 2012). The misstep, likely due to extreme stress and a lapse in execution, resulted in both firefighters being overcome. NIOSH recommended regular and repeated SCBA emergency training to reinforce procedural muscle memory and reduce cognitive overload in such scenarios.

The HFACS framework reinforces the view that these lapses are not simply individual failings but are shaped by conditions such as fatigue, stress, and system design (Shappell & Wiegmann, 2003). This perspective aligns with a growing emphasis in fire service psychology on creating training environments that simulate stress and test the retention of procedural tasks. Near-miss and injury reports increasingly point to the importance of situational awareness, attention management, and routine reinforcement of basic skills as countermeasures to these errors (Gough, 2022).

The incorporation of human factors into fire service operations acknowledges the reality of human limitations while promoting systemic solutions that enhance overall effectiveness. Strategies may include the use of checklists, cognitive aids, peer cross-checks, and realistic simulation-based training to help firefighters sustain high levels of performance in low-margin situations. As skill-based errors remain a leading contributor to operational failure, integrating this understanding into fire service training and safety culture is important for reducing preventable injuries and fatalities.

Perceptual Errors: Five Senses

Human performance is profoundly influenced by perceptual processes, with errors in sensory interpretation, such as those involving visual and auditory input, posing significant risks in high-stakes environments. In the firefighting domain, such perceptual errors are often exacerbated by the complex interplay between environmental stressors and the physical limitations of protective gear. Misjudgments in sensory data can lead to delayed reactions, impaired situational awareness, and ultimately, an increased risk of injury.

Clarke et al. (2021) provide compelling evidence that illustrates how the thermal protection capabilities of firefighter garments may inadvertently contribute to sensory misinterpretation under fireground conditions. Their study explored the relationship between the heat protection performance (TPP) ratings of firefighter garments and the concept of the available safe escape time (ASET). They reported that even garments meeting minimum safety standards may not fully support optimal sensory perception and timely escape, especially under extreme heat flux scenarios simulated through computational fluid dynamics (CFD) models.

By translating TPP values into quantifiable escape times, researchers have demonstrated that protective gear can significantly influence a firefighter's ability to perceive heat exposure risk and make accurate, informed decisions. The study also validated the fire model's capacity to predict the likelihood of injury, reinforcing the importance of integrating garment performance metrics with environmental modeling. This integration helps mitigate perceptual errors by aligning sensory cues with objective safety thresholds (Clarke et al., 2021).

Ultimately, these findings suggest that improving perceptual accuracy in high-risk professions, such as firefighting, depends not only on individual training but also on engineering solutions that enhance the fidelity of sensory input in extreme environments.

Routine Violations: Normalized Rule Deviations in the Fire Service

Within the HFACS framework, routine violations refer to habitual, intentional deviations from established procedures that are often tolerated or even implicitly reinforced within an organizational culture (Shappell & Wiegmann, 2003). In the fire service, these violations often arise from operational habits developed over time, influenced by peer behavior, time pressures, or skepticism about the practicality of specific rules and regulations. Examples include neglecting to wear seatbelts in an apparatus, failing to complete personal protective equipment (PPE) during overhaul, or skipping accountability check-ins. While these actions may seem minor or justified by efficiency, they erode the integrity of safety systems and contribute to cumulative risk exposure.

NIOSH (2016) identified several incidents in which routine violations contributed to firefighter fatalities, such as failure to follow standard communication protocols or the use of unauthorized equipment. These actions were often not the result of ignorance or defiance but rather a reflection of *normalized* deviance—a condition in which unsafe practices become routine owing to the absence of immediate negative consequences (Vaughan, 1996). Over time, such practices become embedded in department culture, particularly when leadership fails to model or enforce procedural compliance. DeJoy et al. (2004) argue that when personnel perceive a disconnect between policies and the operational realities of the job, they are more likely to adapt rules informally to match what they see as practical or realistic.

From a fire service psychology standpoint, routine violations are not just behavioral missteps but also indicators of cultural and organizational drift. Addressing them requires more than discipline; it demands interventions that clarify the relevance of procedures, ensure that they are contextually appropriate, and reinforce them through leadership modeling and peer accountability. Safety messaging, behavior-based coaching, and inclusive policy reviews can help reduce the gap between written standards and day-to-day practices. Recognizing the psychological and cultural underpinnings of routine violations is critical to fostering a safety culture that supports consistent rule adherence in operational environments.

Exceptional Violations

Exceptional violations are defined in HFACS as rare, atypical deviations from standard procedures that occur under unusual or extreme circumstances (Shappell & Wiegmann, 2003). These acts typically arise when personnel face unexpected or rapidly evolving events, often making split-second decisions that conflict with established policy. In the fire service, exceptional violations might include entering a structure alone without command authorization, initiating a high-risk rescue outside one's scope of training, or improvising tactics in a way that bypasses safety checks. While these acts may be motivated by urgency, perceived moral duty, or a desire to help others, they still involve intentional departures from the protocol.

Investigations from the NIOSH Fire Fighter Fatality Investigation and Prevention Program (FFFIPP) frequently document exceptional violations during high-stress operations. In one case, a firefighter died during a water rescue training event after attempting maneuvers beyond the parameters of the assigned drill (NIOSH, 2020). Although the intent was not reckless, the deviation from the training scope ultimately contributed to the fatal outcome. These kinds of violations are psychologically complex and often involve a mix of emotional responses, identity constructs, and momentary judgments.

Fire service psychology recognizes that exceptional violations often reflect value-laden decisions rather than conscious risk-taking for its own sake. Firefighters operating in life-threatening situations may override protocols because they feel an internal obligation to act, even when doing so violates formal guidance. This highlights the need for psychologically grounded training that emphasizes situational awareness, decision-making under pressure, and structured risk–benefit evaluation. As Reason (1997) and DeJoy et al. (2004) suggest, safety systems should be designed not only to enforce compliance but also to support good judgment in ambiguous, high-risk situations.

Culturally, departments need to distinguish between well-intentioned actions that deviate from policy in rare contexts and more routine actions that disregard procedures. The goal is not to suppress initiative but to ensure that firefighters are trained and empowered to act decisively within a framework that supports safety. Integrating HFACS into post-incident analysis helps identify when exceptional violations reflect breakdowns in training, supervision, or procedural clarity, thus informing improvements without assigning unjust blame.

Preconditions for Unsafe Acts

Within the HFACS framework, preconditions for unsafe acts refer to the situational and human factors that shape the context in which errors or violations are more likely to occur (Shappell & Wiegmann, 2003). These are not the unsafe acts themselves but rather the underlying conditions, psychological, physiological, environmental, or organizational, that increase the probability of performance breakdown. In the fire service, such preconditions include factors such as inadequate teamwork, stress, fatigue, equipment design issues, and individual limitations in skill or knowledge. These elements often interact dynamically, creating a high-risk operational environment even before a specific decision or action takes place. Understanding and addressing these preconditions is important for proactive safety management, as it allows organizations to identify vulnerabilities that precede and precipitate unsafe behaviors on the fireground.

Environmental Factors in the Fire Service

In the HFACS model, preconditions for unsafe acts represent the latent factors that shape the operational context in which human errors and violations are likely to occur (Shappell & Wiegmann, 2003). These are not the unsafe acts themselves but the conditions that make such acts more probable. Within fire and emergency services, understanding these preconditions is crucial for identifying systemic vulnerabilities and designing interventions that reduce the likelihood of errors. One critical set of preconditions falls under environmental factors, which include both the physical environment, the tangible operating space and conditions, and the technological environment, tools, systems, and design interfaces that firefighters interact with during operations.

Physical Environment: Operational Hazards and Uncontrollable Conditions

The physical environment refers to the immediate, external conditions in which firefighters operate. This includes variables such as weather, visibility, terrain, building construction, and the condition or arrangement of equipment. In many fireground situations, the physical environment is unpredictable and constantly evolving, often introducing unanticipated hazards that contribute to slips, trips, exposure, or spatial disorientation. For example, dense smoke, unstable structural elements, or icy surfaces can rapidly degrade firefighter performance and increase the risk of accidents (NIOSH, 2017). These environmental challenges are often beyond the direct control of personnel but interact with individual behavior and decision-making in ways that contribute to unsafe acts.

In one case investigated by NIOSH (2017), a firefighter died after falling through a floor weakened by fire damage, a hazard not visible during initial size-up due to smoke and cluttered conditions. Although the firefighter's actions did not violate the policy or protocol, the fatal event illustrates how environmental preconditions can set the stage for tragedy. Fire service psychology must account for these external stressors by promoting enhanced risk assessment practices, environmental scanning techniques, and decision-making models that integrate sensory limitations and uncertainty into operational planning and decision-making processes.

Technological Environment: System Design, Equipment Interface, and Human–Machine Interaction

The technological environment involves systems, tools, and equipment that firefighters rely on to perform their duties. Poorly designed interfaces, malfunctioning equipment, or a lack of standardization can introduce cognitive and physical burdens that contribute to unsafe acts. From SCBA configurations and radio communication systems to fire apparatus controls and thermal imaging cameras, the usability and reliability of technology can directly affect firefighter safety.

Research on human factor engineering emphasizes the importance of designing equipment that supports intuitive use under stress and degraded visibility, conditions common in fireground operations (Reason, 1997). Unfortunately, technological shortcomings are frequently cited in firefighter fatalities and near-miss reports. For example, NIOSH (2013) documented a case in which radio communication failures, linked to building construction and system limitations, contributed to a delayed mayday response and ultimately to a fatality. In such cases, the failure is not due to human error in isolation but to a technological precondition that impedes effective performance.

Poor design can also contribute to mode confusion, where firefighters may mistakenly believe that they have activated a device (e.g., a PASS alarm or pump panel function) when they have not, especially under stress or with limited sensory feedback. The HFACS framework allows investigators to identify these latent conditions and trace their influence on unsafe acts. A fire service psychology approach must therefore emphasize human-centered design in equipment procurement, realistic equipment training, and user feedback loops to identify and resolve usability issues before they contribute to incidents.

Condition of Operators

Adverse Mental States

Adverse mental states, characterized by stress, distraction, emotional fatigue, and psychological trauma, can significantly impair situational awareness and decision-making in emergency responders. Firefighters operate under persistent cognitive and emotional stress, often with insufficient systemic support to buffer against its cumulative impact.

Psychological trauma remains a critical concern. In a study of firefighters responding to the 2023 Pazarcik and Elbistan earthquakes, Bakirci et al. (2024) reported high trauma levels, with those exhibiting severe symptoms also demonstrating lower resilience and elevated rates of depression, anxiety, and PTSD. These findings underscore the need for proactive psychological support strategies and resilience training designed explicitly for high-exposure roles.

Senger et al. (2023) further explored this dimension through a structural equation modeling approach and reported that resilience was more strongly associated with reductions in PTSD symptoms and chronic pain, whereas hope was a more potent predictor of posttraumatic growth and overall well-being. These psychosocial factors together accounted for up to 33% of the variance in mental and physical health outcomes. This highlights the potential for integrating resilience-building interventions into firefighter mental health programs.

Cognitive impairment resulting from emotional strain or mental fatigue is often interwoven with physiological deficits. For example, the cognitive effects of sleep deprivation, slower reaction times, and diminished executive functioning can also stem from mental overload (Stout et al., 2021). In this context, physiological and mental states interact in complex ways, often compounding risk.

These insights underscore that firefighter mental readiness is not only a matter of individual resilience but also an organizational investment in psychological safety, trauma-informed leadership, and supportive team dynamics. Addressing adverse mental states is important for safeguarding not only health but also operational effectiveness.

Adverse Physiological States

Adverse physiological states, such as fatigue, physical overload, and disrupted recovery cycles, pose significant threats to human performance in emergency response occupations. In firefighting, these states often arise from long-duration shifts, demanding physical exertion, and the physiological costs of protective gear and environmental stressors.

Sleep disruption is a well-documented issue within fire and emergency services. Stout et al. (2021) reported that firefighters averaged just over 5 h of sleep during 24-h shifts, resulting in significant reductions in processing speed, reaction time, and visual–motor coordination. These impairments directly increase the risk of operational error. Complementary findings from Fletcher et al. (2022) indicate that structured opportunities for napping, particularly during low-activity duty periods, could mitigate such risks, challenging the existing assumption that sleep is unachievable during shifts.

Physiological recovery also presents a challenge. Lyytikäinen et al. (2017) monitored heart rate variability and the cortisol response across multiple shifts and rest days and concluded that full autonomic recovery after a 24-h shift can take several days. Without adequate recovery, responders are at risk of developing cumulative physiological strain, which degrades performance and increases their susceptibility to injury.

Physical workload and biomechanical strain are further contributors to adverse physiological states. Drain et al. (2016) reviewed models for predicting acceptable load carriage durations. They reported that traditional workload guidelines for unloaded tasks are insufficient for roles involving sustained physical exertion under load, such as firefighting. Similarly, reasearch suggests postural stability deteriorates over prolonged shifts, increasing the risk of slips and falls, despite initial improvements in proprioceptive stability from wearing turnout gear and the SCBA (Kollock et al., 2021).

Movement dysfunctions, often unnoticed until an injury occurs, also warrant attention. Bock and Orr (2015) reviewed the use of the Functional Movement Screen (FMS) in tactical populations and concluded that FMS scores reliably predict injury risk. Firefighters with suboptimal scores may be more prone to musculoskeletal injuries under operational stress, suggesting that the Functional Movement Screen (FMS) may be a helpful screening and training tool.

Taken together, these studies emphasize the importance of acknowledging and addressing the physiological boundaries of responders through evidence-informed fatigue management, task design, and conditioning protocols.

Physical and Mental Limitations: Human Capability and Operational Demands

Under the HFACS framework, physical and mental limitations are preconditions for unsafe acts that stem from inherent or acquired constraints in an individual's knowledge, skills, or cognitive and physical capacities (Shappell & Wiegmann, 2003). In fire and emergency services, these limitations can manifest in various ways, from gaps in procedural knowledge or technical proficiency to decreased mental acuity under stress or even physical exhaustion. These are not character flaws but rather natural human limitations that, if unaddressed by training, staffing, or task design, increase the likelihood of unsafe acts.

From a psychological standpoint, one key contributor to performance breakdowns is cognitive overload, which occurs when task demands exceed a firefighter's working memory or attentional capacity. Under extreme time pressure or high-stress scenarios, even skilled individuals can forget steps, misinterpret cues, or default to inappropriate behaviors. This is especially relevant during low-frequency, high-consequence events, where proficiency may degrade due to a lack of recent practice (Gough, 2022). Research indicates that when firefighters are physically fatigued or cognitively taxed, their error rates increase, particularly for tasks that require sustained attention, decision-making, or fine motor control (Le et al., 2020).

Another critical factor is insufficient knowledge or skill acquisition, particularly among newer personnel or those who have not received adequate training in specialized tasks. NIOSH investigations have repeatedly identified cases where firefighters were placed in roles or environments that exceeded their level of training or preparedness, contributing to fatal outcomes. These findings highlight the importance of aligning task complexity with individual competence and ensuring that training is both current and scenario relevant.

It is equally important to recognize physical limitations; not all firefighters have the same baseline capacity for exertion, heat tolerance, or mobility. When physical demands outpace individual capability, risk increases substantially. Tasks such as advancing charged hose lines up stairwells, dragging victims, or operating heavy equipment require not only strength but also endurance and fine motor control, all of which can be impaired by fatigue, dehydration, or musculoskeletal limitations. Fire service psychology must advocate for a systems approach that incorporates ongoing physical assessments, recovery protocols, and realistic staffing to prevent overload and mitigate risk.

Addressing physical and mental limitations requires more than selection or screening; it necessitates continuous monitoring, support, and adaptation of expectations to align with the capacities of the workforce. Training programs must strike a balance between skill acquisition and cognitive load management, and departments should foster a culture in which recognizing one's limitations is viewed as a strength, not a weakness. In doing so, the fire service can reduce the frequency of errors born not from recklessness but from being placed in situations that exceed human capability.

Personnel Factors

In the HFACS framework, *Personnel Factors* represent the cognitive, physical, and behavioral characteristics of individuals who influence their performance in operational environments. This category includes elements such as crew resource management, personal readiness, adverse mental states, adverse physiological states, and routine violations, each of which can significantly affect the safety and effectiveness of firefighting operations.

In the fire service, personnel factors are particularly critical due to the unpredictable and high-risk nature of the work. Individual conditions such as fatigue, stress, distraction, or complacency have been shown to impair decision-making, reduce situational awareness, and increase the likelihood of procedural errors (Ghasemi et al., 2022). Similarly, physical readiness, including sleep adequacy, hydration, fitness, and recovery, plays a central role in sustaining performance under pressure (Stout et al., 2021; Lyytikäinen et al., 2017). When fire service personnel operate without sufficient physical or psychological preparedness, they are more vulnerable to both acute injuries and long-term occupational illness.

Furthermore, effective team coordination, a central aspect of crew resource management, is often influenced by individual attitudes toward communication, leadership, and peer support. Research shows that personnel factors can either enhance or undermine team effectiveness, depending on how well individuals are trained, supported, and integrated into cohesive operational units (Heinemann et al., 2024a, 2024b).

Addressing personnel factors requires a holistic approach that includes physical conditioning, mental health support, communication skills development, and ongoing performance assessment. By understanding and managing these human variables, fire departments can reduce error rates, improve resilience, and promote safer operational outcomes.

Personnel Factors: Crew Resource Management (CRM)

Within the HFACS framework, personnel factors encompass cognitive and behavioral attributes that influence individual and team performance. Among these, crew resource management (CRM) stands as a pivotal component, addressing the nontechnical skills important to effective teamwork, such as communication, leadership, emotional regulation, and decision-making. In high-reliability organizations, such as fire and emergency services, breakdowns in CRM are frequent precursors to unsafe acts and operational failures.

The complex and dynamic environments in which firefighting teams operate amplify the consequences of even minor teamwork failures. In response to this reality, Heinemann et al. (2024a, 2024b) developed REST-Q Fire, a validated instrument designed to measure the frequency and intensity of team-related stressors and resources during firefighting operations. Through interviews with experienced firefighters and document analysis, the tool provides a diagnostic approach for understanding both harmful and protective factors that affect crew cohesion.

Their study, involving 491 firefighters, revealed a positive correlation between the intensity of teamwork-related stressors and self-reported stress levels ($r = 0.19$–0.27), underscoring the impact of interpersonal dynamics on both psychological and operational performance. Notably, the most prominent stressors included the "behavior of leaders" and "behavior of team members," both of which scored high in frequency and intensity. These findings highlight the crucial role of relational factors, particularly those rooted in communication and interpersonal trust, in shaping team effectiveness (Heinemann et al., 2024a, 2024b).

On the other hand, key resources, such as "reliability of team members," "watching out for/checking on each other," and "knowledge about team members' skills," were reported more frequently and perceived more intensely than the stressors. These protective factors underscore the importance of shared mental models, mutual monitoring, and psychological safety—core elements of CRM that support resilience under stress.

Expanding on these insights, Hobbs (I.S., 2023) examined communication loops, emotional dynamics, and team adaptability during firefighting operations. Their findings revealed that "enriched closed-loop communication," positive emotional exchanges, and "gamma-type" adaptive behaviors were associated with greater team effectiveness. Conversely, open or incomplete communication loops, negative emotional interactions, and rigid adaptation styles (such as "alpha" or "beta" types) were associated with reduced performance. Furthermore, organizational trust and motivation were found to mediate team effectiveness, underscoring the impact of organizational culture on frontline coordination.

These studies collectively highlight the urgent need for structured CRM training programs that extend beyond technical proficiency to encompass nontechnical skills, including assertive communication, emotional regulation, and adaptive coordination strategies. In doing so, organizations can mitigate latent crew-level vulnerabilities and proactively foster high-performing teams.

Moreover, incorporating tools such as the REST-Q Fire into organizational assessments, training evaluations, and post-incident debriefings can help identify emerging threats to team cohesion before they manifest as errors. When personnel factors are systematically evaluated and addressed, fire service organizations are better positioned to reduce human error, optimize team performance, and enhance operational safety.

Personal Readiness

Within the Human Factors Analysis and Classification System (HFACS), Personal Readiness is categorized under Personnel Factors and pertains to an individual's off-duty activities that influence their on-duty performance. This includes adherence to rest requirements, abstention from substances that impair performance, and maintenance of the physical and mental fitness necessary for operational tasks.

In the context of firefighting, personal readiness is paramount due to the physically demanding and high-stress nature of the profession. Research indicates that many firefighters fail to meet the recommended aerobic fitness standards, which can compromise their ability to perform essential tasks safely and effectively. For example, a study by Chizewski et al. (2021) revealed that a 7-week high-intensity functional training (HIFT) program significantly improved recruits' cardiovascular fitness, muscular endurance, and overall firefighting ability.

Similarly, Kamuk (2020) assessed the impact of a 12-week exercise regimen on Turkish firefighters and reported notable improvements in their physical fitness and body mass index (BMI). The study emphasized the importance of regular physical training in enhancing firefighters' readiness and reducing the risk of injury.

In addition to physical fitness, mental preparedness is also a critical component of personal readiness. Firefighters are frequently exposed to traumatic events, and inadequate mental health support can lead to adverse outcomes such as burnout and impaired decision-making. The implementation of comprehensive wellness programs that address both physical and psychological aspects can bolster resilience and operational effectiveness.

In conclusion, ensuring personal readiness through structured fitness programs, adequate rest, and mental health support is important for maintaining high performance standards in firefighting operations. Organizations should prioritize these elements to increase safety and efficiency on firegrounds.

Unsafe Supervision

Within the Human Factors Analysis and Classification System (HFACS), *unsafe supervision* captures the critical role that supervisory personnel play in shaping operational safety. This category includes failures such as inadequate oversight, planned inappropriate operations, failure to correct known problems, and supervisory violations, each of which can significantly increase the risk of human error, procedural noncompliance, and adverse outcomes on the fireground.

In fire and emergency services, supervisors often serve as a bridge between policy and practice. Their decisions influence training quality, task assignments, safety enforcement, and team readiness. Research indicates that breakdowns at this level, whether due to passive oversight, misjudgment, or willful disregard, can have fatal consequences. For example, studies have shown that supervisory inaction in enforcing basic safety policies such as seatbelt use or personal protective equipment compliance has been a recurrent theme in firefighter line-of-duty deaths (NIOSH, 2017, 2018). Additionally, leadership behavior at the supervisory level plays a direct role in shaping the safety climate and influencing the behaviors of subordinates (Smith et al., 2023).

Unsafe supervision is not limited to individual error; it reflects more profound systemic weaknesses in accountability, training, and safety culture. Addressing this layer of human factors requires departments to prioritize leadership development, promote proactive risk management, and ensure consistent adherence to safety protocols at all supervisory levels.

Unsafe Supervision: Inadequate Supervision

Within the HFACS framework, unsafe supervision refers to failures at the supervisory level that contribute to unsafe conditions or behaviors. Specifically, the subcategory of inadequate supervision encompasses the failure to provide personnel with appropriate training, oversight, or resources that enable them to perform safely and effectively. In the fire service, where operational environments are often extreme, inadequate supervisory practices in areas such as heat stress management can directly undermine firefighter health, endurance, and safety.

One critical area where supervisory inadequacy can manifest is in the implementation of recovery protocols during high-heat operations. Firefighting in thermally stressful environments, especially when full firefighting protective clothing (FPC) and self-contained breathing apparatus (SCBA) are worn, poses serious physiological risks, including heat exhaustion and cardiovascular strain. Despite this, cooling and recovery strategies are not always standardized or consistently enforced across departments, which may reflect gaps in supervisory oversight or resource allocation.

Selkirk et al. (2004) investigated the comparative effectiveness of three recovery methods- forearm submersion (FS), misting (M), and passive cooling (PC)- on heat-strained firefighters during intermittent work at 35 °C in a 50% relative humidity (RH) environment. Their findings demonstrated that, compared with passive cooling, active cooling strategies, particularly forearm submersion, significantly improved work tolerance and reduced core temperature, heart rate, and skin temperature. FS resulted in the highest tolerance time (178.7 ± 13.0 min) and total work time (124.7 ± 7.94 min), substantially outperforming both M and PC.

Most notably, during the first rest period, the core temperature (Tre) decreased significantly under FS conditions (~0.4 °C), whereas it increased with passive cooling (~0.2 °C). These differences widened over subsequent rest intervals, revealing that FS is the most effective intervention for thermal recovery (Selkirk et al., 2004). Despite the availability of such evidence-based strategies, their adoption and integration into fireground rehab procedures often depend on supervisory initiatives and training mandates.

Failure to incorporate proven cooling methods, such as FS, into operational protocols constitutes a clear example of inadequate supervision. Supervisors are responsible not only for ensuring that personnel have access to practical recovery tools but also for training crews in their correct application and enforcing their use during operations. The consequences of neglecting this responsibility may include reduced operational endurance, an increased incidence of heat-related illnesses, and avoidable injuries.

To address this gap, supervisory frameworks must evolve to incorporate evidence-based physiological recovery protocols as a standard component of firefighter rehab. This requires not only the dissemination of best practices but also a culture of accountability, where the supervisory chain actively champions health-preserving procedures on the fireground.

Planned Inappropriate Operations

Within the Human Factors Analysis and Classification System (HFACS), planned inappropriate operations refer to supervisory decisions that assign tasks or roles without fully accounting for associated risks. In the fire service, this often manifests during fireground operations, where the failure to consider environmental hazards, resource availability, or personnel capability can lead to catastrophic outcomes. This subcategory of unsafe supervision is particularly relevant to incident commanders and supervisors, who must make time-critical decisions under uncertainty and pressure.

Several case studies from the National Institute for Occupational Safety and Health (NIOSH) illustrate how planned inappropriate operations have led to firefighter fatalities. In a 2023 Maryland incident, both a lieutenant and a probationary firefighter died after experiencing thermal degradation of their self-contained breathing apparatus (SCBA) facepiece lenses. The NIOSH investigation determined that crews were deployed under extreme heat conditions without adequate situational awareness or understanding of the limitations of thermal imaging cameras and SCBA gears. Supervisors have failed to incorporate this critical knowledge into operational decisions, exposing personnel to untenable heat and ultimately contributing to fatalities.

A second case in Illinois, also in the same year, involved a firefighter who fell into a light or air shaft while conducting rooftop ventilation on a four-story mixed-use building. The firefighter had been assigned to perform vertical ventilation without sufficient information about the building's structural design or hazards. NIOSH concluded that the incident stemmed from a lack of supervisory preplanning, ineffective communication, and inadequate hazard identification during task assignment.

These cases highlight the role of fireground supervisors in conducting dynamic risk assessments and aligning task assignments with current conditions and the readiness of firefighters. Assigning firefighters to roles without accounting for physical hazards, crew qualifications, or shifting fire behavior not only violates incident command principles but also exemplifies planned inappropriate operations.

To mitigate supervisory failures, fire departments must ensure that incident commanders are equipped with the critical competencies necessary to support safe and effective operations. These include the ability to perform real-time hazard identification, understand the operational limits of both personnel and equipment, provide clear and continuous communication throughout assignments, and apply standard operating procedures (SOPs) as a decision-making framework under pressure. When these supervisory functions are neglected, the risk of task misallocation and preventable tragedy increases significantly. Institutionalizing these risk-aware supervisory practices across all levels of command enhances operational safety and reduces the likelihood of unsafe fireground tasking.

Failure to Correct Problems

Within the Human Factors Analysis and Classification System (HFACS), failure to correct problems is categorized under unsafe supervision. It refers to instances where supervisors neglect to address known safety hazards, recurrent violations, or organizational deficiencies. In fire service, this failure is not limited to individual oversight; it often reflects a systemic tolerance for unsafe practices that persist despite prior warnings or incidents. Several recurring issues, including seatbelt non-compliance, equipment maintenance failure, and inadequate training, exemplify this supervisory breakdown and have contributed to firefighter fatalities nationwide.

Seatbelt Noncompliance: A Persistent and Preventable Hazard

Despite long-standing awareness of the life-saving benefits of seatbelt use, enforcement remains inconsistent across many fire departments. In a 2017 incident, a volunteer firefighter in Iowa died after being ejected from a fire department pickup truck during a rollover crash. The firefighter was not wearing a seatbelt due to a medical waiver granted by the department, which allowed for policy noncompliance. NIOSH investigators cited this waiver and the department's failure to correct known seatbelt enforcement issues as a direct contributor to the fatality (NIOSH, 2017).

A similar tragedy occurred in 2018 in West Virginia, where two firefighters were killed and three others were injured in an apparatus crash while responding to an emergency. None of the vehicle occupants wore seatbelts at the time of the incident. NIOSH concluded that the department's supervisory personnel failed to enforce its seat belt policy, despite national standards and internal protocols requiring the use of restraints (NIOSH, 2018). These cases demonstrate a pattern of supervisory inaction in the face of known risk, a textbook example of failure to correct problems as defined by HFACS.

Equipment Maintenance and Inspection Deficiencies

Supervisory oversight also plays a critical role in ensuring the reliability of firefighting equipment. In a 2012 investigation, NIOSH reported that a firefighter experienced a malfunction of their self-contained breathing apparatus (SCBA) during an interior fire attack. The cause was traced to improper maintenance and a lack of routine inspection. Although the department had documented previous maintenance issues, corrective action had not been taken, ultimately resulting in the firefighter sustaining injury due to oxygen deprivation (NIOSH, 2012).

Such failures in equipment oversight are compounded by the fact that many fire departments operate under constrained budgets or rely heavily on volunteer staff. However, HFACS emphasizes that limited resources do not absolve supervisors from responsibility. When known equipment issues become unresolved, operational integrity is compromised, and personnel are exposed to avoidable hazards.

Inadequate and Outdated Training

Another recurring supervisory failure involves a lack of updated and recurrent training. In a 2010 line-of-duty death investigation, NIOSH concluded that a department failed to provide firefighters with adequate SCBA training, particularly in recognizing facepiece failure and understanding emergency air supply procedures. This training gap can directly contribute to fatality during a structural fire in which the firefighter becomes disoriented and runs out of air (NIOSH, 2010).

Supervisors are responsible not only for initial onboarding but also for sustaining operational readiness through continuous education. The failure to mandate refresher courses, skills recertification, or scenario-based drills reflects a broader unwillingness to address deficiencies once identified, again fitting squarely within HFACS's definition of failure to correct problems.

Organizational Implications

What links these varied examples (seatbelt noncompliance, poor equipment maintenance, and inadequate training) is a shared theme of supervisory inaction. These are not isolated or unpredictable events. Instead, they are repeated safety issues that have been thoroughly documented in the fire service literature, national standards, and prior incident reports.

Fire departments must implement proactive supervisory systems that monitor compliance, act on safety recommendations, and hold personnel accountable for their actions. This includes regular internal audits, follow-through on incident action items, and a commitment to enforcing safety policy without exception. Where known hazards persist without correction, the integrity of the entire organization is compromised.

Supervisory Violations

Within the Human Factors Analysis and Classification System (HFACS), Supervisory Violations represent instances in which supervisors intentionally disregard established rules, procedures, or safety policies. Unlike errors born of ignorance or oversight, these actions are characterized by a willful decision to bypass protocols, often under the guise of operational urgency or cultural norms. In fire and emergency services, such decisions can undermine safety culture, degrade crew trust, and significantly increase the risk of injury or fatality during emergency operations.

One of the most tragic and well-documented cases of supervisory violation occurred during the 2007 Charleston Sofa Super Store fire in South Carolina, where nine firefighters lost their lives. Investigations conducted by the Canton-Tompson et al. (2008) and the National Institute of Standards and Technology (NIST) revealed systemic failures in supervision during the incident. Supervisors failed to implement a functional incident command system and neglected to adjust tactics despite early indicators of deteriorating structural conditions. Notably, the decision to continue aggressive interior fire attacks, despite visible signs of collapse risk, constituted a willful deviation from the standard risk-based firefighting strategy. These actions reflected not just procedural lapses but also deliberate departures from accepted safety doctrine, placing personnel in preventable peril.

Supervisory violations also occur when commanders override or ignore well-established federal safety standards, such as the Occupational Safety and Health

Administration's (OSHA) two-in/two-out rule. This standard mandates that no interior firefighting in Immediately Dangerous to Life or Health (IDLH) environments occurs unless two personnel are inside with at least two stationed outside for rapid intervention. When supervisors neglect or intentionally bypass this regulation, whether due to workforce shortages or pressure to act quickly, they expose personnel to unacceptable risks and open their organizations to liability and legal consequences.

The culture of disregarding safety practices is sometimes rationalized under "get-the-job-done" mentalities, where expediency is placed above the protocol. However, research and incident analysis have repeatedly shown that deliberate noncompliance with risk management principles leads to catastrophic outcomes. Supervisors who ignore risk assessments, suppress dissenting safety concerns, or model unsafe behavior create environments in which procedural violations are normalized (U.S. Fire Administration, 2016).

To reduce supervisory violations, organizations must take deliberate steps to reinforce accountability and hold individuals accountable. This includes clearly articulating the consequences of rule violations, integrating supervisory decisions into post-incident reviews, and conducting regular audits of fireground leadership behavior. Furthermore, a sustained commitment to leadership development and ethics training is important for cultivating a command culture that views adherence to safety procedures not as optional but as foundational to professional integrity and firefighter survival.

Organizational Influences

In the HFACS framework, *organizational influences* refer to broad systemic conditions, such as leadership commitment, safety culture, resource allocation, and structural policies, that shape how individuals and teams operate within high-risk environments. These foundational elements set the tone for operational expectations and can directly impact the likelihood of human error at every level of the organization. Within fire and emergency services, inadequate organizational alignment with safety values can erode compliance, increase stress, and normalize risky behavior.

Research has consistently shown that organizational climate and leadership behavior are upstream predictors of safety outcomes in firefighting environments (Geczik et al., 2022). Specifically, low perceived management commitment to safety and passive leadership approaches have been linked to increased injury risk, diminished safety behavior, and deteriorated job satisfaction among firefighters (Smith et al., 2023; Geczik et al., 2024). These findings highlight the critical role of organizational systems in either mitigating or enabling the latent conditions that lead to unsafe acts.

Organizational Climate

Within the Human Factors Analysis and Classification System (HFACS), organizational climate is a foundational layer of influence, encompassing leadership attitudes, cultural norms, and policy frameworks that shape how safety is perceived, prioritized, and practiced. In the fire service, the organizational climate operates as a systemic force, reinforcing or eroding safety behaviors across all levels, from the firehouse floor to administrative leadership. When the climate lacks a clear safety commitment or tolerates disengaged leadership, the conditions are set for breakdowns in both compliance and resilience.

Passive Leadership and Psychological Risk

One critical component of organizational climate is leadership behavior, particularly the role of safety-specific leadership in shaping day-to-day operations. Smith et al. (2023) examined the effects of passive leadership on firefighter safety outcomes in a study involving 708 professional firefighters. Their findings revealed that passive leadership, defined as a lack of engagement or failure to intervene in safety-relevant issues, was significantly associated with elevated stress levels. This stress, in turn, increased anxiety, which directly undermined safety compliance and PPE use. The result is a cascading effect where leadership disengagement contributes to psychological strain and ultimately diminishes frontline safety behavior.

This dynamic illustrates how leadership attitudes extend beyond influence, functioning as active predictors of behavioral risk. In high-stakes professions such as firefighting, passivity in leadership is not benign; it contributes to systemic vulnerability.

Safety Climate and Structural Differences

The broader climate of safety in fire departments has also been evaluated through tools such as the Fire Service Organizational Culture of Safety (FOCUS) survey. Geczik et al. (2022, 2024) utilized this validated instrument to assess perceptions of Management Commitment to Safety and Supervisor Support for Safety among thousands of firefighters in both volunteer and career departments. The results revealed a consistent trend: career departments reported significantly lower scores in Management Commitment to Safety and higher injury rates than volunteer departments did. These findings highlight a disconnect between administrative leadership and perceived frontline support, suggesting that organizational type plays a moderating role in shaping climate.

Crucially, across both waves of the FOCUS survey, firefighters consistently rated supervisor support for safety higher than management commitment to safety (Geczik et al., 2024). This suggests that while policy and funding decisions originate from leadership at the top, firefighters perceive immediate supervisors as more directly responsible for ensuring safe practices. The implications are clear: frontline leadership behaviors often carry greater weight in shaping culture and influencing adherence to safety protocols.

International Perspectives: The Role of Stress and Cohesion

Complementary research conducted in Sweden supports these findings while adding new dimensions to the conversation. Lindén et al. (2023) analyzed safety climate outcomes among Swedish firefighters and reported that individual-level factors, including personal risk-taking, emotional exhaustion, and work pressure, were powerful predictors of noncompliance and error rates. However, group-level dynamics such as supervisory support and team cohesion also emerged as significant influences on safety behavior. These findings confirm that the organizational climate is not merely a top-down phenomenon; it is constructed through the interplay of individual stress, peer influence, and leadership engagement.

Emotional exhaustion, in particular, was identified as a predictor of mistakes and unsafe behaviors, aligning with earlier research linking chronic psychological stress to deteriorating safety performance (Ghasemi et al., 2022). These outcomes underscore the importance of fire service organizations recognizing psychological well-being as an integral component of safety management rather than a separate concern.

Toward a Safer Organizational Climate

Together, these studies highlight the multifaceted nature of the organizational climate and its impact on firefighter safety. Passive leadership, inadequate management commitment, and a failure to mitigate chronic psychological stress create a climate in which risk tolerance increases and compliance erodes. Critically, firefighters rate supervisor support higher than executive-level commitment does, suggesting that frontline leadership has greater perceived influence on safety behavior than does top-level management (Geczik et al., 2024).

To improve the organizational climate and reduce systemic vulnerability, fire departments must take deliberate action to cultivate a culture that prioritizes both psychological and operational safety. This begins with leadership development, which focuses on active safety engagement, ensuring that leaders model and reinforce safe behaviors. Departments should also formally recognize stress and mental health as integral components of safety rather than separate concerns. Continuous assessment of the safety climate, using validated tools such as the Firefighter Organizational Culture of Safety (FOCUS) survey, can provide valuable insights into emerging risks and organizational blind spots. Additionally, implementing cross-rank communication strategies helps align the safety priorities of frontline personnel with those of management. Enhancing the organizational climate is not a passive endeavor; it requires intentional leadership, cultural accountability, and the sustained integration of evidence-based practices to support firefighter well-being and resilience.

Operational Process

Within the HFACS framework, the operational process refers to systemic failures in planning, logistics, scheduling, or resource management that set the stage for unsafe acts (Shappell & Wiegmann, 2003). These deficiencies are often embedded in an organization's infrastructure and decision-making systems. In the fire service, operational process failures may manifest as inefficient deployment strategies, inadequate maintenance of apparatus and equipment, delayed decision-making structures, or poor alignment between staffing and risk levels. Although not directly visible in moment-to-moment operations, these systemic inefficiencies create latent conditions that increase the likelihood of errors or violations on the fireground.

For example, inadequate pre-incident planning has been cited in numerous firefighter fatality investigations by the National Institute for Occupational Safety and Health (NIOSH). In cases where building layouts were unknown, hydrant access was unclear, or preplans were outdated, crews were left without critical information at pivotal moments (NIOSH, 2014a, 2014b). Similarly, insufficient resource allocation, such as assigning an understaffed engine company to a high-risk structure fire, can lead to overextension of personnel and rushed, uncoordinated operations. These organizational-level decisions do not directly cause unsafe acts but create a high-risk environment in which individual decisions are made under suboptimal conditions.

Maintenance failures are another key concern. When a fire apparatus or life-saving equipment is not maintained according to the manufacturer's standards or is subjected to prolonged usage without inspection, the risk of malfunction increases. One NIOSH investigation documented a fatal incident in which a firefighter's PASS device failed to activate during a mayday, an outcome linked to irregular maintenance and a lack of inspection protocols (NIOSH, 2014a, 2014b). In this case, the breakdown of the operational process did not stem from firefighter behavior but from a systemic lapse in accountability for equipment readiness.

From a psychological perspective, inefficient operational processes undermine trust, increase stress, and impair performance. Firefighters who repeatedly encounter broken equipment, inconsistent staffing, or unclear directives may become disengaged, frustrated, or more prone to error due to fatigue and cognitive overload (DeJoy et al., 2004). The organizational psychology literature highlights the connection between operational reliability and worker resilience. When systems are predictable and well maintained, responders can allocate their cognitive resources to situational decision-making rather than compensating for upstream inefficiencies.

To mitigate these risks, fire service leaders must prioritize integrated planning, logistical foresight, and continuous quality assurance in operations. This includes conducting regular audits of equipment, validating and updating response protocols, and using data to align resources with incident demands. Departments should also foster a culture of reporting where frontline personnel can flag systemic concerns, such as recurring shortages, outdated plans, or infrastructure problems, without fear of reprisal. By viewing operational processes as human factors, organizations can shift from reactive firefighting to proactive system management, reducing the underlying vulnerabilities that compromise safety.

Resource Management

Under the HFACS framework, resource management is one of the core organizational influences that shapes the operational environment in which firefighters act (Shappell & Wiegmann, 2003). It refers to how an organization allocates its financial, human, and material resources, including funding, staffing levels, apparatus, equipment, and training infrastructure. Inadequacies in these areas do not typically lead directly to unsafe acts, but they set the stage for operational vulnerabilities by limiting personnel's capacity to perform safely and effectively. When fire departments are underserved, firefighters are more likely to operate under fatigue, take procedural shortcuts, or improvise in ways that increase risk.

Staffing shortages are among the most frequently cited resource management challenges in fire service fatality investigations. NIOSH (2014a, 2014b) reports repeatedly identified incidents where inadequate crew size delayed rescue operations, reduced task coverage, or forced firefighters to operate without the support of a rapid intervention team (RIT). For example, sending a two-person engine company into a structure fire significantly limits the ability to perform fire attack, search and rescue, and backup simultaneously. These conditions not only heighten physical strain but also reduce team communication and coordination, increasing the likelihood of slips, lapses, or decision errors under pressure.

Funding deficiencies further exacerbate these challenges. Budget constraints often result in an aging apparatus, deferred maintenance, outdated PPE, or reductions in training opportunities, all of which diminish operational readiness. DeJoy et al. (2004) emphasize that organizational constraints such as underfunding and understaffing are not merely administrative issues; they are latent conditions that increase error vulnerability across all operational levels. For example, a department that cannot afford annual SCBA fit testing or thermal imaging cameras is inherently less prepared to detect and mitigate evolving fireground hazards. Firefighters in such departments may also experience elevated psychological stress, knowing that they lack the same safety resources available in better-funded jurisdictions.

Equipment availability and reliability are equally central to firefighter safety. When critical tools (e.g., radios, PASS devices, and hose lines) are missing, incompatible, or unreliable, firefighters are forced to adapt on the spot, often with reduced efficiency and increased exposure. One NIOSH (2014a, 2014b) report documented a fatal incident where incompatible radio systems between mutual aid departments contributed to a breakdown in communication during a rapidly evolving structure fire. The inability to coordinate across agencies due to equipment incompatibility is a textbook example of a resource management failure cascading into operational risk. These failures are not caused by frontline personnel but by decisions at higher organizational levels that leave responders with insufficient tools to manage dynamic threats.

From a psychological perspective, persistent resource shortfalls degrade morale and increase cognitive strain. Firefighters may feel unsupported by leadership or forced to choose between mission success and personal safety. Over time, this may contribute to the normalization of risk, burnout, or disengagement from safety protocols. Organizational psychology emphasizes that perceptions of fairness, trust, and support are vital to workforce motivation and performance, which are factors that are directly shaped by how resources are allocated (Maslach & Leiter, 2016).

Addressing resource management issues requires proactive investment and strategic foresight from organizational leaders. Fire service administrators must advocate for sustainable budgets, equitable staffing models, and standardized procurement practices that ensure that every crew is equipped and trained to meet the demands of their service area. Departments should also integrate risk-informed decision-making into budget and staffing processes, prioritizing investments that have the most significant impact on firefighter and civilian safety. By recognizing resource management as a foundational element of system safety, departments can reduce the likelihood of unsafe acts and build operational environments that support resilience, efficiency, and long-term firefighter well-being.

Future Directions

As the operational demands and safety expectations of fire and emergency services continue to evolve, the tools and frameworks used to understand and mitigate risk must also evolve. The Human Factors Analysis and Classification System (HFACS) has proven effective in diagnosing latent organizational weaknesses and mapping the chain of errors that precede critical incidents. However, the future of firefighter safety lies not only in retrospective analysis but also in proactive, predictive, and integrative approaches to human factor management.

Development of Proactive Safety Models

Future research and operational practice should focus on developing proactive safety models that can identify root causes before adverse events occur. Studies have demonstrated the value of hybrid analytical methods that combine HFACS with quantitative risk modeling tools such as fuzzy fault tree analysis (FFTA) (Sarıalioğlu et al., 2020) and fuzzy cognitive mapping (FCM) (Soner et al., 2015). These integrated approaches provide deeper insights into the complex interplay between human errors, technical failures, and systemic deficiencies, enabling fire service agencies to prioritize interventions on the basis of probabilistic risk assessments and real-world operational data.

Such models move beyond static incident reconstruction and offer dynamic, scenario-based assessments that can inform real-time decision-making, safety drills, and resource allocation. For example, Sarıalioğlu et al. (2020) demonstrated how the HFACS-FFTA model successfully identified the likelihood and underlying contributors to fire-explosion scenarios aboard aging vessels, offering a blueprint for fire departments to assess their risks related to equipment age, material compatibility, and maintenance practices.

Leveraging Machine Learning for Human Factor Analysis

Another promising avenue for advancement lies in the application of machine learning to accident analysis. Automation has the potential to streamline the classification of human error and the identification of causal patterns across large datasets. Qi et al. (2024) explored the use of ensemble learning models to extract and categorize accident causation from unstructured report narratives and reported that algorithmic tools can support human analysts by reducing subjectivity and processing time. The incorporation of such tools into HFACS-based investigations may allow fire service agencies to detect trends earlier and implement targeted safety interventions more effectively.

This direction aligns with broader efforts in safety science to leverage artificial intelligence (AI) for pattern recognition, predictive modeling, and adaptive training environments, ultimately contributing to more robust safety management systems within high-risk professions, such as firefighting.

Establishing the Best Practices for HFACS Integration in the Fire Service

Despite its demonstrated utility, HFACS remains underutilized in routine fire service operations. The future should include the formal integration of HFACS into after-action reviews, training programs, and strategic planning processes. The best practices should draw from system-based accident analyses such as those applied to the Tianjin Port explosion (Zhang et al., 2018) which used HFACS alongside AcciMap and STAMP to provide a multilayered understanding of causation. These comparative analyses highlight HFACS's strength in practice; its structured taxonomy allows for repeatable and transparent investigations, which are critical for both operational learning and institutional accountability.

To further embed HFACS, agencies should adopt cross-sector strategies from maritime, chemical, and offshore industries, where the system is increasingly paired with Bayesian networks, fuzzy logic, and other advanced tools to model uncertainty and causal probability (Ma et al., 2022; Gordon et al., 2005).

Bridging Human Factors, Psychology, and Systems Thinking

Together, these emerging directions reflect a necessary shift toward bridging psychological insights, organizational dynamics, and systems-level safety engineering. To address chronic stress and fatigue (Orosa et al., 2011) or foster a climate of active leadership and accountability (Smith et al., 2023), human factors must be considered both operational and cultural priorities. Only by developing holistic, data-driven safety strategies can fire departments keep pace with the evolving risks of modern emergency services.

As fire service organizations increasingly face complex hazards, constrained resources, and dynamic operational environments, integrating HFACS into a broader, forward-thinking safety framework is imperative for health, safety, and longevity.

Chapter Review

Assignment: Applying Human Factors Analysis in Fire Service Safety

Designing a Human Factors–Informed Strategy for Fireground Safety Improvement

Assignment Overview (2500–3000 words)

Act as a human factors consultant for a fire department seeking to reduce firefighter injuries. Using this chapter and the HFACS model, evaluate current investigative practices, apply theoretical insights, and propose interventions to enhance safety culture and operational effectiveness.

Assignment Components

1. Literature Synthesis (20%)

   (a) Compare traditional Root Cause Analysis with human factors approaches (e.g., HFACS, Swiss Cheese Model).
   (b) Briefly trace the evolution from Skinner's behaviorism to systems-based psychology.
   (c) Explain why a multidisciplinary approach is essential in fire service safety.

2. HFACS Case Mapping (25%)

Choose a real or realistic incident and analyze it using HFACS.

Identify:

   (a) Unsafe acts
   (b) Preconditions for errors
   (c) Supervisory failures
   (d) Organizational factors
   (e) Describe how systemic variables contributed to the outcome.

3. Behavioral & Cultural Analysis (20%)
   (a) Explain how reinforcement, identity, and fire service culture shape risk-taking and decision-making.
   (b) Discuss barriers that impact behavioral accountability within the fire service context.
   (c) Suggest one method (e.g., behavioral audit) to assess the department's cultural norms.
4. Intervention Plan (25%)
Propose a practical, multilevel intervention strategy:
   (a) Organizational (e.g., SOP changes)
   (b) Supervisory (e.g., CRM training)
   (c) Individual (e.g., fatigue/resilience support)
   (d) Investigative (e.g., HFACS in post-incident reviews)
5. Ethical and Cultural Considerations (10%)
   (a) Address ethical and political challenges in applying human factors analysis, especially when fatalities occur.
   (b) How can departments balance honoring firefighters with promoting learning and change?

Formatting
   (a) Word count: 2500–3000
   (b) APA 7 format
   (c) Use at least 8 academic references

Chapter 9
Suicide in the Fire Service and the Role of Psychological Autopsies for Prevention

Understanding the underlying causes of firefighter suicides requires careful, in-depth investigation, and psychological autopsies offer an important method for doing so. These structured inquiries reveal that the complex interplay of mental health struggles, cultural pressures, and organizational factors contributes to suicide risk among firefighters. Firefighters face distinct challenges, including elevated rates of posttraumatic stress disorder (PTSD), sleep disturbances, and access to firearms, all of which increase vulnerability to suicide. Despite national advocacy for improved mental health services in fire and emergency services (Jahnke et al., 2012*), there is currently no dedicated psychological autopsy program designed specifically for firefighters. Implementing such a program would provide valuable data to guide evidence-based interventions, promote early detection of at-risk individuals, and strengthen mental health support within the fire service, ultimately aiming to reduce suicide rates among firefighters.*

Conceptualization of Suicide

Suicide is a deliberate act taken by an individual to end their own life, and it occurs within a complex web of interacting biological, psychological, social, and cultural factors (Turecki & Brent, 2016). Cultural norms significantly influence both the prevalence and methods of suicide. For example, suicide by firearms is more common in countries where guns are widely accessible, whereas in nations with stricter firearm regulations, alternative means are more prevalent (Florentine & Crane, 2010).

The language surrounding suicide is also critical and has become increasingly scrutinized within academic and clinical communities. Using terms such as "committed suicide" may imply criminality or immorality, thereby reinforcing stigma and potentially contributing to negative public perceptions of both the deceased and those struggling with suicidal ideation (Silverman, 2006). In response, mental

K. Wheldon, *Fire Service Psychology*,
https://doi.org/10.1007/978-3-032-02126-7_9

health advocates and researchers encourage the use of alternatives such as "died by suicide" to shift the narrative toward understanding suicide as a public health concern rather than a moral failure (Silverman, 2006).

However, framing suicide purely as the inevitable result of mental illness carries risks. Conceptualizing suicide as an uncontrollable consequence of pathology may inadvertently diminish individuals' perceived agency and resilience, potentially fostering a sense of helplessness among those experiencing suicidal thoughts (O'Connor & Kirtley, 2018). This highlights the importance of maintaining a nuanced perspective that recognizes the profound suffering underlying suicidal behavior while preserving a person's capacity for agency and recovery.

Suicide as a Line of Duty Death

Amid growing concerns about the mental health crisis among first responders, recent federal policy initiatives have expanded support for cases involving suicide within the first responder community. In 2022, the Biden Administration extended the Public Safety Officers' Benefits (PSOB) Program to include deaths by suicide, provided that suicide was the direct result of duty-related trauma, such as posttraumatic stress disorder (PTSD) or acute stress disorder. While this policy change represents an important step in acknowledging the psychological sacrifices of public safety personnel, it also introduces potential ethical concerns. Specifically, there is a risk of unintentionally valorizing suicide by equating it with deaths incurred during acts of physical bravery, potentially reinforcing dangerous narratives around PTSD and martyrdom (Stanley et al., 2016b).

Such framing may distort public and organizational understanding of PTSD, mistakenly portraying it as a "badge of honor" rather than recognizing it as a chronic condition characterized by persistent hyperactivation of the sympathetic nervous system (Shalev et al., 2024). Effective treatment for PTSD targets this maladaptive fear-based conditioning through approaches such as prolonged exposure therapy, cognitive processing therapy, and counterconditioning techniques.

Labeling suicide as a line-of-duty death introduces a complicated risk, the normalization of deviance (Vaughan, 1996). Suicide is typically excluded from major insurance policies because it is viewed legally and ethically as an intentional act. While firefighters and EMS personnel experience elevated exposure to potentially traumatic events, which increases vulnerability to posttraumatic stress (Berger et al., 2012), suicide itself is understood as a behavioral outcome influenced by a complex interplay of risk and protective factors, including mental health, social support, impulsivity, and cognitive distortions (Klonsky et al., 2016). These factors may impair judgment, but suicide remains, fundamentally, a decision. Framing it as a line-of-duty death risks oversimplifying this reality and may unintentionally shift cultural norms around accountability and prevention within the fire service.

Under the Public Safety Officer Support Act of 2022, a public safety officer's death by suicide may qualify for public safety officers' benefits (PSOB) if specific criteria are met. First, the officer should have been exposed to one or more traumatic events while on duty. A traumatic event is defined as experiencing or witnessing a homicide, suicide, violent or gruesome death, a harrowing circumstance posing extraordinary danger to life or serious bodily harm, or an act of criminal sexual violence (Public Safety Officer Support Act of 2022, n.d.).

Second, the officer should have developed posttraumatic stress disorder (PTSD), acute stress disorder, or another trauma and stress-related disorder, diagnosed by a licensed medical or mental health professional. The law presumes that such disorders are personal injuries sustained in the line of duty if the exposure is a substantial factor in causing the disorder.

In cases of suicide, the officer must have taken an action intended to bring about their death, and it should be demonstrated that duty-related traumatic exposure directly and proximately caused this action. If suicide occurs within 45 days of the traumatic event, there should also be evidence that the action was not inconsistent with a psychiatric disorder. If suicide occurs more than 45 days after exposure, it should still be shown that traumatic exposure is a substantial factor in the officer's decision to act.

Additionally, the law and PSOB guidance state that intentional actions and substance use do not automatically disqualify eligibility in suicide cases, provided the statutory criteria are otherwise met and duty-related traumatic exposure is shown to be a substantial factor. (Public Safety Officer Support Act of 2022, n.d.).

Given the complexities of trauma-related suicides, due diligence should be applied to demonstrate a clear and supported link between occupational trauma exposure and suicide before classifying such deaths as line-of-duty deaths. While this change represents a significant step in acknowledging the psychological risks inherent to public safety work, the PSOB maintains a high evidentiary standard. Detailed documentation, clinical evidence, and a clear linkage between duty-related trauma and suicide are all needed to meet the program's strict guidelines (Bureau of Justice Assistance, 2022).

Psychological Autopsies Data on Other Populations

Psychological autopsies provide valuable insights into the complex dynamics that lead to suicide. These investigations examine sociocultural factors, mental health challenges, operational dynamics, and organizational issues that influence suicide risk across different populations (Pouliot & De Leo, 2006). Findings from psychological autopsy studies emphasize the need to tailor suicide prevention efforts to the specific needs of distinct groups.

Despite calls for improved mental health initiatives in fire and emergency services, there is currently no psychological autopsy program dedicated to understanding the specific factors contributing to firefighter suicide. Although suicide was formally recognized as a potential line-of-duty death in 2022, the field still lacks a system with the specificity needed to guide effective prevention strategies (Stanley et al., 2016a, 2016b). Implementing a psychological autopsy system tailored to fire and emergency services would strengthen suicide prevention and intervention efforts by providing better data on risk factors specific to firefighters.

Compared with the general population, firefighters face increased risks for PTSD and suicidal ideation (Healy & Vujanovic, 2021; Stanley et al., 2019). Sleep disturbances further contribute to this risk, and systemic operational practices related to shift work often prevent adequate sleep. Research shows that aspects of sleep quality, such as sleep efficiency and perceived sleep disruption, moderate the relationship between PTSD symptoms and suicide risk, highlighting the importance of addressing sleep issues (Healy & Vujanovic, 2021).

Firearm ownership and unsafe storage practices are also relevant concerns within fire and emergency services, increasing the potential for firearm-related suicides (Stanley et al., 2024). Promoting secure firearm storage represents a necessary step toward reducing this risk (Robison et al., 2025). Furthermore, interorganizational collaboration can play a critical role in enhancing suicide prevention by ensuring that multiple agencies work from shared frameworks. Research in Sweden has shown that when fire services, police, ambulance personnel, and municipal actors adopt joint intervention plans and maintain open channels for cooperation, the result is faster mobilization, greater trust among professionals, and more coordinated use of resources during crises. These collaborative structures—ranging from common action plans to interagency working groups—enable communication to flow more effectively across organizational boundaries, which in turn supports timely and coordinated responses to suicidal crises and strengthens post-incident support for affected individuals and families (Hedman, 2023).

With regard to specific at risk groups, compared with their male counterparts, female firefighters may face different stressors and report higher rates of suicidal ideation, suggesting the need for specialized support services (Hom et al., 2018). Additionally, exposure to traumatic events throughout a firefighting career has been associated with higher rates of mental health symptoms and suicidal thoughts, reinforcing the importance of early detection and targeted intervention (Herzog et al., 2023). Developing population specific strategies (even sub populations), may enhance suicide prevention and intervention strategies.

Mindfulness-based practices may help reduce suicide risk among firefighters by moderating the effects of PTSD symptoms, and these strategies could be considered alongside other evidence-based approaches (Stanley et al., 2019). However, more research is needed to explore how organizational dynamics, such as perceived betrayal or institutional failure, might contribute to suicide risk within this population.

International studies offer additional insights. Psychological autopsies conducted in Nepal identified poverty, lack of education, family conflict, and gender-based violence as prominent factors (Hagaman et al., 2018). In Australia, research focused on LGBTQ populations has revealed that internalized homophobia, a lack of acceptance, and early experiences are significant contributors to suicide risk (Skerrett et al., 2012). In rural China, chronic illnesses such as cancer and stroke are strongly associated with suicide, underscoring the need to integrate suicide prevention with healthcare services (Mo et al., 2020).

In military populations, psychological autopsies help identify factors such as traumatic brain injury (TBI), relationship stress, and substance abuse as contributors to suicide, providing important information for developing prevention programs (Litz & Gray, 2002). Correctional settings have also benefited from psychological autopsy studies, which have identified operational shortcomings and gaps in mental health care as factors linked to inmate suicides (Skerrett et al., 2012).

Conducting psychological autopsies requires trained mental health professionals with expertise in forensic assessment. These investigations typically involve reviewing medical and mental health records, interviewing key informants, and reconstructing the decedent's psychological state prior to death (Pouliot & De Leo, 2006). Data collected through psychological autopsies can support the development of population-specific risk assessment tools that evolve in response to changes in identified risk factors.

Given the known challenges facing firefighters, including trauma exposure, sleep disruption, firearm access, and systemic occupational stress, developing a National Psychological Autopsy Program (NPAP) for fire and emergency services would strengthen efforts to prevent suicide. A tailored program would provide the empirical foundation needed for early intervention, policy development, and improved support for firefighters and EMS professionals.

Research on Suicide in the Fire Service

Suicide within fire and emergency services is an increasingly recognized but still under-researched issue, with underreporting further complicating accurate understanding (Henderson et al., 2016). Firefighters experience elevated suicide risk due to high rates of posttraumatic stress disorder (PTSD) and substance abuse. However, mental health providers face challenges in addressing these concerns because of limited empirical research and cultural stigma within the profession (Henderson et al., 2016). Low reporting rates, the absence of a national tracking database, and a lack of firefighter-specific assessment tools contribute to widespread misunderstanding of both suicide attempts and completed suicides among this population (Henderson et al., 2016).

Research has identified specific risk factors that exacerbate vulnerability among firefighters. Histories of physical or sexual abuse are significant predictors of suicidality; among a sample of 309 firefighters, 45.9% reported career suicide ideation, 18.3% reported suicide planning, and 14.6% reported suicide attempts, with significant percentages experiencing depression and severe PTSD symptoms (Hom et al., 2015). Cumulative exposure to suicide attempts and deaths has also been linked to increased suicidal behavior; firefighters reported an average of 13.1 such exposures, and those with 12 or more were significantly more likely to screen positive for suicide risk (Kimbrel et al., 2016).

Subgroup differences in suicide risk within the fire and emergency services have emerged as a critical area of inquiry. Compared with their nonwildland peers, wildland firefighters report greater suicide risk, with thwarted belongingness rather than perceived burdensomeness, statistically explaining the association (Stanley et al., 2018). Enhancing social connectedness may be a promising avenue for suicide prevention efforts within this subgroup (Stanley et al., 2019).

Additionally, firefighters from specific demographic groups face disproportionately high suicide risk. American Indian/Alaskan Native (AI/AN) firefighters were found to be 16.31 times more likely to report a career suicide attempt than their non-AI/AN counterparts were, with exposure to painful and provocative events identified as a significant mediator of this increased risk (Stanley et al., 2020). Among women firefighters, suicide rates are also notably high, with precareer and career suicidal ideation and attempts significantly associated with psychiatric symptoms and occupational harassment.

Moral injury, a construct traditionally associated with military populations, is increasingly considered a relevant factor in first responder suicides, including among firefighters. Moral injury refers to emotional, psychological, and spiritual distress arising from actions that violate deeply held moral beliefs. The evidence suggests that greater exposure to morally injurious events is significantly linked to increased suicide risk, highlighting the need for research beyond military samples to include first responders (Jamieson et al., 2023).

Recent studies further underscore the urgent need for structured suicide prevention and postvention strategies in fire and emergency services. The suicide postvention guidelines developed for fire and emergency services aim to support survivors and mitigate the risk of further adverse outcomes following suicide death (Gulliver et al., 2016, 2023). Moreover, the COVID-19 pandemic has been associated with an increase in suicide attempts among the general public, including cases attended by fire departments, emphasizing the ongoing relevance of firefighters' roles in suicide response and the risks they may face themselves (de Almeida et al., 2022).

Injury and the recovery process have also been shown to impact firefighters' mental health and potential suicide risk. Barriers such as communication breakdowns, lack of confidence in returning to operational duties, and detachment from teams ("watches") have been identified as critical psychosocial factors influencing successful recovery and return to work (Noll et al., 2022). Consistency in support processes is critical to promoting firefighter wellness during recovery, which could, in turn, reduce long-term mental health risks, including suicidality (Noll et al., 2022).

Collectively, these findings demonstrate that firefighter suicide is a multifaceted issue influenced by personal history, cumulative occupational exposure, social connectedness, and organizational support structures. Targeted, evidence-based interventions that consider demographic differences, subgroup vulnerabilities, and broader constructs, such as moral injury, are necessary to address this growing public health concern within fire and emergency services.

What Psychological Autopsy Data from Other Populations Could Teach Us About Firefighter Suicide?

Psychological autopsies have provided important insights into suicide risk across various populations, often revealing factors that traditional research methods overlook. Applying lessons from these investigations to fire and emergency services could significantly expand our understanding of firefighter suicides beyond what is currently captured through epidemiological studies and retrospective analyses.

Psychological autopsies offer a multidimensional view of suicide, assessing psychiatric diagnoses alongside sociocultural influences, organizational dynamics, and interpersonal stressors (Pouliot & De Leo, 2006). Unlike survey-based studies, which often narrowly focus on PTSD or depression, psychological autopsies can reveal underexplored factors specific to fire and emergency services, such as perceived betrayal by leadership, institutional failure, or social isolation, issues suggested in existing firefighter mental health research but not yet systematically studied (Healy & Vujanovic, 2021; Stanley et al., 2019).

Findings from military psychological autopsies demonstrate that moral injury, feelings of guilt, shame, and anger after the violation of personal moral codes are potent predictors of suicide risk (Jamieson et al., 2023; Litz & Gray, 2002). Firefighting often demands rapid, high-stakes decisions under traumatic conditions, making moral injury a likely, although underinvestigated, contributor to suicide within the fire service. Psychological autopsies could illuminate the true prevalence and impact of moral injury among firefighters, offering a new dimension for prevention efforts.

Psychological autopsy studies from international civilian populations reveal how suicide risk varies across cultural and contextual factors, including poverty, family conflict, and systemic discrimination (Hagaman et al., 2018; Mo et al., 2020; Skerrett et al., 2012). Similar dynamics may affect subgroups within U.S. fire and emergency services, such as American Indian/Alaskan Native firefighters and women, who face disproportionate suicide risk due to systemic and cultural stressors (Stanley et al., 2020). Tailoring psychological autopsy protocols to firefighters could better capture how identity-related stressors, including minority status and gender-based discrimination within the firehouse, contribute to suicide risk.

Operational and organizational contributors to suicide risk are also critical to investigate. Factors such as chronic sleep deprivation, unsafe firearm storage practices, and cumulative exposure to traumatic events have been individually linked to increased suicide risk among firefighters (Healy & Vujanovic, 2021; Robison et al., 2025). Psychological autopsies could move beyond examining isolated factors to explore how these risks accumulate and interact over time, thereby increasing vulnerability.

Studies from other high-risk occupations further reinforce these insights. In the military, psychological autopsies have identified cumulative trauma, traumatic brain injuries, relational strain, and organizational stigma surrounding mental health as major suicide risk factors (USSOCOM, 2017). These parallels are striking compared with the experiences of firefighters. Research on correctional officers shows that chronic occupational stress, exposure to violence, and institutional barriers to mental healthcare are major contributors to suicide, mirroring the organizational challenges experienced in fire and emergency services (Stack & Tsoudis, 1997). Similarly, in healthcare populations, compassion fatigue, moral distress, and prolonged exposure to suffering have been associated with increased suicide risk (Davidson et al., 2020), a pattern also observed among firefighters who are routinely exposed to death and serious injury.

By systematically integrating psychological autopsy findings from diverse occupational groups, fire and emergency services can better identify critical risk factors, including trauma exposure, organizational culture, relational strain, and systemic barriers to accessing care. Psychological autopsies not only enhance the understanding of suicide risk but also directly inform prevention strategies, fostering organizational change grounded in empirical evidence.

Additionally, psychological autopsy investigations could generate firefighter-specific risk profiles and inform the development of tailored prevention programs. Current initiatives often adapt to the general population or military-based models, which may fail to fully address the unique operational realities and cultural dynamics of firefighting. Insights from psychological autopsies could drive the development of specialized postvention protocols (Gulliver et al., 2016, 2023) and mental health interventions specifically designed for fire and emergency services.

While existing firefighter suicide research has revealed important correlates such as PTSD, substance abuse, and cumulative trauma exposure (Henderson et al., 2016; Kimbrel et al., 2016; Hom et al., 2015), psychological autopsies could reveal deeper, hidden patterns, and underappreciated risk factors. Establishing a National Psychological Autopsy Program (NPAP) specifically for firefighters would bridge critical knowledge gaps, strengthen early detection efforts, and support meaningful systemic reforms to reduce suicide rates within the profession.

Steps in Psychological Autopsy

Psychological autopsy is a structured method for reconstructing the psychosocial circumstances leading to an individual's death, particularly when suicide is suspected. Although various models exist, the core steps consistently supported in peer-reviewed literature include (1) collecting all available case records, such as medical, psychiatric, and legal documents; (2) conducting structured interviews with family members, friends, coworkers, and healthcare providers; (3) assessing the individual's mental health status, coping mechanisms, and exposure to psychosocial stressors; (4) analyzing circumstances surrounding the death to determine intent; and (5) synthesizing all findings into a comprehensive case formulation (Cavanagh et al., 2003; Pouliot & De Leo, 2006).

While peers can play a valuable role in supporting mental health initiatives within the fire service, assigning them to conduct psychological autopsies presents significant ethical and clinical challenges. Psychological autopsies require a high level of expertise in trauma-informed interviewing, forensic analysis, and clinical judgment to piece together the complex interplay of psychological, social, and environmental factors that may have contributed to a suicide. Peers, despite their lived experience and good intentions, are not trained to navigate the nuanced ethical boundaries, confidentiality standards, and potential re-traumatization risks involved in such investigations. Involving them in this capacity may inadvertently cause harm to themselves and to the bereaved by reinforcing inaccurate narratives or misinterpreting sensitive psychological data. For these reasons, psychological autopsies are best conducted by licensed mental health professionals with specialized training in suicide assessment and postvention, who can ensure the process is clinically sound, ethically managed, and trauma-informed.

Conclusion

In our society, suicide is a leading cause of death. It causes devastation to families, friends, workplaces, and communities. According to the American Psychological Association (APA), suicide is defined as the act of killing oneself (American Psychological Association, 2023). While this problem continues to persist across the country, there is particular concern within our fire service community about how factors within the job (specifically, exposure to potentially traumatic events) can impact suicide rates among the population (Berger et al., 2012; Bartlett et al., 2018).

Regrettably, no national database or psychological autopsy program has been established to identify specific risk and protective factors unique to firefighter and emergency medical provider groups (Bartlett & Schmitz, 2023). As such, we speculate. In our efforts to understand this issue, there is a common assumption that the job itself can cause suicide.

Suicide occurs when a person decides to end their life and takes action to fulfill the intention. As psychologists know, behavior is an outcome of underlying beliefs, thoughts, and emotions, which ultimately translate into specific actions (Benight & Bandura, 2004). Many factors may influence belief systems, thought processes, and emotional experiences, including trauma history, workplace stressors, and perceived lack of alternatives (Behnke et al., 2020).

In our attempt to understand this phenomenon, we should be careful not to assume that the job caused the suicide. Variables within the job can increase risk, whereas others can serve as protective factors (Berger et al., 2012). Some may tie suicide to the job as a way of refraining from moral judgment about the behavior, as if to say it was something beyond their control. To preserve the deceased's reputation, we might inadvertently send the wrong message. If suicide is seen as being beyond one's control, one becomes helpless to change the outcome. Helplessness can increase risk when an individual is vulnerable and may believe that they do not have any other options (Benight & Bandura, 2004; Arbona et al., 2016).

The moral dilemma of how to respect the deceased without reinforcing the behavior of suicide is a challenge for anyone confronted with the aftermath of suicide. Notably, major fire service stakeholders advocated including suicide as a line-of-duty death in 2022 without consulting the American Psychological Association or the American Psychiatric Association to explore how that action may or may not increase suicide rates within the fire service (Bartlett & Schmitz, 2023).

People who have died by suicide may not believe that they have had another option. Our job is to raise ambivalence and connect them with appropriate resources, including mental health professionals, who can assist them in reorganizing the underlying belief system that leads them to view suicide as the only way to address the psychic pain they are currently experiencing (Benight & Bandura, 2004; Arbona et al., 2016). Let us show our respect to the person who lived without reinforcing the way they died. It is important to do both.

Chapter Review

Assignment: Suicide Prevention in the Fire Service Through Psychological Autopsies

Assignment Overview (2500–3000 words)

You are advising the US Fire Administration through a national task force exploring the development of a National Psychological Autopsy Program (NPAP) for fire and emergency services. Your role is to synthesize psychological theories, suicide prevention research, and operational realities to produce a clear strategy for implementation, education, and ethical messaging within the fire service.

Assignment Components

1. Conceptual Foundations of Firefighter Suicide (20%)
   (a) Summarize the multifactorial model of suicide, including psychological, cultural, and occupational components.
   (b) Critically analyze the pros and cons of framing suicide as a line-of-duty death.
   (c) Explain how this framing can influence stigma, help-seeking, and cultural norms.

2. Application of Psychological Autopsies (25%)
   (a) Explain what psychological autopsies are, how they work, and how they differ from traditional postvention methods.
   (b) Propose a plan for how a fire service-specific psychological autopsy program could be designed and implemented.
   (c) Address training needs, protocols, and the kind of data it should collect.
3. Risk and Protective Factors (20%)
   (a) Identify the most salient fire service-specific risk and protective factors (e.g., PTSD, sleep disruption, firearm access, moral injury, family, peer support, etc).
   (b) Discuss demographic subgroup vulnerabilities (e.g., female, AI/AN, and wildland firefighters).
   (c) Propose targeted prevention strategies informed by psychological theory and empirical evidence.
4. Ethical and Organizational Considerations (20%)
   (a) Reflect on the ethical tensions in post-suicide communication, such as honoring the deceased without normalizing suicide.
   (b) Discuss institutional barriers to suicide prevention (e.g., stigma, policy inertia, and legal risk).
   (c) Propose messaging and leadership strategies to support a healthy organizational climate around mental health.
5. Integration and Prevention Framework (15%)
   (a) Design a brief model integrating psychological autopsy findings into existing prevention, intervention, and postvention efforts.
   (b) Include data feedback loops, training, leadership engagement, and evaluation methods.

Formatting Guidelines

- Word count: 2500–3000 words
- APA 7 citation format
- Include at least 8 scholarly references (beyond the chapter)

Learning Goals

- Apply psychological theory to complex occupational mental health issues
- Evaluate the role of institutional policy and ethics in suicide postvention
- Propose actionable strategies grounded in empirical and cultural realities

Chapter 10
Occupational Trauma Risk Management in the Fire Service

Trauma exposure is an inherent part of fire service work, but the psychological consequences are not uniform, nor are they always immediately visible. While many firefighters demonstrate remarkable resilience, a significant subset experiences lingering distress, moral conflict, and mental health challenges, which, if unaddressed, can escalate into clinically substantial conditions such as posttraumatic stress disorder (PTSD), depression, or even suicide. Traditional models of intervention have often emphasized acute care or diagnostic labeling; however, contemporary trauma risk management requires a more nuanced, preventative, and culturally informed approach. The fire and emergency service professions should embrace a multidimensional framework for supporting firefighter mental health, emphasizing the integration of peer support, psychological triage, and trauma-informed leadership. Drawing from evidence-based strategies such as Trauma Risk Management (TRiM) within a Psychological First Aid (PFA) model, fire departments can promote adaptive recovery without overpathologizing natural stress responses. Additionally, it confronts more complex psychological phenomena, such as moral injury and organizational betrayal, which often underlie unrecognized suffering and resistance to help-seeking. By examining the intersections of stress physiology, behavioral health outcomes, and occupational culture, there are practical and ethical processes of building systems that not only respond to trauma but also prevent it from becoming a silent burden.

Peer Support Team Development

Firefighters, by and large, are remarkably resilient and typically do not require clinical intervention after every potentially traumatic incident. Instead of defaulting to pathologize natural recovery, systems that can identify when someone does require clinical support may be needed. Psychological triage comes in here, and it could be

K. Wheldon, *Fire Service Psychology*,
https://doi.org/10.1007/978-3-032-02126-7_10

a core part of firefighter training. Psychological triage could emphasize an understanding of how posttraumatic stress symptoms emerge and evolve, incorporating knowledge of PTSD development and the various factors that contribute to increased risk. Research has identified several variables, such as prior trauma exposure, cumulative stress, and especially alcohol use (Jakupcak et al., 2010), moral distress (Litz et al., 2009), lack of social support (Ozer et al., 2003), and emotional suppression (Gross & John, 2003). Significantly heighten the likelihood of acute stress responses progressing into diagnosable PTSD (Berger et al., 2012; Marmar et al., 2006). Integrating these insights into triage practices enables more targeted and informed peer support, as well as timely clinical intervention when necessary. When peer support teams are trained in this way, they are not only able to walk alongside someone through the normal recovery process but also better equipped to recognize when a situation is outside their scope and requires a clinical referral. Clarity is important for protecting both the firefighter and the integrity of the peer support team.

In recent years, fire and emergency services have made important cultural strides, PTSD and suicide are no longer taboo topics, and we are seeing more open dialog around behavioral health. Peer support and critical incident stress management (CISM) teams have helped move the needle, but they are not enough in regard to addressing PTSD in a sustained, clinically informed way. Firefighters have elevated PTSD rates relative to the general population (Berger, 2012). One model that has shown real promise is Trauma Risk Management (TRiM), initially developed by the British Armed Forces. TRiM is effective because it aligns with the body's natural recovery process while also encouraging timely access to psychological care without jumping straight to pathologizing normal reactions to trauma (Greenberg et al., 2015). Studies have shown that TRiM reduces both PTSD symptoms and the stigma associated with seeking help, especially in high-risk occupations such as military and law enforcement (Jones et al., 2017; Greenberg et al., 2015). Given its established utility, TRiM is a relevant model for the incorporation of fire and emergency services into its behavioral health framework.

The fire service, as a whole, has not traditionally emphasized soft skills such as active listening, de-escalation, or emotional regulation, which are crucial in behavioral health work. While specific specialized roles, such as SWAT medics or behavioral health units, may receive this type of training, it is not the norm across the profession (Klimley et al., 2018). If we are aware of the need to integrate a model such as Trauma Risk Management (TRiM) into fire and emergency services, soft skills training must first be provided. Training could start with helping members understand the distinctions between morals, ethics, and values. When a firefighter turns to peer support following a potentially traumatic event, the peer team member should be able to stay grounded, recognizing when their own moral or emotional responses are being activated so that they do not lose effectiveness in their role (Dean et al., 2019). Understanding that not everyone shares the same value system is important. If someone is emotionally reactive, they often reveal something core about their values, not just the content of the trauma. It does not require the peer support member's job to change or challenge but rather to recognize it, validate it, and use ethical grounding to respond appropriately. When signs of moral distress or moral injury emerge, peer support members need to know when it is time to seek clinical support (Williamson et al., 2020).

Trust is foundational to the function of any peer support team. In fire and emergency services, trust is not a vague concept; it is often broken down into specific dimensions that firefighters intuitively recognize, even if they do not always label them formally. One practical framework distinguishes between character and competence (Mayer et al., 1995). Character involves both intent and integrity. Intent encompasses qualities such as caring, openness, and transparency, whereas integrity is rooted in fairness, honesty, and authenticity.

On the other hand, competence refers to both the capability and the results achieved. Capability includes skills, training, and experience, whereas results are related to reputation, credibility, and past performance (Dirks & Ferrin, 2002). Research on fire and emergency services suggests that firefighters make these exact distinctions when discussing trust. When someone says that they "trust" a peer, there is often a follow-up question: "Trust them with what?" This concept highlights that trust is not one-size-fits-all; it is situational and built on both who the person is and what they can do (Adams et al., 2004).

To provide adequate peer support within any team, maintaining a clear understanding of professional boundaries is important. While these boundaries may seem less pressing in professions where team members live, work, and eat together, peer support should still be held to a higher standard of ethics. This concept is fundamental because individuals may share some of the most vulnerable aspects of their lives in these interactions (Corey et al., 2011).

Boundaries reflect both the formal role of peer support within the department and the informal dynamics of the team itself. One critical factor is rank, which can significantly influence interpersonal relationships. For example, a firefighter may hesitate to disclose their struggles following a traumatic event to someone in a leadership position, particularly if a person plays a role in promotions or fitness-for-duty evaluations. In such cases, the peer support relationship lacks true peer-to-peer equality, which can hinder trust and openness (SAMHSA, 2015).

These relationships can also become complicated if either the supporter or the recipient changes roles within the department. A shift in rank or responsibility can lead to concerns about bias or the perception of bias, which may erode trust or professionalism.

Additionally, the concept of overfamiliarity should be taken seriously. It may be unethical for someone to provide peer support to a close friend, especially since they may become emotionally invested in the situation. In such cases, personal closeness can compromise objectivity and create unintended emotional entanglements. Overfamiliarity becomes even more concerning when it involves sexual contact between peer support team members. Such interactions introduce severe power imbalances that can lead to perceived or actual exploitation, conflicts of interest, or breaches of trust. These dynamics not only jeopardize the emotional safety of those receiving support but also undermine the integrity of the peer support program as a whole. The presence of sexual involvement between team members may be viewed as unethical, potentially exploitative, and deeply unprofessional (Corey et al., 2011).

Ultimately, peer support programs should be built on ethical foundations, with careful attention given to boundaries, rank dynamics, and the potential pitfalls of overly personal or romantic relationships. Organizations could provide clear policies, ethics training, and supervisory support to help peer supporters navigate these complex interpersonal dynamics effectively (National Institutes of Health, 2023).

In any operational setting, we recognize that specific skills are perishable and that peer support is no different. Core competencies, such as active listening and strategic thinking, can fade without consistent practice and reinforcement. Peer support teams must also be intentional about managing internal dynamics, particularly bias and potential conflicts of interest, which can quietly undermine effectiveness if left unaddressed (Everly et al., 2014). Like any functioning team, there needs to be a clear framework for measuring performance. However, those metrics must extend beyond surface-level data, such as contact hours or the number of people seen. An analogy would be measuring the effectiveness of a fitness program by only counting attendance without looking at changes in weight, fitness goals, improved stamina, or lifting abilities. Meaningful performance indicators reflect whether the team is genuinely helping people move forward. Additionally, peer support programs should plan for sustainability through structured recruitment and succession planning. Without a system in place onboard and retaining qualified members, a team's longevity and credibility can be compromised (Woodman et al., 2021).

Peer support teams could implement a clear and transparent informed consent process. While peer support is not a form of clinical treatment, it often involves sensitive disclosures and emotional vulnerability. As such, individuals engaging with peer support should understand what the interaction entails and what it does not. This responsibility entails clarifying that peer supporters are not licensed therapists and that the support being offered is nonclinical (Solomon, 2004; Chinman et al., 2014).

The informed consent process could address several important components:

- ***Training:*** Defining the scope and limitations of the training that peer support team members have received is essential, as this contributes to trust and role clarity (Repper & Carter, 2011).
- ***Potential Conflicts of Interest:*** In tight-knit environments such as fire departments, being transparent about dual relationships or overlapping roles can help reduce bias and improve team functioning (Davidson et al., 2012).
- ***Appropriate Referrals:*** Informed consent should highlight that peer support is not a substitute for clinical care and should outline the referral process to mental health professionals when symptoms exceed the scope of peer support (Gidugu et al., 2015).
- ***Time:*** Clear boundaries around availability and interaction length help maintain role expectations and avoid burnout for peer supporters (Salzer, 2002).
- ***Confidentiality and Its Limitations:*** Individuals could be informed about what remains private and what should be disclosed, particularly in cases of harm to

themselves or others, which is consistent with ethical frameworks (SAMHSA, 2015).

Establishing informed consent in peer support protects both the individual seeking help and the peer supporter while reinforcing ethical boundaries and setting appropriate expectations.

Building an effective referral base goes far beyond pulling names from a list. It requires a deliberate investment in understanding the quality and fit of the mental health resources available in the community. Factors such as provider competency, cultural fit, accessibility, and responsiveness all play a role in determining whether a referral is applicable (SAMHSA, 2015). In many cases, particularly in rural or underserved areas, there are often limited behavioral health options. It is not enough to dismiss an Employee Assistance Program (EAP) as inadequate if it is the only local resource, especially if the main issue is that providers lack cultural competency or familiarity with the fire service context. Instead of walking away from those services, peer support teams and fire service leaders can choose to invest in them, engage with providers, offer education on firefighter culture, and help them grow professionally. Development of a foundation now creates a more robust, culturally attuned network of support for the future.

Firefighters often hear the word "stress" and immediately associate it with something negative. However, not all stress is harmful. What is often overlooked is the distinction between eustress (positive, performance-enhancing stress) and distress (debilitating stress) and how the brain's cognitive appraisal determines which of the two we experience (Lazarus & Folkman, 1984). When the mind perceives a situation as a threat, the sympathetic nervous system kicks in, activating the body's survival response. This fight-or-flight mode prioritizes immediate physical readiness over cognitive processes, such as impulse control, decision-making, and problem-solving (McEwen, 2007; Thayer & Lane, 2000).

Understanding the physiology of stress can help firefighters effectively regulate their responses in real time. By learning and practicing arousal control techniques, such as controlled breathing, mindfulness, and reframing through intentional cognitive appraisal, they can shift from the reactive survival mode to a more focused and effective state (Merrigan et al., 2023). Additionally, becoming aware of early-learned coping strategies allows firefighters to evaluate whether their responses are helpful or harmful and choose healthier, proactive methods instead (Compas et al., 2001). Training in these areas not only boosts performance but also builds psychological resilience over time.

Through training, firefighters can begin to recognize various behavioral health outcomes as byproducts of multiple factors, including substance abuse, relationship conflict, absenteeism, interpersonal violence, workplace conflict, workplace violence, risk-taking behavior, relationship satisfaction, job satisfaction, gambling addiction, sexual addiction, gaming addiction, and even opportunities for growth and wisdom. Research indicates that individuals at increased risk for behavioral addictions, including gambling, sex addiction, and internet use, often experience co-occurring issues with substance abuse and other mental health disorders (İzci et al., 2022).

Behavior is the result of underlying thoughts, emotional processes, and cognitive decision-making mechanisms. The somatic marker hypothesis, for example, posits that motions play a critical role in guiding decisions by linking bodily responses with expected outcomes (Bechara et al., 2000). Furthermore, emotions significantly influence cognitive evaluations and the selection of behavior, especially in high-stress professions such as firefighting (Lerner et al., 2015).

By understanding these processes, individuals become more empowered to make alternative and healthier behavioral choices. Moreover, organizations are better positioned to implement evidence-based strategies to protect and promote the psychological health and safety of their members (Substance Abuse and Mental Health Services Administration [SAMHSA], 2014).

Diagnostic and Statistical Manual of Mental Disorders

The Diagnostic and Statistical Manual of Mental Disorders, Fifth Edition, Text Revision (DSM-5-TR) was developed to establish a standardized language for mental health professionals to describe specific clinical presentations. This standardization of diagnostic criteria provides a foundation for clinical communication, enabling consistent research and treatment planning (American Psychiatric Association, 2022).

Despite its clinical utility, many individuals remain hesitant to receive a formal diagnosis because of the stigma historically associated with mental illness. Mental illness has often been misunderstood as a sign of personal weakness, unpredictability, or dangerousness, which can lead individuals to avoid treatment out of fear of judgment or discrimination (Corrigan et al., 2014). Unfortunately, this reluctance to seek care can increase suffering, as untreated mental health conditions are associated with worsened outcomes across multiple life domains, including relationships, employment, and overall functioning (Henderson et al., 2013).

A formal diagnosis, when delivered appropriately, is often the first step in establishing an effective and evidence-based treatment plan. For many individuals, it represents the beginning of a healing process and a pathway to recovery. However, in high-stigma environments such as fire service environments, there has been a push to shift language from “disorder” to “injury” in an attempt to reduce stigma and encourage help-seeking (Jones et al., 2017). While this language shift may have merit in reducing shame, it also risks clinical ambiguity, potentially obscuring whether someone is experiencing natural stress recovery, meets the criteria for PTSD, or is dealing with another issue entirely. Without an accurate diagnosis, individuals may not receive proper treatment, highlighting how even well-meaning cultural practices can unintentionally lead to harm (Corrigan et al., 2014).

Given the hands-on nature of their work, firefighters often respond better to tangible, skill-based approaches in the otherwise abstract world of soft skills and mental health support. Foundational peer support competencies could include active listening, the behavioral influence stairway model (BISM) used in crisis de-escalation, guided problem-solving, and psychological first aid (PFA), which includes frameworks such as trauma risk management (TRiM) (Greenberg et al., 2008).

Active Listening Skills

Active listening is a cornerstone of adequate peer support and crisis intervention. It requires focusing entirely on the speaker, demonstrating empathy, and reflecting understanding—skills that have been shown to improve rapport and reduce distress in high-pressure environments (Weger et al., 2014). Because these are perishable skills, they should be practiced regularly and reinforced through training and supervision.

Effective active listening also involves integrating tools summarized by the acronym "MORE PIE(S)", which stands for:

- Minimal encouragement (e.g., nodding, "uh-huh").
- Open-ended questions
- Reflections
- Effective pauses
- Paraphrasing
- I-messages (statements focus on the speaker's experience)
- Emotional labeling
- Summarizations

These techniques help listeners clarify content, convey empathy, and deepen their understanding of important components in crisis communication and emotional support (Weger et al., 2010).

Before someone can effectively practice active listening, they can be trained to do the following:

- Build Trust and Rapport
- Recognizing and managing personal biases and anecdotal interpretations
- Avoid taking responsibility for the other person's actions
- Recognizing both content and emotional levels of communication
- Understand that people attribute value differently
- Maintaining a nonjudgmental stance
- Avoid imposing their feelings, values, and opinions

The Behavioral Influence Stairway Model (BISM)—developed in crisis negotiation—emphasizes active listening → empathy → rapport → influence → behavioral change and has been described for use in high-stakes contexts, with elements adaptable to peer support (Vecchi et al., 2005).

Psychological First Aid as a Method to Manage Occupational Trauma

Psychological first aid (PFA), an evidence-based, modular approach, is designed to reduce initial distress and promote adaptive functioning following exposure to traumatic events (Brymer et al., 2006). It emphasizes principles of safety, calming, connectedness, self-efficacy, and hope, offering immediate, practical support without pathologizing normal stress reactions. Owing to its scalable and flexible nature, PFA has become the internationally endorsed standard for early psychological intervention in crisis contexts. PFA is widely promoted in international guidance for early response (e.g., NCTSN Field Operations Guide; WHO PFA Guide; VA/DoD CPGs encourage early practical support and discourage routine debriefing). PTSD 2006 (Greenberg, et. al., 2008). Within the framework of PFA, trauma risk management (TRiM) has emerged as a peer-delivered strategy that equips personnel to identify and support colleagues experiencing early signs of trauma-related distress. TRiM has been associated with increased help-seeking and reduced stigma, with emerging evidence on symptom benefits (Greenberg et al., 2008; Jones et al., 2017). The integration of TRiM within a PFA framework supports a trauma-informed organizational culture and enhances early intervention without overmedicalizing adaptive stress responses.

Posttraumatic Stress Disorder

Currently, the fire service has acknowledged and accepted that behavioral health outcomes can be linked to the job. Posttraumatic stress disorder and suicide were once considered signs of weakness and fallibility, but have become symbols of sacrifice and honor, as those affected have been seen enduring suffering behind the work of service to others. There have been no studies revealing whether these cultural shifts have changed the frequency of these behavioral health outcomes.

Posttraumatic stress is a frequently observed psychological reaction following exposure to traumatic events. However, distinguishing this normative stress response from posttraumatic stress disorder (PTSD), which is a diagnosable mental health condition, is important. According to the American Psychiatric Association's Diagnostic and Statistical Manual of Mental Disorders, Fifth Edition (DSM-5), PTSD is defined by the fulfillment of multiple diagnostic criteria (A-H) necessary to meet the threshold for diagnosis (American Psychiatric Association, 2022).

Criterion A stipulates that an individual should have been exposed to actual or threatened death, serious injury, or sexual violence. This exposure can occur through direct experience, witnessing the traumatic event, learning a close relative or friend was subjected to trauma, or through repeated or extreme indirect exposure to aversive details of traumatic events, typically in the context of professional responsibilities (e.g., first responders, medics) (American Psychiatric Association, 2022).

Criterion B pertains to persistent re-experiencing of the traumatic event, which may manifest as intrusive and distressing memories, nightmares, dissociative reactions (e.g., flashbacks), emotional distress in response to trauma-related cues, and marked physiological reactivity following exposure to such reminders (American Psychiatric Association, 2022).

Criterion C involves the avoidance of trauma-related stimuli, whether internal (thoughts, feelings) or external (reminders of the traumatic event) (American Psychiatric Association, 2022).

Criterion D describes negative alterations in cognition and mood associated with the traumatic experience. These include the inability to recall important aspects of the trauma, persistent negative beliefs about oneself or others, distorted blame, pervasive negative emotional states, diminished interest in significant activities, feelings of detachment, and anhedonia (American Psychiatric Association, 2022).

Criterion E relates to marked alterations in arousal and reactivity, such as irritability or aggression, reckless or self-destructive behavior, hypervigilance, exaggerated startle response, concentration difficulties, and sleep disturbances (American Psychiatric Association, 2022).

Criterion F requires that the duration of symptoms exceeds one month. Criterion G demands that these symptoms cause clinically significant distress or impairment in social, occupational, or other important areas of functioning. Criterion H clarifies that these disturbances are not attributable to the physiological effects of a substance or another medical condition (American Psychiatric Association, 2022). The DSM-5 also identifies two specifiers: dissociative symptoms and delayed expression (American Psychiatric Association, 2022).

Firefighters, as members of the broader public safety personnel (PSP) community, are repeatedly exposed to potentially traumatic events (PTEs), placing them at heightened risk for a wide range of mental health challenges, most notably posttraumatic stress disorder (PTSD), depression, anxiety, substance misuse, and relational strain (Harvey et al., 2016; Lade et al., 2023). Moreover, PTSD has traditionally been the focus of research in this field, and an increasing body of evidence suggests that cumulative trauma can contribute to comorbid conditions, including hazardous alcohol use and chronic pain (Miloslavich et al., 2023; Senger et al., 2023). In an extensive study conducted in New South Wales, Australia, current firefighters reported rates of PTSD and depression of 8% and 5%, respectively, whereas heavy alcohol consumption was noted in 4% of participants. Among retired firefighters, these rates more than doubled, with 18% reporting PTSD and depression and 7% engaging in heavy drinking (Harvey et al., 2016). These findings underscore the enduring impact of trauma across the firefighter career lifespan.

Notably, PTSD symptoms are further exacerbated by operational stressors, such as involvement in postmortem inquiries and negative media attention following critical incidents. Regehr et al. (2003) reported that firefighters involved in formal review processes experienced significantly higher levels of traumatic stress and depressive symptoms, with many requiring mental health-related leave. These findings suggest that post-incident organizational procedures can unintentionally exacerbate distress rather than alleviate it.

Modifiable psychological resources such as resilience, hope, and a sense of coherence have emerged as key protective factors. In a U.S.-based study, Senger et al. (2023) reported that resilience was negatively associated with both PTSD symptoms and chronic pain, whereas hope was strongly linked to posttraumatic growth (PTG) and overall well-being. Similarly, Egberink et al. (2020) validated the Sense of Coherence-Revised (SOC-R) scale in a Dutch sample of firefighters, confirming its utility in screening for resilience potential and its inverse relationship with psychopathology. These tools support primary and secondary prevention strategies focused on psychological fortification prior to and following exposure to trauma.

In addition to PTSD, the intersection of anger and substance use has received attention. Miloslavich et al. (2023) demonstrated that anger, an often overlooked but clinically relevant emotional state, predicts alcohol use severity among firefighters. This association remained significant even after controlling for general negative affect. Moreover, drinking motives related to social enhancement and mood improvement moderated this relationship, indicating that emotion regulation-informed interventions could play an important role in addressing alcohol misuse in fire service populations.

Relational dynamics also intersect with mental health outcomes. In a recent study of married or cohabiting firefighters, those with low relationship satisfaction demonstrated significantly higher levels of PTSD, depression, and other mental health symptoms than their satisfied counterparts did (Zegel et al., 2024). These findings suggest that promoting relational health could serve as a protective buffer against occupational stress.

Despite increased mental health awareness, numerous barriers to care persist. Firefighters often face stigma, anticipate negative occupational consequences, or encounter logistical barriers to accessing mental health services. Johnson et al. (2020) emphasize the importance of culturally competent care that is informed by an understanding of fire service norms, including group cohesion, stoicism, and perceived invulnerability. Carleton et al. (2020) similarly reported that PSP personnel overwhelmingly preferred informal support networks, especially spouses, over formal services and that engagement in any mental health training program was associated with lower mental disorder rates. However, access to professional resources remains underutilized.

Global events further demonstrate the psychological toll of firefighting. Following the 2023 earthquakes in Turkey, firefighters presented high levels of PTSD symptoms, depression, anxiety, and reduced resilience, as measured by validated psychometric scales (Bakirci et al., 2024). These outcomes underscore the pressing need for pre-incident resilience training and scalable post-incident interventions specifically designed for first responders.

Taken together, the literature reveals a multifaceted picture of PTSD in firefighter populations, where cumulative trauma, emotional dysregulation, organizational dynamics, and cultural barriers converge. Effective mitigation requires multilevel strategies encompassing individual resilience-building, relationship support, culturally sensitive mental health services, and systemic changes to reduce stigma and increase access to care. Such approaches are important in safeguarding the mental health and operational readiness of firefighters across all phases of their careers.

Given the high frequency of trauma exposure inherent in firefighting duties, these professionals are at elevated risk for developing PTSD and other psychopathologies (Pinto et al., 2015). From a cognitive psychological perspective, it is not the objective traumatic event itself but rather the subjective interpretation of the trauma that predominantly contributes to PTSD development (Pinto et al., 2015). A study conducted among Portuguese firefighters examined the role of perceived threat in PTSD symptomatology and reported that perceived threat accounted for a unique proportion of the variance in PTSD symptoms (Pinto et al., 2015). These findings underscore the potential benefit of interventions aimed at modifying threat perception in mitigating PTSD risk among firefighters.

PTSD has been one of the most extensively examined psychological conditions among firefighter populations. However, it is imperative to differentiate between posttraumatic stress, posttraumatic stress symptoms (PTSS), and the clinical diagnosis of PTSD. In some instances, research conflates these distinct constructs, leading to an overestimation of PTSD prevalence within this occupational group. Moreover, it is important to acknowledge other relevant psychological concerns, including domestic violence exposure, suicide risk, homicide involvement, and various forms of substance abuse beyond alcohol, to obtain a comprehensive understanding of the mental health challenges faced by firefighters.

In addition to trauma exposure, sources of occupational stress in emergency service professions can be categorized as operational or organizational. Research by Armstrong et al. (2016) suggests that organizational stress, stress derived from the organizational structure, culture, and management practices, may have a more profound effect on adverse mental health outcomes than operational stress does. While operational stress is directly associated with PTSD symptoms, organizational stress is indirectly related to posttraumatic growth via the mediating influence of organizational belongingness (Armstrong et al., 2016). These findings advocate the development of psychosocial interventions to foster organizational belongingness to support firefighters' psychological adjustment posttraumatic exposure.

A study conducted in Greece explored the psychological consequences of a devastating 2007 wildfire, which resulted in forty-three fatalities, including three firefighters. Among the study participants, 18.6% met the diagnostic criteria for PTSD (Psarros et al., 2018). The key predictors of PTSD included the fear of dying during the incident, insomnia, elevated levels of neuroticism, and concurrent depression. Notably, career firefighters presented a 70% lower likelihood of developing PTSD than their seasonal counterparts did (Psarros et al., 2018).

Somatic correlates of PTSD were investigated in a study involving Australian firefighters. Milligan-Saville et al. (2017) reported that firefighters with probable PTSD reported higher levels of neurological, gastrointestinal, and cardiorespiratory symptoms than did those without PTSD. Furthermore, the severity of total somatic symptoms is significantly greater among individuals with PTSD, irrespective of age (Milligan-Saville et al., 2017).

Posttraumatic stress symptoms are prevalent among municipal firefighters and are predictive of maladaptive coping strategies and alcohol-related consequences. Tomaka et al. (2017) reported that approximately 32.4% of firefighters experienced significant levels of PTSS. These symptoms were associated with at-risk drinking behaviors, alcohol-related problems, and the utilization of maladaptive coping strategies, including substance use. Importantly, substance use coping and drinking-to-cope were identified as mediators in the relationship between PTSS and problematic alcohol use (Tomaka et al., 2017).

In South Korea, Lee et al. (2017) investigated the relationship between duty-related traumatic events and PTSSs. Their findings indicated that exposure to multiple potentially traumatic events (PTEs) and heightened peritraumatic suffering significantly increased the likelihood of PTSS, even after adjusting for demographic variables, depressive symptoms, and childhood trauma. Notably, colleague-related PTEs and indirect exposures are particularly associated with elevated PTSD symptoms (PTSSs) (Lee et al., 2017). The combination of PTE exposure and peritraumatic suffering emerged as a stronger predictor of PTSS than either factor independently (Lee et al., 2017).

Few studies have examined the biological underpinnings of PTSD among firefighter populations. One such study conducted in South Korea explored the associations between adiponectin, a hormone involved in neurobiological pathways of fear extinction, and PTSD severity (Na et al., 2017). The findings indicated that compared with control participants, male firefighters with PTSD presented significantly lower plasma adiponectin levels. Furthermore, adiponectin levels are inversely correlated with PTSD severity, whereas no such correlation was found with depression symptoms (Na et al., 2017).

Early-life victimization has also been identified as a risk factor for adverse mental health outcomes among first responders. Komarovskaya et al. (2014) examined police officers and firefighters who responded to Hurricane Katrina and reported that early physical victimization was modestly associated with PTSD symptoms, depression, sleep disturbances, and peritraumatic dissociation. These findings highlight the enduring impact of early-life trauma on later psychological resilience in high-stress professions (Komarovskaya et al., 2014).

Firefighters and paramedics are routinely exposed to life-threatening emergencies, mass casualty events, and critical incident stress, all of which increase the risk for posttraumatic stress disorder (PTSD) and other mental health conditions. While the role of trauma exposure is well documented, recent research has emphasized the importance of coping mechanisms, personality traits, and workplace dynamics in shaping psychological outcomes in fire service personnel (Beaton et al., 1999; Meyer et al., 2021).

A foundational study by Beaton et al. (1999) revealed that among urban firefighters and paramedics, self-reported PTSD symptoms were more strongly related to coping styles, as measured by the Coping Responses of Rescue Workers Inventory (CRRWI), than to years of service or frequency of trauma exposure. This finding underscores the importance of psychological flexibility and emotion regulation in post-incident recovery. Similarly, a large-scale cross-sectional study of more than 1300 Chinese firefighters demonstrated that an imbalance between occupational effort and reward, particularly when compounded by negative coping styles, was significantly associated with increased depressive symptoms (Yu et al., 2023). These findings suggest that coping is not only a personal skill set but also a factor embedded in organizational culture.

Personality factors further compound these vulnerabilities. Meyer et al. (2021) conducted a 3-year prospective study of firefighters. They reported that negative emotionality (NEM) assessed at entry into the fire academy predicted the development of PTSD symptoms over time. NEM also moderated the impact of trauma exposure on clinical symptomatology, demonstrating the need for early psychological screening and targeted support for recruits at greater psychological risk.

Network analyses have advanced our understanding of symptom patterns associated with PTSD. An et al. (2022) used partial correlation modeling to identify irritability and negative emotional states as central and predictive symptoms in Chinese firefighter populations. These findings suggest that key treatment targets may interrupt the broader symptom network and reduce overall distress. Similarly, Steinberg and Vujanovic (2024) found support for a unidimensional model of the PTSD Checklist for DSM-5 (PCL-5) using a firefighter sample, confirming that PTSD symptoms among this group can be reliably conceptualized along a single latent continuum, which may enhance assessment precision in clinical settings.

Despite their clinical needs, many firefighters do not access mental health care. In a landmark population-based study in South Korea, Kim et al. (2018) reported that only 9.7% of firefighters with probable PTSD sought treatment within the previous month. The most commonly cited barriers were stigma (33.8%) and concerns about accessibility (29.3%). Notably, those with the most severe symptoms were both more likely to seek help and more likely to perceive stigma. These results emphasize the dual role of symptom severity and institutional culture in shaping treatment engagement.

Interpersonal and motivational dynamics also affect mental health outcomes. In a recent large-scale study, Pan (2024) reported that admiration, particularly when linked to internal motivation, was associated with decreased PTSD symptoms. In contrast, external motivation was associated with greater symptom severity, suggesting that interventions fostering intrinsic purpose and identity within the fire service may be protective. Likewise, relational health is emerging as a buffer; firefighters who reported dissatisfaction in romantic relationships presented significantly greater levels of depression, anxiety, and PTSD symptoms than did those in satisfying partnerships (Zegel et al., 2024).

From a systems-level perspective, understanding treatment barriers and drivers of resilience is critical. Carleton et al. (2019) reported that although most public safety personnel (PSPs) report access to professional and nonprofessional support networks, they overwhelmingly turn to spouses and colleagues first. Training for these informal support systems may therefore enhance the overall effectiveness of intervention strategies. Additionally, Johnson et al. (2020) argued that culturally tailored approaches, which respect firehouse norms, operational realities, and stigma, are crucial for enhancing help-seeking and long-term care engagement. Resilience scores are closely tied to symptom severity (Bakirci et al., 2024). These findings underscore the importance of resilience-building as a fundamental component of trauma-informed preparedness training.

The psychological impacts of large-scale disasters offer further insights into how firefighters experience cumulative stress. In the aftermath of the 2023 earthquake in

Turkey, firefighters demonstrated significantly elevated PTSD, depression, anxiety, and stress levels, with lower social support emerging as a critical buffer against the psychological toll of trauma exposure among firefighters and other first responders. Recent findings emphasize that perceived social support, not merely receipt, plays a central role in mitigating the development and severity of posttraumatic stress disorder (PTSD) symptoms (Prati & Pietrantoni, 2010). Among firefighters, higher levels of perceived support are linked to reductions in intrusive rumination and feelings of entrapment, both of which mediate the relationship between trauma exposure and PTSD symptomatology (Lee, 2019). This protective function extends beyond PTSD, as social support also mediates the impact of occupational stressors on depression and anxiety in first responder populations (Kshtriya et al., 2020). The importance of support systems is further underscored by their positive association with coping self-efficacy and quality of life (Noda et al., 2024). These findings suggest that enhancing social connectedness not only buffers against distress but also fosters psychological resilience and functional well-being. Moreover, active coping strategies and resilience-building, often fostered through strong social networks, are positively associated with improved mental health and life satisfaction among emergency workers (Noda et al., 2024). The high prevalence of sleep disturbances in firefighters, reported by more than half of the study participants, also correlates with psychological distress and highlights the need for comprehensive approaches to occupational health that incorporate mental wellness and sleep hygiene (Vargas de Barros et al., 2013). Particularly vulnerable are volunteer firefighters, who face increased PTSD risk due to the cumulative burden of traumatic exposure, including high-threat situations such as entrapment or assault (Milligan-Saville et al., 2018). These findings collectively support a systemic emphasis on social support structures within fire service organizations as critical elements of trauma risk management.

Taken together, these studies reinforce a multifaceted understanding of PTSD and mental health risk in fire and emergency services. Trauma exposure alone does not affect outcomes; coping strategies, emotional regulation, organizational support, and interpersonal relationships shape the trajectory of psychological wellness. A comprehensive model of firefighter mental health must account for individual predispositions, occupational demands, and the sociocultural framework in which firefighters operate.

Critical Incident Stress Management in the Fire Service

Critical incident stress management (CISM) was introduced to the emergency services field in the early 1980s as a structured, group-based method intended to mitigate psychological harm following exposure to traumatic incidents (Mitchell, 1983). Drawing from psychoanalytic traditions, the model posited that open expression and discussion of traumatic experiences could facilitate emotional catharsis, normalize stress responses, identify individuals at risk, and enhance group cohesion. Central to this approach was critical incident stress debriefing (CISD), a postevent intervention typically led by a trained facilitator within 72 hours of a critical incident. The model gained traction rapidly, becoming a staple of behavioral health programming in fire departments across the United States (Mitchell & Everly, 1995). Note that CISD was only one component of a broader, multielement CISM program; however, because it was often implemented as a routine, single-session group debrief soon after an event, it became the focal point of later empirical scrutiny and the subsequent shift toward needs-based models (e.g., Psychological First Aid).

However, as empirical scrutiny increased, so did skepticism regarding its efficacy. Multiple meta-analyses have shown that CISM, particularly single-session debriefings administered shortly after trauma exposure, may not prevent PTSD and could even impede natural recovery. Rose et al. (2003) reported that participants who underwent CISM had worse psychological outcomes than did those who received no intervention or non-CISM alternatives. Similarly, van Emmerik et al. (2002) concluded that early debriefing failed to prevent posttraumatic distress and was not significantly more effective than naturalistic coping was. Gersons et al. (2000) reported that Dutch police officers who participated in debriefings presented more PTSD symptoms one week posttrauma than did those who did not, suggesting that premature emotional processing may exacerbate distress. Consistent with these reviews, randomized trials in civilian samples found that single-session debriefing conferred no benefit and, in some cases, worse outcomes at follow-up (e.g., Bisson et al., 1997; Mayou et al., 2000).

In parallel, national and international health agencies have revised their recommendations. The National Institute of Mental Health (2002), the U.K. National Institute for Health and Care Excellence—NICE (2005), and the World Health Organization's Psychological First Aid: Guide for Field Workers (2011; 2014 facilitator/orientation materials) endorse Psychological First Aid (PFA) over prescriptive, single-session group debriefing, emphasizing flexibility, self-determination, and supportive presence without compelled disclosure.

Real-world evaluations support these conclusions. Jahnke et al. (2014) conducted focus groups with U.S. firefighters, revealing mixed responses to CISD. While some appreciated the opportunity to share experiences, others reported feeling forced to confront distressing events prematurely, sometimes experiencing increased emotional discomfort. In contrast, informal peer support and spontaneous conversations with trusted colleagues were viewed as more beneficial and culturally aligned with the values of the fire service.

More recently, Sarabia et al. (2024) explored firefighter preferences for post-critical incident interventions and examined how these choices were related to coping self-efficacy. In a sample of 241 firefighters, 46.9% preferred CISD; however, this group also reported significantly lower levels of fire service coping self-efficacy (FFCSE) and trauma coping self-efficacy (CSE-T) than did those who preferred no intervention. Similarly, individuals who favored one-on-one counseling also exhibited lower self-efficacy, suggesting that personal confidence in coping may influence help-seeking behaviors. These findings underscore the need to align post-incident interventions with individual readiness and psychological resilience rather than applying uniform approaches.

The cultural context remains central. Despite mounting evidence against the universal application of the CISM, it remains widely used in U.S. fire and emergency services, likely due to its long-standing institutional familiarity and the perceived value of structured group discussions. Nevertheless, growing concerns about psychological harm have shifted the focus toward more flexible and individualized models. Psychological first aid (PFA), now widely endorsed, allows individuals to receive support on the basis of their unique needs and readiness without requiring full emotional disclosure immediately following trauma (Brymer et al., 2006).

Overall, the evolution of trauma care in fire and emergency services reflects a broader paradigm shift from structured debriefings toward adaptive, peer-led, and person-centered strategies. While CISM represents a progressive step in addressing emergency responders' mental health, contemporary best practices increasingly favor approaches that respect individual coping trajectories and emphasize psychological safety over forced expression. As research and practice continue to evolve, fire departments must critically evaluate legacy practices in light of emerging evidence and prioritize interventions to enhance recovery without compromising the well-being of those affected.

Moral Injury in the Fire Service

While trauma in fire and emergency services has traditionally been conceptualized through the framework of posttraumatic stress disorder (PTSD), emerging research highlights the significance of moral injury (MI) as a distinct yet sometimes overlapping psychological phenomenon. Moral injury refers to the profound emotional, psychological, and spiritual distress that arises when an individual participates in, witnesses, or is unable to prevent actions that violate deeply held moral beliefs or ethical codes (Litz et al., 2009; Nash & Litz, 2013; Nash, 2021). For firefighters and emergency medical personnel, whose work often entails making triage decisions, operating under constrained conditions, and frequently exposing them to suffering, the risk of moral injury is both substantial and historically underrecognized (Barrett, 2023; Roth et al., 2022).

Unlike PTSD, which is rooted in fear-based responses to life-threatening situations, moral injury centers on guilt, shame, betrayal, and moral dissonance. These reactions may not meet diagnostic criteria for a mental disorder but can still result in considerable psychological impairment, professional dysfunction, and existential distress (Jinkerson, 2016; Nash, 2021). In fire service, moral injuries may emerge from perceived failure to save lives, survivor guilt after a colleague's death, or the provision of life-sustaining aid to individuals who have caused harm to others (Barrett, 2023; Roth et al., 2022). These experiences can deeply challenge a firefighter's sense of moral identity and provoke ongoing internal conflict over personal integrity and self-worth.

Barrett (2023) classified moral injury along multiple dimensions, including loss of trust, guilt, and damage to one's moral virtue. Trust may be eroded when firefighters perceive leadership decisions as unjust or negligent, particularly when such decisions result in preventable harm. Guilt may follow when firefighters are unable to act owing to procedural constraints or when they feel complicit in systemic shortcomings, such as failure to report misconduct within their teams. Encounters that provoke dissonance between professional obligations and personal values, such as delivering care to a violent offender, can likewise destabilize a firefighter's belief in their capacity for ethical action.

Recent empirical studies have begun to clarify the psychological and developmental correlates of moral injury in public safety personnel (PSPs). In a cross-sectional analysis of 294 Canadian and American PSPs, Roth et al. (2022) reported that adverse childhood experiences (ACEs) significantly predict adult symptoms of PTSD, depression, and dissociation, with moral injury acting as a key mediating factor. Emotional regulation skills emerged as a protective buffer, suggesting that psychological flexibility and coping capacity may moderate the severity of moral distress (Roth et al., 2022).

Given the potentially debilitating effects of moral injury and its distinction from traditional trauma, researchers have emphasized the importance of contextualized assessment tools. The development of the Emergency Services Moral Injury Scale-Firefighter Version (EMIS-F) represents a significant step forward in acknowledging the unique ethical challenges faced by firefighters. This tool enables departments to screen for betrayal-based, perpetration-based, and omission-based injuries that are unique to first responders (DeMoulin et al., 2023). When incorporated into routine annual wellness assessments, alongside instruments such as the Firefighter Coping Self-Efficacy Scale (FFCSE) and the Firefighter Assessment of Stress Test (FAST), the EMIS-F can help identify early signs of moral distress and support targeted, proactive intervention (Lambert et al., 2012; Schuhmann et al., 2022).

These assessments, particularly when administered confidentially through secure digital platforms or wellness clinics, provide scalable and non-pathologizing ways to support firefighter mental health. Participation should remain voluntary and non-punitive, reinforcing the message that mental health monitoring is a shared professional responsibility, not an indicator of personal weakness. Moreover, aggregated and de-identified data from these tools can provide leaders with important organizational insights, surfacing systemic stressors such as shift fatigue, operational overload, or breakdowns in trust that may otherwise be unreported (Lambert et al., 2012).

The consequences of unaddressed moral injury can be severe. A recent systematic review by Jamieson et al. (2023) identified morally injurious experiences as significant predictors of suicide risk in military populations, independent of PTSD symptomatology. Although data on firefighters are still emerging, the similarity of occupational stressors suggests that these findings are relevant and urgently applicable to fire service contexts.

In response to the increasing recognition of moral injury, several evidence-based therapeutic models have been developed. Litz, Lebowitz, Gray, and Nash (2016) introduced adaptive disclosure, a structured intervention originally designed for military personnel, which facilitates moral repair through guided narrative, accountability, and the integration of values such as honor and forgiveness. Other interventions, including spiritually integrated cognitive processing therapy and forgiveness-based models, have also shown promise, particularly for those whose recovery is rooted in meaning-making and moral clarity (Jinkerson, 2016).

Ultimately, recognizing and addressing moral injury represents a necessary evolution in how firefighter mental health is conceptualized and understood. Firefighters may struggle not only with what they have witnessed or survived but also with what they were unable to prevent or with systems that failed to uphold ethical standards. Effective care must go beyond symptom reduction and address the moral and relational dimensions of distress. By integrating culturally validated assessments, ethically grounded practices, and strengths-based interventions into routine care, departments can better support the moral resilience of their members and foster a culture where psychological integrity is protected as fiercely as physical safety.

Organizational Betrayal in the Fire Service

In high-risk occupational environments, factors such as firefighting, trust in leadership, team cohesion, and institutional integrity are crucial for both psychological safety and operational effectiveness. Organizational betrayal occurs when individuals perceive that their institution or leadership has violated their expectations of fairness, support, or ethical responsibility, particularly following exposure to trauma (Smith & Freyd, 2013). Within the fire service, organizational betrayal may manifest as inadequate response to mental health needs, failure to support injured personnel, toleration of discrimination or harassment, or punitive responses to help-seeking behavior.

According to the theory of betrayal trauma, first introduced by Freyd (1996), the impact of trauma is compounded when the source of harm is someone or something the individual depends on for safety or support. When firefighters experience betrayal by their department, such as being denied resources, facing retaliation after reporting misconduct, or being ostracized following a mental health disclosure, this betrayal can intensify posttraumatic stress, depression, and occupational disengagement (Smith & Freyd, 2013).

Research has shown that institutional betrayal is strongly associated with increased symptoms of PTSD and depression, especially among individuals who report high levels of organizational trust prior to betrayal (Platt et al., 2009; Smith & Freyd, 2013). In public safety professions, this betrayal may arise when departments fail to validate or respond to traumatic exposures, delay mental health referrals, or mismanage fitness-for-duty evaluations. In their study of police officers, Papazoglou et al. (2020) reported that perceived betrayal by leadership was a stronger predictor of emotional distress than exposure to critical incidents themselves.

Within the fire service, betrayal by the organization can be particularly damaging due to the paramilitary hierarchy, high occupational loyalty, and cultural stigmas around vulnerability. Firefighters who report feeling unsupported after a traumatic event or who are punished for seeking help may internalize this treatment as confirmation that their psychological injury is a personal weakness rather than an occupational hazard. This can lead to increased suicide risk, decreased help-seeking, and moral injury, particularly when values such as loyalty and courage are undermined by institutional behavior.

To address organizational betrayal, fire departments must adopt trauma-informed leadership practices that prioritize psychological safety, transparency, and accountability. Smith and Freyd (2013) recommend strategies including acknowledging harm when it occurs, supporting whistleblowers, and creating confidential, nonpunitive pathways to access mental health services. Peer support teams, if adequately trained, can also act as intermediaries to rebuild trust and bridge the gap between firefighters and department leadership.

In sum, organizational betrayal is not merely a breakdown in trust; it is a profound psychological breach that can exacerbate trauma, damage morale, and erode the very foundation of public safety organizations. Recognizing, preventing, and addressing this phenomenon are critical components of comprehensive trauma risk management in fire and emergency services.

Moral Injury and Suicide Risk: Implications for Fire Service Behavioral Health

Within trauma-exposed occupational groups, including military and emergency responders, conventional risk factors such as posttraumatic stress disorder (PTSD) do not fully account for the increasing incidence of suicide. A growing body of research suggests that moral injury (MI), defined as the psychological, spiritual, and social conflict resulting from transgressions of deeply held moral beliefs, may serve as an additional, salient correlate of suicidality suicide risk (Jamieson et al., 2023). While not classified as a formal mental health disorder, moral injury is frequently comorbid with PTSD and has been shown to profoundly affect emotional, behavioral, and existential functioning (Jamieson et al., 2023). In a systematic review of 12 studies examining moral injury and suicidality among active-duty and veteran military populations, Jamieson et al. (2023) reported consistent evidence linking morally injurious experiences, such as betrayal by leadership, perpetration of violence, or failure to prevent harm, to increased rates of suicidal ideation, planning, and attempts. These findings are particularly significant for public safety personnel, including firefighters, who face similar moral and ethical stressors in high-stakes environments. The review recommends expanding this research to include first responders, medical professionals, and allied health workers, whose roles often involve making morally ambiguous decisions under intense pressure (Jamieson et al., 2023). For trauma risk management in fire and emergency services, this emerging evidence underscores the necessity of assessing moral injury as a unique factor contributing to suicide risk, which traditional PTSD-focused frameworks may not capture. Integrating MI-informed assessments and interventions into behavioral health protocols could increase prevention efforts by addressing the complex interplay between ethical conflict, emotional distress, and self-harm.

Trauma Risk Management (TRiM): A Peer-Led, Risk-Based Framework for Recovery Support

TRiM is a structured, peer-delivered process designed to identify, monitor, and respond to psychological risk following exposure to a potentially traumatic event (PTE). Unlike the legacy term critical incident, which implies inherent trauma, PTE reflects a more accurate and trauma-informed conceptualization: no incident is inherently traumatic; trauma is defined by an individual's subjective response, not the objective nature of the event. This distinction is significant in high-risk professions, such as fire and emergency services, where multiple individuals can experience the same event with vastly different psychological outcomes (Figley & Nash, 2007; Greenberg et al., 2010).

The British Armed Forces developed TRiM as an alternative to debriefing-centered approaches, such as critical incident stress debriefing (CISD), which have been criticized for their potential to impede natural recovery when used prematurely or universally (Bisson et al., 1997; Mayou et al., 2000; Rose et al., 2002/2003). TRiM emphasizes the early identification of individuals at psychological risk, the normalization of acute stress responses, and the facilitation of clinical care when appropriate, all while supporting the natural recovery process in those who do not require formal intervention (Greenberg et al., 2008; Figley & Nash, 2007).

The TRiM process typically includes the following steps:

- An initial structured screening within 72 hours to one week of a PTE was conducted by a trained peer supporter using a semistructured tool to assess the individual's experience, functional impact, and perceived psychological distress.
- A follow-up screening approximately 28–30 days later was completed by the same peer supporter to evaluate the recovery trajectory and symptom persistence or emergence.
- A third follow-up may be necessary in some cases, particularly when delayed or evolving symptoms warrant additional monitoring.

TRiM screenings help identify four common psychological trajectories following trauma:

1. **Natural Recovery**: The most frequent outcome, in which symptoms are present initially but resolve spontaneously by 30 days without formal treatment.
2. **Resilient:** Characterized by minimal or no symptom development at either time point, indicating adaptive stress response mechanisms.

3. **Chronic:** Marked by persistent and impairing symptoms at both the initial and follow-up assessments, often requiring clinical referral.
4. **Delayed Presentation:** Where the individual initially appears asymptomatic but distress emerges at the follow-up screening.

This staged, data-informed approach enables fire departments to integrate psychological triage into standard operations. Departments can predefine certain PTEs, such as pediatric deaths, firefighter injuries, or large-scale disasters, as triggers for TRiM activation, thereby building mental health responsiveness into the organizational structure (Greenberg et al., 2010; Whybrow et al., 2015; Jones et al., 2017).

Importantly, TRiM equips peer supporters with clear criteria for clinical escalation, enhancing ethical boundaries and role clarity. The ongoing nature of the intervention, led by the same trained peer over time, provides continuity and trust, moving away from the outdated "one and done" model commonly associated with CISD (Greenberg et al., 2010; Whybrow et al., 2015; Jones et al., 2017). TRiM's non-pathologizing framework affirms that most individuals will recover naturally with appropriate support while ensuring that those on a trajectory toward clinical impairment are identified early and connected with professional care. Consistent with international guidance, group formats should prioritize psychoeducation and practical support rather than compelled disclosure (NICE, 2005; WHO, 2011/2014; Rose et al., 2002/2003).

The Risks of Group Debriefing and the Value of Individualized Support

Unlike CISD, which emphasizes group emotional processing, effective TRiM strategies should explicitly avoid premature, unstructured disclosure. Psychological trauma is experienced individually, even when the event is shared. Group debriefings, particularly those conducted too soon after an event, carry significant risks.

Maladaptive narratives can be unintentionally shared, leading to secondary traumatization among participants who may not have been initially distressed. Some individuals may shift their attention toward relieving others' pain rather than attending to their recovery. Creating emotional entanglement can hinder self-regulation and resilience. The social dynamics of group settings may amplify feelings of comparison, guilt, or inadequacy, primarily if participants differ in their emotional responses. In contrast, TRiM emphasizes individual check-ins to ensure psychological safety, emotional containment, and role clarity. In other words, psychoeducation, a core component of TRiM, can be delivered in group settings, provided that the group is homogeneous (e.g., members of the same team or unit). In such cases, a structured discussion can be used to provide information about typical stress responses, expected recovery trajectories, and when to seek help without pressuring participants to disclose sensitive information.

When the group composition is homogeneous and trust is well established, the TRiM screening itself can be conducted in a group format with careful facilitation. This can potentially foster shared understanding and reduce assumptions about who was "most affected," which often complicates unstructured post-incident conversations. Ideally, however, TRiM screenings should be conducted one-to-one. When trust and homogeneity are high, group sessions should be used for structured psychoeducation and sign-posting, with private, individual screenings scheduled as needed.

Ultimately, TRiM offers a flexible, culturally attuned approach to post-incident support that prioritizes safety, accuracy, and sustainability. By embedding TRiM within a department's behavioral health strategy, fire service leaders can shift from reactive interventions to a proactive, systematized method of psychological risk management, one that preserves operational integrity while honoring the individual nature of trauma.

Conclusion

Effective trauma risk management in fire and emergency services requires a deliberate shift from a reactive crisis response toward proactive, evidence-based, and culturally competent systems of support. Exposure to potentially traumatic events (PTEs) is inherent to the profession, but psychological outcomes are shaped by far more than the events themselves; they are influenced by individual coping capacity, peer and organizational support, and the availability of timely, informed intervention. Tools such as psychological triage, resilience training, and peer-led interventions can empower departments to identify at-risk individuals early and support recovery without overpathologizing normal stress responses.

Trauma risk management (TRiM), a structured peer-delivered screening protocol, is one such tool. As the screening component within a broader psychological first aid (PFA) framework, TRiM enables departments to track recovery trajectories after PTEs, identify when clinical referrals are warranted, and provide follow-up care that respects both individual privacy and the cultural context. This model stands in contrast to "one and done" approaches, such as critical incident stress debriefing, which offers instead a system of continued, structured, and monitored support.

At the same time, addressing deeper and more complex forms of distress, such as moral injury, organizational betrayal, and stigma, requires ethical leadership, clear boundaries, and sustained investment in behavioral health infrastructure. When peer support programs are appropriately structured, adequately trained, and ethically grounded, they become a critical bridge between the firehouse and professional mental health care.

In recognizing the potential for psychological impacts related to firefighting and emergency medical services, we affirm that protecting the mental health of firefighters and EMS providers is not an adjunct to operational success; it is imperative. Trauma-informed leadership ensures that firefighters are not only physically protected in the line of duty but also psychologically supported throughout their careers.

Chapter Review

Assignment: Building a Trauma-Informed Fire Service: Psychological Triage, Peer Support, and Moral Injury Mitigation

You are advising a leadership council on developing a department-wide trauma risk management framework for a large metropolitan fire agency. Your task is to integrate scientific insights into peer-led psychological triage, identify ethical tensions in trauma support, and address culture-specific barriers to behavioral health engagement.

Learning Objectives

- Analyze trauma from both clinical and occupational perspectives
- Propose trauma-informed, ethical systems for fire service leadership
- Evaluate peer support and behavioral health integration strategies

Assignment Components

1. Conceptualizing Occupational Trauma (15%)

(a) Define occupational trauma and contrast acute stress vs. Post-Traumatic Stress Disorder (PTSD).
(b) Explain how subjective threat appraisal, moral injury, and organizational betrayal influence recovery.

2. Trauma Risk Management (TRiM) & Peer Support Strategy (25%)

(a) Summarize the TRiM model and explain how it functions within a Psychological First Aid (PFA) framework.
(b) Propose how peer support teams can be ethically structured to deliver triage, monitor trajectories, and escalate care.

3. Prevention through Culture & Training (20%)

(a) Describe key elements of trauma-informed leadership and their importance in high-risk organizations.
(b) Recommend training priorities (e.g., active listening, moral sensitivity, and soft skills) to enhance peer team capacity.

4. Boundaries, Trust, and Ethical Risk (20%)

(a) Discuss risks of overfamiliarity, boundary violations, and dual relationships within peer teams.
(b) Propose a clear informed consent model and explain how peer teams can navigate rank dynamics and referral ethics.

5. Risk Factors and Resilience Targets (15%)

(a) Identify modifiable risk factors (e.g., alcohol use, cumulative stress, and relationship distress).
(b) Recommend resilience-building strategies and prevention tools, such as the EMIS-F, SOC-R, and relational health interventions.

6. Critique of Legacy Models (CISM) (5%)

(a) Briefly evaluate the limitations of Critical Incident Stress Management (CISM) and why models like TRiM may be better suited to address occupational stress within the fire service.

Format Requirements

- Length: 2500–3000 words
- APA 7 formatting
- At least eight scholarly references (beyond the chapter)

Chapter 11
Fire Service Cultural Competency Training Program

Firefighters occupy a professional domain defined by extreme occupational demands, high psychological risk, and a unique cultural identity rooted in hierarchy, stoicism, and collective resilience. Despite these challenges, and perhaps in part because of them, fire service personnel often underutilize behavioral health services, citing concerns such as stigma, confidentiality, and a lack of culturally competent clinicians who understand their lived experiences. The Fire Service Cultural Competency Training Program was developed in direct response to this need. It aims to bridge the divide between mental health professionals and fire service members by equipping clinicians with the knowledge, skills, and experiential understanding necessary to deliver ethical, effective, and culturally congruent care. The program fosters clinical proficiency and relational trust through a structured curriculum that includes academic instruction, live-fire simulations, ride-alongs, and supervised consultation. Grounded in the ethical mandates of cultural responsiveness (APA, 2017), the program's rationale, structure, and expected outcomes are of critical importance in advancing behavioral health services for fire and emergency service populations.

There is an ongoing need to develop culturally competent mental health clinicians for firefighters. Firefighters face greater risks for psychological issues such as depression, anxiety, PTSD, and substance abuse, but are less likely to seek mental health services because of a lack of culturally competent clinicians and stigma. This program includes classroom training, practical fire operation experiences, and ride-alongs to help clinicians understand fire service culture. The participants learned about unique stressors, work environments, and challenges that firefighters face. The program emphasizes the importance of self-care for clinicians to manage risks such as vicarious trauma and burnout. By fostering interdisciplinary relationships, the program seeks to bridge the gap between firefighters and mental health services, ensuring that firefighters receive the support they need.

Compared with the general population, fire service personnel are at increased risk for a range of psychological health issues, including depression, anxiety,

K. Wheldon, *Fire Service Psychology*,
https://doi.org/10.1007/978-3-032-02126-7_11

posttraumatic stress, substance use disorders, and suicidality. Notably, Stanley et al. surveyed over 1000 firefighters and reported that 47% had experienced suicidal ideation at some point during their careers. This rate is markedly higher than estimates for the general population, which suggests that approximately 15% have similar experiences. Despite the higher prevalence of psychological challenges, firefighters are less likely to access professional health services.

Gulliver et al. (2019) surveyed 2156 professional firefighters to examine their access to and attitudes toward health care. The majority (81%) reported access to mental health services through their departments; however, disparities were noted among personnel in smaller or rural departments, who were less likely to have the same access. Interestingly, 67% indicated that they would turn to nonprofessional support, such as a spouse or family member, before considering clinical services. Only 60% said they would pursue private, professional intervention even when services were available. A notable trend emerged wherein newer firefighters were more likely to confide with peers or family, whereas more seasoned members tended to prefer professional services.

Although stigma is often cited as a deterrent to help-seeking behavior in public safety professions, Gulliver et al. (2019) reported that while few firefighters explicitly named stigma a barrier, 68% said that they would not recommend professional behavioral health services to a colleague, suggesting that stigma remains a significant underlying factor. A common concern was the lack of clinicians genuinely understanding the unique culture and occupational realities of fire and emergency services. Johnson et al. (2020) further underscored this point, identifying stigma, negative expectations about treatment outcomes, and structural obstacles as key deterrents to care seeking. These factors do not operate in isolation but intersect in ways that inhibit firefighter engagement with mental health services.

Additional layers of complexity arise from the heterogeneity of the fire service itself. Stanley et al. (2017) compared volunteer and career firefighters and reported that volunteer firefighters reported higher levels of depression, posttraumatic stress symptoms, and suicidal ideation. In contrast, career firefighters presented higher levels of problematic alcohol use. Structural barriers, including cost and limited availability of services, disproportionately affect volunteer personnel, potentially contributing to their heightened symptomatology.

Pennington et al. expanded on this research by examining the perceived availability of services and barriers to care in volunteer versus career firefighters. Volunteer firefighters were less likely to report access to substance abuse treatment or couples/family counseling, but were more likely to report the availability of trained peer support and follow-up care. Volunteers were also five times more likely to identify cost as a barrier, although they were less likely to report concerns about leadership support or confidentiality. Both volunteer and career firefighters expressed similar concerns about stigma. These findings emphasize the importance of tailored, population-specific mental health interventions that reflect not only the fire service's shared culture but also the nuanced differences between its subgroups.

Johnson et al. (2020) emphasized the importance of understanding fire culture and its implications for treatment. They argued that mental health care for firefighters must be adapted on the basis of unique subcultural contexts, such as geographic location (urban vs. rural) and functional role (career, volunteer, wildland, or aircraft rescue). Cultural nuance matters because it influences mental health outcomes and the likelihood of seeking help. Consequently, clinicians working with firefighters must go beyond generalized cultural competence to develop population-specific insights and treatment approaches.

Despite the growing awareness of mental health needs within fire and emergency services, research on effective behavioral health interventions remains limited. Nevertheless, the literature points to promising directions, including peer support, telehealth services, mindfulness-based practices, digital storytelling, work-recovery strategies, and critical incident stress management. Importantly, many of these modalities must be adapted to align with the fire service's cultural values, such as camaraderie, stoicism, and task orientation.

The overarching issue remains: many firefighters are reluctant to engage in care because they doubt that mental health professionals can truly understand their lived experience. The American Psychological Association (APA) defines culture as "the distinctive customs, values, beliefs, knowledge, art, and language of a society or community" and recognizes that culture includes professional groups. Cultural competence, therefore, is not a peripheral skill. Ultimately, improving firefighter mental health outcomes depends on reducing stigma, increasing access, addressing structural barriers, and, critically, ensuring that providers are culturally competent. Cultural competence means having a deep understanding of the fire service's values, structure, stressors, and support systems. It is not enough to be a trained clinician; one must be a clinician who understands the fire service. By investing in this competence, the fire service can better support its members and improve individual well-being and organizational resilience. As Smith et al. (2011) contend, culturally informed care is a prerequisite for effective and ethical practice.

According to the American Psychological Association (2023), "cultural competence" is defined as "1. Possessions of skills and knowledge are appropriate for and specific to a given culture. 2. The ability to collaborate effectively with individuals from different cultures in personal and professional settings. This usually involves recognition of the diversity both between and within cultures, a capacity for cultural self-assessment, and a willingness to adapt personal behaviors and practices. Cultural competence, also known as intercultural competence, has become a central concept in business, education, health care, government, and many other areas."

Cultural competence, the ability to effectively navigate cultural differences in service of meaningful interpersonal and organizational goals, is foundational to ethical and practical practice in high-stakes professions, including fire and emergency services. While often discussed conceptually, cultural competence can also be operationalized and measured through various tools designed to assess awareness, knowledge, attitudes, and skills. Several established instruments offer models for such evaluation, particularly within healthcare and education. The Cultural Diversity Questionnaire for Nurse Educators (CDQNE), for example, assesses six dimensions of cultural competence in educational settings: cultural awareness, cultural knowledge, cultural skill, cultural encounters, and culturally responsive teaching behaviors (Majnoon et al., 2023). Similarly, the Cultural Competence Assessment (CCA) tool measures healthcare providers' experiences and behaviors across four domains: cultural diversity exposure, awareness, sensitivity, and competence-related behaviors (Schim et al., 2023). Another widely used evaluative model is the cultural competence continuum, which conceptualizes cultural competence development as a staged process (Cross, 2020). This framework outlines six progressive phases: cultural destructiveness, cultural incapacity, cultural blindness, cultural pre-competence, cultural competence, and cultural proficiency. It provides a diagnostic roadmap for institutions seeking to understand and advance their organizational cultural responsiveness.

Collectively, these tools share a common foundation rooted in four primary components of cultural competence:

Awareness of one's cultural worldview and assumptions
Attitudes toward cultural differences
Knowledge of diverse cultural practices and worldviews
Cross-Cultural Skills for effective interaction in multicultural settings

While none of these instruments were developed specifically for the fire service, they offer valuable frameworks that can inform the creation of field-specific assessment tools. Given the distinct cultural environment of fire departments, characterized by hierarchy, tradition, peer solidarity, and occupational exposure to trauma, tailoring cultural competence measures to reflect these realities is crucial for fostering inclusive, effective behavioral health support systems within fire and emergency services.

The development of a culturally competent healthcare workforce is crucial for ensuring that firefighters and emergency medical providers have access to mental health resources that are equipped to address their specific needs. Although no specific research is available on the topic, according to the United States Fire Administration. The U.S. Fire Administration has highlighted ongoing gaps in access to culturally competent behavioral health support for firefighters and the limitations of many local EAPs in meeting first-responder needs (U.S. Fire Administration, 2023).

Generally, a culturally competent healthcare workforce can deliver high-quality, continuous patient care. Given the closed system of fire and emergency services, a culturally competent clinician would need to demonstrate competence across areas of complex cultural, ethnic, gender, age, or language differences in addition to the specific cultural dynamics of fire and emergency services. Research indicates that integrating culture into clinical care remains a challenging task. A study in Australia revealed that clinical supervisors struggled to define and teach cultural competence in hospital settings (Berger & Peerson, 2015).

Despite the increased emphasis on cultural competence across healthcare and behavioral fields, a critical gap remains in tools specifically designed to assess the unique cultural dynamics of fire and emergency services. Measuring cultural competence itself presents conceptual and practical challenges, as there is no existing instrument tailored to capture the norms, values, and interpersonal dynamics that shape firefighter culture. Nonetheless, cultural competence is not only a best-practice standard but also an ethical imperative. According to the American Psychological Association's Ethics Code, integrating cultural responsiveness into practice is essential for providing ethical and practical service delivery (APA, 2017).

Domenech Rodríguez et al. (2022) developed a general population measure of cultural competence on the basis of three foundational dimensions—awareness, knowledge, and skills—and addressed the broader need for empirically validated assessment tools. Their initial 81-item scale underwent expert review and was tested on a nationally representative sample of 204 adults. Factor analysis revealed four key components, awareness of self, awareness of others, proactive skills development, and knowledge, all of which demonstrated strong internal reliability ($\alpha = .87$–$.92$). The final 37-item instrument, known as the awareness, knowledge, skills-general (ASK-G) scale, showed high overall reliability ($\alpha = .94$) and robust validity across multiple domains.

Although designed for general application, ASK-G offers a valuable foundation for future adaptation to specialized professional groups. Given the fire service's distinct cultural characteristics, paramilitary structure, group cohesion, hierarchical leadership, and stoic norms, a compelling need exists to develop or adapt tools to assess cultural competence within this context reliably. Doing so would provide not only a means to evaluate training effectiveness but also a pathway to promote inclusivity, trust, and ethical care within fire departments.

Potential for Biases

Cultural competence must be distinguished from personal familiarity. Being related to a firefighter (whether as a spouse, sibling, or parent) does not automatically translate into cultural competence. Personal connections may introduce unconscious biases or role conflicts that compromise objectivity and clinical effectiveness (APA, 2023). Familiarity can provide a window into the fire service lifestyle, but it must be supplemented with formal training, ethical grounding, and cultural humility to be clinically helpful (APA, 2017). Clinicians must critically examine their assumptions and receive feedback from the fire service community to avoid overidentification, misinterpretation of experiences, or inappropriate application of therapeutic models (APA, 2017).

Similarly, clinicians who are former firefighters bring invaluable firsthand experience to their practice, offering a unique capacity to build rapport and trust with clients who are also firefighters. An intimate understanding of the demands of fire and emergency services can enhance therapeutic alliances. However, this dual identity may also present challenges. Former firefighters might inadvertently project their own experiences onto clients, leading to overidentification or assumptions that hinder objective assessment and intervention. Such clinicians must continuously self-reflect and seek supervision to navigate potential biases (APA, 2017). Open discussions about these dynamics in therapy can foster transparency and empower clients to share their experiences without fear of judgment.

While clinicians with direct fire service experience may offer lived insight, those without such backgrounds bring equally valuable perspectives to the therapeutic process. A psychologist who has never served as a firefighter may approach fire service culture with fresh eyes, characterized by genuine curiosity, openness, and humility. This outsider vantage point can facilitate a more deliberate cultural learning process, free from overidentification or assumptions shaped by personal experience (Sue, 2006). In many cases, such psychologists ask clarifying questions and invite clients to reflect more deeply on the nuances of their work, helping uncover themes that the firefighter may take for granted or feel are too embedded in to articulate.

Moreover, the lack of prior affiliation allows the clinician to maintain clinical neutrality, reducing the risk of shared trauma exposure or unconscious alignment with firehouse norms such as stoicism or emotional suppression. When supported by structured cultural competency training, mental health professionals can combine evidence-based practice with culturally responsive care, earning trust through respectful inquiry rather than assumed familiarity (APA, 2017). Research suggests that client perceptions of clinician authenticity and empathic engagement often matter more than shared identity alone (Sue, 2006). When adequately prepared, a non-firefighter clinician can build meaningful therapeutic relationships and validate the firefighter's lived experience while introducing new perspectives on coping, resilience, and recovery.

Cultural competency is a term used to describe the stages of development a provider undergoes to deliver professional services to a diverse population effectively (APA, 2023). Using a transtheoretical approach, fire service cultural competency enables the identification, assessment, and tracking of knowledge, skills, attitudes, and values, which are grounded in the foundation of various professional competencies within the fire service. Psychologists could be prepared to explore fire service-specific values, experiences, and sensitivities regarding individual and cultural differences within systems, as well as ethical and legal standards of practice, current coping strategies, scientific knowledge, and methods used in assessment, intervention, consultation, and operational work (APA, 2017). This preparation could also encompass evidence-based practices for clinical intervention and other relevant topics.

Mental Health Clinician Designations

Understanding the structure, scope, and qualifications of various mental health professionals is important for delivering culturally competent care to firefighter populations. Firefighters often seek services during periods of heightened stress or crisis, and the ability to communicate the clinician's role, licensure, scope of practice, and professional limitations is a foundational element of informed consent. In a culture that values clarity, trust, and operational transparency, clinicians must be equipped to explain their therapeutic approach, professional training, and legal responsibilities. This transparency fosters trust, reduces confusion, and empowers firefighter clients to make informed decisions about their care. Moreover, given the complexity of mental health licensures and varying scopes of practice, particularly across state lines, fire service personnel benefit from understanding the distinct qualifications among psychologists, psychiatrists, social workers, marriage and family therapists, and counselors. Ensuring that clinicians can articulate these distinctions enhances ethical practice and affirms the clinician's cultural respect for the fire service's structured and hierarchical environment. In accordance with the APA's Ethical Principles of Psychologists and Code of Conduct, psychologists are required to obtain informed consent using language that is reasonably understandable to clients. This includes providing information about the nature and anticipated course of therapy, fees, the involvement of third parties, and the limits of confidentiality, among other pertinent details.

Psychiatrists are medical doctors (M.D. or D.O.) who specialize in the prevention, diagnosis, and treatment of mental health disorders. Their scope of practice includes prescribing medications, conducting psychotherapy, and engaging in clinical research. Psychiatrists may work in private practice, hospitals, or clinical settings. To practice, they must earn a medical doctorate, complete supervised clinical training, and pass both a national board examination and a state licensure exam (ACGME, 2023; ABPN, n.d.).

Psychologists are doctoral-level professionals (Ph.D. or Psy.D.) trained to assess, diagnose, and treat emotional, cognitive, and behavioral issues. They may provide individual, group, couples, or family therapy and often perform psychological testing for purposes such as pre-employment screenings or fitness-for-duty evaluations. Psychologists have also developed, implemented, and evaluated behavioral health programs. Their roles span assessment, intervention, consultation, and operational support. Licensure requires the completion of a doctoral program, supervised practice hours, a research component (such as a dissertation), a national examination, and a state-specific licensing exam (ASPPB, n.d.).

Marriage and Family Therapists (MFTs) are master's-level clinicians trained to address relational and family dynamics. They provide psychotherapy to individuals, couples, and families, with a focus on interpersonal relationships and systemic issues. Licensure requires a master's degree, supervised clinical hours, and successful completion of national and state examinations. In many jurisdictions (e.g., California), use of the title 'psychologist' is legally restricted to individuals licensed as psychologists; holding a different mental health license—even with a doctorate—does not authorize that title (California Business & Professions Code § 2903).

Licensed Clinical Social Workers (LCSWs) provide therapy and case management services across diverse settings, including hospitals, community agencies, and private practices. In addition to providing counseling, LCSWs help clients access critical social resources. They must complete a master's degree in social work, obtain supervised experience, and pass both national and state licensure exams.

Educational Psychologists (EPs) typically work in school systems or private practices, specializing in assessments and interventions related to academic performance, learning challenges, and behavioral issues. Licensure requires a master's degree, supervised practice hours, and the passage of national and state examinations relevant to educational psychology. In the United States, this role is often licensed (where available) as a Licensed Educational Psychologist (LEP)—for example in California—with a scope focused on educationally related assessment and consultation (California Board of Behavioral Sciences, n.d.). Licensed Educational Psychologist (LEP). https://www.bbs.ca.gov/

Professional Clinical Counselors (PCCs) are licensed master's-level clinicians trained to provide therapeutic services for individuals facing emotional, cognitive, or behavioral difficulties. Their scope includes treatment for personal development, adjustment to disability, trauma, and environmental stressors. PCCs must earn a master's degree in counseling or a related field, complete a specified number of supervised hours, and pass national and state licensing examinations. Professional counselors are commonly titled Licensed Professional Counselors (LPCs); in some states (e.g., California) the title is Licensed Professional Clinical Counselor (LPCC) (California Business & Professions Code § 4999.20).

Mental Health Trainee Designations

Understanding the various stages of clinical training is crucial for providing culturally competent care, particularly when working with high-risk, high-accountability populations such as firefighters. Many fire service professionals may encounter student clinicians while caring for individuals practicing under supervision as part of their educational and licensure requirements. Mental health trainees and their supervisors must communicate the trainee's role, level of training, scope of practice, and supervision structure as part of the informed consent process. This transparency respects the cultural value that fire and emergency services place on hierarchy, competence, and trust. According to the American Psychological Association's (2017) *Ethical Principles of Psychologists and Code of Conduct*, psychologists must obtain informed consent using language understandable to clients and disclose all aspects of treatment, including the involvement of trainees and their supervisory arrangements. Establishing this clarity not only builds rapport but also enhances clinical credibility and ethical integrity.

Practicum Students

Practicum students are typically in the early stages of their clinical training. They are enrolled in a graduate program in psychology, social work, marriage and family therapy, counseling, or a related field. They engage in supervised clinical work as part of their academic coursework, often within university clinics, community mental health centers, or hospitals. Their responsibilities may include conducting intake assessments, facilitating therapy under supervision, and assisting with group sessions. Practicum students operate under the close oversight of licensed mental health professionals and are not independently licensed to practice.

Doctoral-Level Psychology Interns (APA-Accredited Internships)

Doctoral psychology interns complete their final year of training before earning their doctorate (Ph.D. or Psy.D.). These individuals have completed all coursework and comprehensive examinations and are engaged in full-time clinical work at an approved internship site. Accredited by the American Psychological Association or other governing bodies, internships are structured to provide diverse and intensive clinical experiences. Interns provide therapy, conduct psychological testing, and participate in multidisciplinary teams under the supervision of licensed professionals. Although they have advanced clinical skills, they are considered pre-licensed and must practice under formal supervisory arrangements.

Master's-Level Clinical Interns

Students pursuing licensures such as licensed clinical social workers (LCSWs), marriage and family therapists (MFTs), or professional clinical counselors (PCCs) also complete a clinical internship during their graduate training. These interns are typically in the final phase of their master's programs and must accrue a specified number of supervised hours across different client populations and settings. Like doctoral interns do, they work under licensed supervision and may conduct therapy, facilitate psychoeducational groups, and provide case management services. Interns should introduce themselves as trainees and identify their supervisor's role in the care process.

Postdoctoral Fellows (Psychology)

Postdoctoral fellows have completed their doctoral degree and internship in psychology and are now accumulating the supervised hours required for licensure as a psychologist. Postdoctoral training often includes advanced clinical specialization in trauma, neuropsychology, or mental health for first responders. Fellows function at a high level of competence but are still under the supervision of a licensed psychologist. In fire service settings, postdocs can offer valuable services such as assessment, individual and group therapy, and consultation, always within the ethical bounds of supervision and informed consent.

Medical Training Pathway for Psychiatrists

Psychiatrists are medical doctors (M.D. or D.O.) who complete a structured and rigorous training process in general medicine and psychiatric care. While they do not hold designations such as "practicum students" or "postdoctoral fellows" as psychologists do, their training includes multiple supervised stages equivalent in depth and intensity:

Medical School (Years 1–4)

Psychiatrists begin their journey with 4 years of medical education, where they complete both classroom-based education in medical sciences and clinical rotations across various specialties, including surgery, pediatrics, internal medicine, and psychiatry. During the psychiatry rotation, students may conduct supervised psychiatric evaluations, participate in team discussions, and observe the planning of treatment.

Psychiatry Residency (Years 1–4 Post-M.D.)

. In the U.S., general psychiatry residency typically spans 48 months (four years) under ACGME accreditation before optional subspecialty fellowship training (ACGME, 2023). This period is fully supervised and includes rotations in general psychiatry, child and adolescent psychiatry, addiction, forensic psychiatry, emergency psychiatry, and consultation-liaison psychiatry. Residents gradually increase their responsibilities under the supervision of board-certified attending psychiatrists. They are not yet independently licensed and must work under supervision, although they are designated "residents" rather than "students."

Fellowship (Optional, Post-Residency)

Some psychiatrists choose to subspecialize through fellowships, which involve an additional 1–2 years of specialized training in child and adolescent psychiatry, forensic psychiatry, addiction medicine, or psychosomatic medicine. Fellows hold medical licenses and often practice under minimal supervision while pursuing board certification in their chosen specialty (ABPN, n.d.).

Fire Service Cultural Competency Program: Training Stages

The Fire Service Cultural Competency Training Program was developed as a structured pathway for mental health professionals at the master's or doctoral level to develop the cultural fluency required to serve firefighter populations across individual, couple, family, and organizational contexts. This program emphasizes experiential learning, clinical application, and interdisciplinary collaboration (Fire Service Psychology Association, 2023).

Classroom training introduces participants to fire service-specific language, shift structures, organizational hierarchies, and the psychosocial demands of emergency work. Upon completion, clinicians are expected to understand trauma exposure, interpersonal relationship challenges unique to the profession, and trends in peer support and mental health service delivery within departments. These foundations are reinforced through immersive experiences, such as Practical Fire Operations 101 and a 40-h Ride-Along and Task Book component, which enable clinicians to observe, participate in, and debrief on fire service activities in real-world contexts.

By combining academic rigor with applied learning, the program provides a comprehensive framework for clinicians to develop and evaluate their fire service cultural competence, addressing risks such as vicarious trauma and burnout through ongoing consultation and reflective practice (Fire Service Psychology Association, 2023).

Introduction: Understanding the Fire Service Culture Course

The introductory course, *Understanding Fire Service Culture*, offers participants a comprehensive overview of the fire service, including its operational demands and psychological dynamics. The participants earn 1 h of continuing education credit per hour of instruction. All coursework is sponsored by the American Psychological Association, ensuring high academic standards and qualifying hours toward licensure requirements.

Upon successful completion, clinicians will be able to do the following:

Identify core cultural components of the fire service, such as shift work, terminology, and operational performance standards.
Describe the complexity of fire and EMS work, including exposure to trauma and its impact on mental health.
Identify unique relational challenges faced by firefighters.
Explain the structure and stressors of a paramilitary work environment.
Summarize emerging trends in peer support, psychological services, and barriers to treatment within fire departments.

Practical Fire Operations 101

This immersive, 1-day training uses scenario-based learning to expose clinicians to real-world hazards that firefighters encounter. The day begins with hands-on instructions on how to carry out structural firefighting gear (turnouts) and use a self-contained breathing apparatus (SCBA). Clinicians learn basic fireground tasks, including forcible entry via the Halligan tool, CPR techniques, and oxygen delivery protocols.

The afternoon features live-fire exercises conducted in a burn building under the supervision of trained instructors. The participants experienced the heat, darkness, and disorientation typical of fireground operations. This exercise introduces them to the cognitive, emotional, and physical stressors that firefighters face. Such exposure is foundational to understanding the fire service mindset and work culture. Similar programs are offered to Congressional staff by the Congressional Fire Services Institute and the Maryland Fire and Rescue Institute (Congressional Fire Services Institute & Maryland Fire and Rescue Institute, 2023). In October 2024, the Fire Service Psychology Association collaborated with the Washington D.C. Fire and Emergency Medical Services Department to deliver cultural competency training for mental health professionals (Fire Service Psychology Association, 2024).

Ride-Along and Task Book: 40 Hour Field Experience

Clinicians will complete 40 hour of field immersion through ride-alongs and in-station observations, scheduled collaboratively with a host fire department. During this period, clinicians gain firsthand exposure to the following:

- Fire service equipment, apparatus, and operational procedures.
- Organizational structure and leadership.
- Team dynamics and shift routines.
- Emergency and nonemergency response environments.

This experience enables mental health professionals to deepen their contextual understanding of fire and emergency services, thereby enhancing their ability to support firefighters through culturally sensitive interventions. It also allows firefighters and officers to become more familiar with the role of professional psychology, fostering mutual trust and collaboration.

The Fire Service Psychology Association (FSPA) emphasized the importance of these shared experiences for building effective, reciprocal relationships between clinicians and fire service personnel. The time spent in the station environment enables both groups to exchange knowledge and break down barriers to communication and service delivery.

Task Book Objectives

Throughout their 40-h experience, clinicians are expected to meet the following competencies:

- Articulate the primary responsibilities and roles of fire companies.
- Describe the physical and emotional stress of wearing structural firefighting gear.
- Explain the effects of operating in high-stress and low-visibility environments.
- Describe the response and coordination required during emergency scenarios.
- Understand and explain the firefighter "MAYDAY" emergency call process.
- This study demonstrates how NIOSH line-of-duty death (LODD) reports inform training and safety protocols.
- (Optional) Experience and articulating the impact of working in a live-burn scenario contingent upon facility availability and clinician readiness
  (Taskbook Developed by Battalion Chief Avsec (Retired) and Dr. Burt Clark, Fire Service Psychology Association, 2023*).*

Consultations with Experienced Fire Service Psychologists

Given the emotional toll of working with high-risk populations, clinicians are encouraged to consult with experienced psychologists from fire and emergency services. These consultations support the development of cultural competence and help clinicians manage the risks associated with vicarious trauma, compassion fatigue, and burnout.

As noted by Corey et al. (2011), clinicians working in "practice in extremis" contexts, such as trauma, emergency response, and public safety, are at heightened risk of emotional erosion, empathy fatigue, and loss of clinical effectiveness. Structured consultation serves as both a safeguard and a reflective tool, helping clinicians refine their approach and remain grounded in ethical, culturally responsive care.

Evaluation

To complete certification, participants are assessed via formative and summative methods. They must:

Conduct case evaluations of two firefighter scenarios and identify key cultural variables.

Demonstrate cultural competency in written or oral formats for review by the FSPA certification committee.

Complete a pre- and post-assessment to gauge gains in cultural knowledge, awareness, and application skills.

Conclusion

The mental health needs of firefighters are complex, urgent, and shaped by a unique occupational culture that is often misunderstood by those outside the fire service. The Fire Service Cultural Competency Training Program offers a rigorous, multidimensional approach to closing the cultural gap between clinicians and the fire service community. By combining foundational academic knowledge with immersive operational experiences and structured reflection, the program equips mental health professionals to provide ethical, relevant, and effective care. This cultural competence is not ancillary. As the literature has shown, access alone does not translate into utilization; firefighters must trust that clinicians understand their realities, language, and values. This trust is built not through assumption or proximity but through structured learning, humility, and sustained engagement. When clinicians are trained to meet firefighters, emotionally, organizationally, and culturally, they can become meaningful partners in prevention, intervention, and resilience-building. The continued development and support of culturally competent clinicians will be pivotal in reducing stigma, improving outcomes, and fostering psychologically safe environments within fire and emergency services. As such, programs such as this are not just educational offerings but moral and professional imperatives.

Chapter Review

Assignment: Advocating for Fire Service Cultural Competency in EAP Systems

Title: Designing a Strategic Outreach Plan for Culturally Competent Fire Service Behavioral Health

Assignment Overview (2500–3000 words): You are the newly appointed psychologist for a metropolitan fire department. Your task is to draft a strategic proposal to the EAP provider, fire chief, and city administrators, advocating for the inclusion of culturally competent clinicians on the department's referral list and recommending specialist pay for those who complete formal cultural competency training.

Assignment Objectives

Your proposal should include:

1. Justification for Cultural Competency (20%)
   (a) Explain why fire service members underutilize traditional mental health resources.
   (b) Identify key cultural, structural, and psychological barriers to care.
   (c) Use empirical data to frame why culturally competent care is ethically and operationally essential.
2. Overview of the Fire Service Cultural Competency Model (25%)
   (a) Describe the structure of the proposed training program (e.g., classroom modules, live-fire simulations, and ride-alongs).
   (b) Highlight the rationale for experiential learning and the outcomes this model aims to achieve in clinician performance and trust-building.
3. Integration with EAP Systems (20%)
   (a) Propose how trained clinicians would be vetted, added to referral lists, and matched with firefighter clients.
   (b) Suggest workflow changes to accommodate consultation between the department psychologist and EAP.
4. Financial Model: Specialist Pay Justification (15%)
   (a) Advocate for increased pay rates or stipends for clinicians who complete the fire service cultural competency program.

   (b) Address issues of recruitment, retention, and the high-risk nature of the population served.

5. Ethical and Political Considerations (10%)
   (a) Discuss any ethical challenges (e.g., dual relationships and trust boundaries) and potential pushback from stakeholders.
   (b) Anticipate concerns from city or EAP leadership and provide mitigation strategies.

6. Implementation Plan Summary (10%)

Provide a clear 6–12 month rollout plan, including:

   (a) Recruitment goals.
   (b) Evaluation metrics (e.g., referral uptake, satisfaction).
   (c) Ongoing consultation and supervision support.

Requirements

   (a) Word count: 2500–3000.
   (b) APA 7 format.
   (c) Use at least eight academic references.
   (d) Include citations from assigned readings (e.g., APA ethics code and fire service mental health data).

Chapter 12
Developing a Comprehensive Fire Service Psychology Program Within a Fire Department or EMS Agency

To create a psychology program that has value to a fire department, it is important to ensure that the program includes key elements, including a needs assessment, clear and measurable objectives, appropriate design, adequate resources, and a way of not only collecting relevant data but also interpreting it to determine the effectiveness of the program. The administrator is responsible for managing a comprehensive range of services and oversight mechanisms. They may be qualified to provide the services they are responsible for overseeing, although they are not tasked with providing direct services, as their role is administrative. This is important for quality assurance purposes. The structure and size of the agency determine the amount of resources needed to provide services to the department. For example, in rural departments, the psychologist may be tasked with overseeing a county-wide initiative rather than providing resources to a single organization.

Contract Services

When serving in a contract capacity, fire department psychologists play a pivotal role in overseeing the psychological services that support the operational and emotional health of personnel. This includes contract oversight for pre-employment psychological screenings, fitness-for-duty evaluations, violence risk assessments, annual wellness exams, and psychological autopsies. The psychologist does not necessarily conduct each of these evaluations directly but is responsible for vetting and selecting qualified providers who possess both clinical expertise and cultural competence in fire service settings. They work closely with department leadership and legal counsel to define the scope of services, ensure adherence to professional standards, and clarify expectations regarding documentation, confidentiality, and outcomes.

K. Wheldon, *Fire Service Psychology*,
https://doi.org/10.1007/978-3-032-02126-7_12

When psychological evaluations are completed, the psychologist interprets the findings within the context of fire service culture and operational demands. They meet with the fire chief, human resources, and legal representation to discuss results and provide informed, appropriate recommendations, ensuring that any administrative decisions related to hiring, retention, or duty status are supported by clinically and legally sound reasoning.

In the unfortunate event of a suicide involving a firefighter, dispatcher, or emergency medical provider, the department psychologist leads the coordination of postvention efforts. This includes initiating a referral for a psychological autopsy and working to support the department in navigating the clinical and emotional aftermath. The psychologist ensures that confidential psychological data are securely stored and accessible only to qualified professionals, maintaining ethical standards around privacy and data integrity.

Depending on the size and resources of the department, psychologists may also play a key administrative role in expanding the network of culturally competent mental health providers. This may involve hiring clinicians familiar with the unique demands of the fire service, collaborating with Employee Assistance Programs (EAPs) to identify suitable practitioners, or curating a vetted list of local or telehealth providers who accept the department's insurance, thus reducing financial barriers to care. In regions where culturally competent providers are limited, the psychologist works to build provider capacity by organizing fire service-specific cultural competency training sessions, facilitating networking among clinicians, and promoting access to continuing education that supports more informed and relevant clinical care.

In all of these functions, the psychologist ensures that contracted services align with the department's mission, legal obligations, and commitment to the well-being of its personnel, serving as both a clinical leader and an organizational advisor.

Mandated, Directed, and Self-Referrals

Directed Services and Program Oversight

Owing to the safety-sensitive nature of emergency operations, fire departments are legally and ethically authorized to mandate psychological evaluations when personnel exhibit signs that may impair their ability to perform important duties. Fitness-for-duty (FFD) evaluations are the primary mechanism used to assess whether a firefighter is psychologically capable of performing duties safely in high-risk environments. Courts have consistently upheld this practice. In Watson v. City of Miami Beach (1999), for example, the Eleventh Circuit affirmed the legality of requiring an FFD evaluation when an employee's behavior raised legitimate concerns. Similarly, in Coffman v. Indianapolis Fire Department (2009), the Seventh Circuit found that psychological assessments were justified in response to observable behavioral concerns and department risk.

If a firefighter is found temporarily unfit for duty, mandated treatment may be recommended as part of a structured return-to-duty process. In such cases, the psychologist works in consultation with department leadership, legal counsel, and treating clinicians to ensure that the recommended intervention meets the standard of reasonable accommodation under the Americans with Disabilities Act (ADA), balancing clinical recovery with operational readiness. Attendance and compliance may be monitored administratively, but clinical content remains confidential unless the member voluntarily authorizes disclosure.

In contrast, direct referrals are often initiated by departments following critical incidents, such as traumatic calls, near fatalities, or distressing operational events. These are voluntary in nature: firefighters are encouraged, but not required, to attend a confidential session with a culturally competent clinician. Voluntary referrals may also originate from the individual themselves, without a triggering event, and are handled with full clinical confidentiality unless a release is authorized. Both types of voluntary engagement help reduce stigma, promote early intervention, and reinforce trust in the psychological support system.

Notably, some departments have adopted trauma risk management (TRiM) as an alternative to traditional critical incident stress debriefing models. TRiM is a peer-delivered, evidence-informed framework originally developed within military contexts to assess risk following exposure to trauma (Greenberg, N., Langston, V., Everitt, B., Iversen, A., Fear, N. T., & Jones, N. (2010)). In fire service adaptation, TRiM trains designated personnel to conduct structured, nonclinical risk assessments following operationally significant events. Rather than offering therapy or emotional ventilation, TRiM practitioners assess functional impact and coping to determine whether a referral to clinical services is warranted. This model allows departments to support early identification of stress injuries while maintaining a non-pathologizing, culturally grounded approach to care.

In addition to individual- and peer-level support, psychologists are also responsible for system-wide program development. This includes overseeing crisis intervention protocols, integrating behavioral health into workers' compensation processes (e.g., return-to-work planning), and delivering ongoing education on topics such as trauma, addiction, suicide risk, and performance under stress. In addition, psychologists may support local workforce development by training clinicians in fire service cultural competence, thereby expanding access to responsive and context-informed mental health care.

Needs Assessment and Data-Driven Solutions

A foundational component of developing a fire service psychology program is conducting a comprehensive needs assessment to identify the goals (behavioral health challenges, operational stressors affecting personnel, etc). This process must be both methodical and inclusive, drawing on surveys, interviews, and focus groups to capture insights from firefighters, leadership, and, when appropriate, their families. Key areas of focus can include psychological distress (e.g., PTSD and depression), occupational burnout, substance use, and the cumulative impact of exposure to trauma. Once goals are defined, objectives can be formulated as actionable steps to achieve them. At this stage, it is important to consider the necessary resources and identify the key participants involved. Following this, a well-designed data collection strategy should be implemented to evaluate the program's effectiveness and efficiency, supporting ongoing quality improvement and the integration of evidence-based practices.

Evidence from healthcare and public safety sectors illustrates how structured needs assessments can guide the development of tailored wellness initiatives. For example, Wilkie et al. (2022) conducted a needs assessment with physicians at a Canadian academic mental health hospital, identifying high rates of emotional distress and organizational barriers to wellness. In response, the organization implemented a multilayered wellness framework, including peer support programs, mentorship, and leadership development initiatives, demonstrating the feasibility of comprehensive wellness strategies when frontline staff are actively engaged and their feedback informs system design.

Similarly, within first responder agencies, the Vicarious Trauma Organizational Readiness Guide (VT-ORG) provides a validated tool to assess an organization's preparedness to address the psychological toll of trauma exposure. Hallinan et al. (2019) evaluated the tool in more than 3000 personnel across emergency services and victim support organizations and reported that the VT-ORG subscales strongly predict outcomes such as turnover intention, compassion satisfaction, and organizational resilience. The psychometric reliability (Cronbach's $\alpha = .98$) and predictive validity of the VT-ORG make it a valuable resource for fire departments seeking to build trauma-informed systems of care.

In addition to qualitative and psychometric tools, departments should leverage existing administrative data systems to analyze trends that may reflect underlying wellness challenges. Human resource information systems (HRISs), incident reporting databases, occupational health platforms, and electronic health records (EHRs) provide insight into patterns of absenteeism, injury, burnout, or medical leave. For example, computer-aided dispatch (CAD) systems may reveal operational trends (e.g., increased call volume or high-risk incidents) that correlate with stress-related claims or behavioral health referrals. Similarly, performance management systems can be used to identify associations between reduced operational readiness and spikes in sick leave or peer support utilization.

By triangulating these data sources, psychometric tools, system metrics, and stakeholder input, fire departments can develop evidence-informed behavioral health strategies. These may include targeted prevention programs, leadership training, peer support expansion, or clinical partnerships tailored to the identified needs of the workforce. Moreover, engaging a range of stakeholders in the needs assessment process fosters shared ownership and enhances the legitimacy of subsequent interventions.

Ultimately, embedding a data-driven approach into fire service psychology programs ensures that interventions are responsive, scalable, and sustainable. It also positions the department to continuously monitor and adapt to emerging behavioral health risks, supporting a culture of psychological resilience across all ranks.

Define Goals and Objectives

The development of a comprehensive fire service psychology program begins with articulating clear, measurable goals and supporting objectives that align with the department's mission, operational demands, and cultural values. As Kettner et al. (2008) emphasize, program goals should not be abstract ideals but concrete benchmarks that guide design, implementation, and evaluation. These benchmarks must also reflect the lived realities of personnel, incorporating organizational priorities and the behavioral health needs of the workforce.

Issel and Wells (2017) further argue that goals must be responsive to the ecological systems in which personnel operate, including organizational structures, peer dynamics, and community expectations. In the fire service context, this means setting goals that address both short-term needs (e.g., crisis intervention and stress management) and long-term priorities (e.g., stigma reduction, resilience-building, and cultural transformation).

Objectives act as actionable steps that lead to broader program goals. McDavid et al. (2019) distinguish between outcome objectives, which target changes in behavior, knowledge, or well-being, and process objectives, which focus on the activities used to achieve those outcomes. For example, a goal to reduce mental health-related absenteeism might include process objectives such as training 20% of supervisors in mental health first aid or launching quarterly resilience workshops for high-risk units. These initiatives aim to shift attitudes, reduce stigma, and foster proactive help-seeking behaviors. The underlying theory of change assumes that by improving mental health literacy and cultivating psychological safety, departments can reduce absenteeism over time. Evaluation methods may include pre- and post-training surveys, monitoring referral patterns, and analyzing absenteeism trends across units.

Internal consistency among goals, objectives, and activities is critical for effective programming. As Rossi et al. (2018) note, a logically aligned program ensures that each activity is directly linked to a stated objective, which in turn supports a broader goal. Logic models, endorsed by both Kettner et al. (2008) and McDavid et al. (2019), serve as effective tools to map these relationships, especially in complex systems such as fire departments. They help stakeholders visualize how peer support teams, resilient trainers, or clinical liaisons contribute to measurable outcomes such as reduced burnout, increased morale, or improved utilization of employee assistance programs (EAPs).

To ensure that these efforts are actionable and accountable, departments should adopt SMART goals, those that are specific, measurable, achievable, relevant, and time-bound (Doran, 1981). The SMART criteria transform general aspirations into concrete targets that can be monitored and adjusted as needed. For example, a goal such as "increase participation in department-offered mental health training to 75% within 12 months" is more practical and valuable than a vague commitment to "improving mental health awareness."

Examples of SMART-aligned goals in fire service mental health programming include reducing stigma around help-seeking by 20% (measured via pre/post surveys), ensuring that 100% of personnel are aware of available mental health resources by year-end, and training 15% of the workforce as peer supporters within 2 years. Departments might also aim to reduce burnout scores by 15% via validated tools such as the Maslach Burnout Inventory, increase EAP utilization by 25%, implement a 24/7 mental health crisis hotline, and ensure that all leaders are trained in mental health support strategies within 1 year. Conducting annual wellness surveys further supports outcome tracking and continuous improvement.

By grounding behavioral health programming in evidence-based planning, fire departments can ensure that their goals are not only aspirational but also strategic, measurable, and culturally relevant. This structured approach, rooted in planning literature and adapted to the realities of emergency services, positions departments to proactively promote mental wellness, build organizational resilience, and deliver sustainable psychological support to their workforce.

Program Design

A comprehensive fire service psychology program must be designed as a multifaceted, prevention-oriented system that addresses behavioral health needs across the continuum of exposure, functioning not only as an intervention mechanism but also as an embedded component of operational readiness. Drawing from the public health and program planning literature, a layered prevention framework comprising primary, secondary, tertiary, and quaternary prevention offers a robust structure to organize psychological services in fire and emergency services (Issel & Wells, 2017; Jamoulle, 2024; Kettner et al., 2008).

Prevention: Education, Stress Management, and Resilience-Building Workshops

A foundational component of a comprehensive fire service psychology program is a robust prevention strategy. Prevention corresponds with primary prevention in public health: it targets the entire workforce to reduce the likelihood of psychological distress before it occurs. This includes proactive measures such as behavioral health education, stress management techniques, sleep hygiene, physical wellness, and resilience-building workshops. These initiatives not only reduce stigma but also promote early help-seeking and self-awareness. Cultivating a department-wide culture of psychological safety encourages adaptive coping and peer accountability and normalizes mental health maintenance as a shared operational responsibility (Issel & Wells, 2017; Vujanovic, 2023). Research highlights the value of proactive wellness frameworks in promoting firefighter well-being and reducing long-term risk for behavioral health conditions (Oliveira et al., 2023).

Intervention: Peer Support Teams, Access to Counseling, Crisis Hotlines

Intervention strategies span both secondary prevention and tertiary prevention, each addressing different stages of behavioral health needs. Secondary prevention focuses on early detection and timely support for firefighters beginning to show signs of psychological distress. This includes well-trained peer support teams, who are not therapists but serve as trusted points of contact to recognize early warning signs and guide peers toward appropriate clinical services. Peer support improves engagement, reduces stigma, and increases the likelihood that individuals will seek care when it is needed (Jahnke et al., 2014).

Tertiary prevention, in contrast, involves formal clinical intervention to treat established mental health conditions and mitigate long-term impacts. This includes access to confidential counseling, crisis hotlines, and evidence-based therapies tailored to first responders, such as cognitive behavioral therapy (CBT) for anxiety, depression, and sleep disturbances and eye movement desensitization and reprocessing (EMDR) for trauma-related symptoms. These clinical practices are supported in the fire service literature as effective interventions when culturally adapted for this population (Haugen et al., 2012; Vujanovic, 2023).

Postvention: Support for Recovery and Reintegration After Critical Incidents

Postvention strategies primarily align with tertiary prevention, focusing on recovery and reducing the risk of long-term psychological harm following exposure to potentially traumatic events (PTEs). Crucially, fire service culture must recognize that no incident is inherently traumatic; the psychological impact varies on the basis of individual factors, prior exposure, perceived threat, and available support. Postvention strategies must therefore be responsive and individualized, avoiding one-size-fits-all approaches to distress (Oliveira et al., 2023).

A critical component of postvention is supporting firefighters who are off-duty due to psychological injury, including posttraumatic stress, cumulative stress effects, and diagnosable conditions such as depression or anxiety. These individuals benefit most from structured return-to-work pathways that prioritize recovery and sustainable reintegration rather than merely clearance for duty. The best practices include individualized planning, clinical collaboration, family engagement, reacclimation protocols, and ongoing therapeutic support (Vujanovic, 2023). Such strategies reduce the risk of relapse, protect operational safety, and demonstrate institutional accountability for psychological recovery.

Postvention also includes support for broader organizational needs following suicide, traumatic calls, or line-of-duty deaths. Peers, supervisors, and families often experience secondary trauma, grief, or moral injury, requiring targeted interventions to restore team cohesion and psychological readiness. This may include brief follow-ups, coaching for leadership, or group-based support, depending on the context (Oliveira et al., 2023).

Aligned with quaternary prevention, postvention must also be cautious not to overmedicalize normal emotional responses. Not all firefighters who experience distress need formal clinical treatment, but all deserve nonjudgmental access to support. Peer-led programs such as trauma risk management (TRiM) provide structured, nonclinical risk assessments that help distinguish between transient stress and emerging psychological injury (Greenberg et al., 2017). This approach safeguards autonomy, maintains cultural alignment, and fosters trust in behavioral health systems.

Ultimately, postvention is not merely reactive. It is a proactive investment in firefighter recovery, team integrity, and psychological safety. When grounded in evidence and applied ethically, it can reduce long-term occupational harm and foster a department-wide culture of care.

A comprehensive program must also reflect quaternary prevention, which seeks to avoid unnecessary psychological interventions and the medicalization of normal emotional responses to high-risk work. In fire service settings, this includes careful screening for clinical referral, safeguarding confidentiality, and minimizing the risk of re-traumatization during post-incident processes. Peer-led tools such as TRiM support informed triage and provide structured pathways for clinical referral when needed (Greenberg et al., 2017). By distinguishing between support, stress, and disorder, departments can ensure appropriate, ethical care that upholds dignity and choice.

By embedding all four levels of prevention, primary, secondary, tertiary, and quaternary, into a single, multifaceted design, fire departments can build a behavioral health system that is responsive, ethical, and culturally relevant. These systems must be routinely evaluated via feedback loops, logic models, and utilization data to remain adaptive over time (Kettner et al., 2008; McDavid et al., 2019). Ultimately, an integrated program design ensures that mental health services are not siloed or reactionary but fully embedded into the department's operational mission and culture.

Engaging Stakeholders

An effective fire service psychology program must be codesigned with those it intends to serve. Engaging stakeholders, including union representatives, department leaders, fire officers, rank-and-file personnel, and mental health professionals, is important not only for program success but also for cultural relevance, sustainability, and legitimacy within the department. Early involvement of key stakeholders fosters ownership, trust, and buy-in, which are critical in professions where skepticism toward behavioral health services may exist (Kettner et al., 2008).

Firefighters are more likely to engage with programs that reflect their lived experiences and operational demands. Therefore, establishing structured feedback loops through surveys, focus groups, or pilot initiatives ensures that program components are not only clinically sound but also contextually appropriate. The inclusion of union representatives and informal leaders in the early stages of planning can preempt resistance and help align behavioral health goals with existing workforce values and operational priorities (Issel & Wells, 2017).

Equally important is partnership with licensed mental health professionals who have demonstrated competence in working with first responder populations. Clinicians with this specialization are more likely to understand fire service norms such as hypervigilance, shift schedules, trauma exposure, and the stigma that often surrounds help-seeking behaviors. When clinicians and department leaders work collaboratively, program components, from peer support training to return-to-work planning, can be more precisely tailored to the unique psychological and cultural needs of the workforce (Vujanovic, 2023).

Stakeholder engagement is not a single step but rather an ongoing process of shared ownership and iterative development. As such, departments should create advisory groups or interdisciplinary wellness committees that include mental health experts, firefighters, and leaders to guide implementation and adapt programming in response to new challenges or lessons learned. This approach reflects best practices in both human services and public health program design: programs are most effective when they are participatory, adaptive, and co-produced with those they are meant to serve (McDavid et al., 2019).

Resource Allocation

A sustainable fire service psychology program requires strategic and transparent resource allocation to ensure that the program is not only developed but also maintained over time. Effective resource planning begins with identifying and securing diverse funding sources, including municipal budgets, federal and state grants, foundations, and public safety mental health initiatives. Programs that demonstrate alignment with organizational goals and community wellness outcomes are often more successful in competing for external funding (McDavid et al., 2019).

Beyond acquisition, resource allocation must also include thoughtful budgeting for training, materials, staffing, and community partnerships. Behavioral health services require not only clinicians but also investments in infrastructure, such as peer support training, mental health literacy campaigns, crisis response resources, and digital tools for tracking utilization and impact. Dedicated funding for these components demonstrates organizational commitment and supports long-term program viability (Kettner et al., 2008).

It is also critical to account for cross-sector partnerships, particularly when leveraging expertise from external mental health professionals or institutions. These partnerships may require memoranda of understanding, stipends for clinical services, or shared training resources. Proactively budgeting for such collaborations enables departments to expand service offerings without overextending internal capacity.

Strategic allocation also involves integrating behavioral health considerations into broader operational budgets, for example, embedding wellness into academic training, promotional coursework, leadership development, and return-to-duty protocols. Embedding psychological safety across operational domains, rather than siloing it, increases the likelihood that behavioral health becomes a normalized and expected element of fire service readiness (Issel & Wells, 2017).

Ultimately, the way resources are allocated communicates departmental priorities. When properly aligned with goals and evaluation strategies, resource planning serves not only as a logistical function but also as a vehicle for cultural change and institutional accountability.

Implementation

The successful execution of a fire service psychology program depends not only on design and planning but also on an intentional and adaptive implementation strategy. Rolling out the program in phases allows departments to manage resource demands, pilot-test interventions, gather stakeholder feedback, and make iterative improvements. Phased implementation also reduces disruption and builds momentum by starting with achievable goals and gradually expanding reach (Kettner et al., 2008). This approach aligns with best practices in human services and public health, where adaptive rollout strategies have been shown to increase both program fidelity and sustainability (Issel & Wells, 2017).

A foundational element of implementation is the training of peer support personnel, supervisors, and leaders in the early stages of the program. Frontline responders often turn to peers before clinicians do; therefore, training must focus not only on the recognition of behavioral health symptoms but also on empathic engagement, boundaries, and appropriate referral procedures. Supervisors should be equipped to support personnel during performance fluctuations, exposure to potentially traumatic events, and reintegration after time off for psychological recovery. Research consistently shows that early intervention by well-trained nonclinical personnel can reduce escalation and improve access to care (Vujanovic, 2023).

Effective implementation also requires clear, consistent, and multichannel communication. Personnel must know what services are available, how to access them, and what to expect regarding confidentiality and support. Communication strategies should include in-person briefings, digital platforms, printed materials, and integration into onboarding and promotional training. Embedding the program into existing department workflows reinforces the message that behavioral health is an important component of operational readiness, not an ancillary concern (McDavid et al., 2019).

In short, implementation should be viewed as a process, not a single event. When executed deliberately, with attention to sequencing, training, and communication, implementation becomes a powerful tool for building credibility, fostering engagement, and embedding mental wellness into the culture of the fire service.

Evaluation and Feedback

Ongoing evaluation is important to ensure that a fire service psychology program remains effective, relevant, and aligned with the evolving needs of personnel. Evaluation is not a final step but an integrated component of the program cycle, guiding refinement, resource allocation, and long-term sustainability (McDavid et al., 2019). A well-structured evaluation plan should include clearly defined metrics aligned with the program's goals and objectives.

Common indicators of program impact may include utilization rates of peer support and counseling services, changes in self-reported well-being, reductions in mental health-related absenteeism, stress-related workers compensation claims, feedback from incident debriefs or post-training surveys, and TRiM data tracking systems. These data help assess both process (e.g., whether interventions are being delivered as intended) and outcome (e.g., whether personnel are experiencing improved resilience or reduced distress) (Rossi et al., 2018).

The incorporation of participant feedback is equally critical. Feedback can be collected through anonymous surveys, focus groups, or suggestion systems that allow firefighters to share insights and concerns candidly. This creates a continuous feedback loop that not only promotes program improvement but also enhances trust and psychological safety. Engaging stakeholders in the interpretation of results, such as presenting findings to peer teams or command staff, fosters shared ownership and responsiveness (Kettner et al., 2008).

Importantly, evaluation findings should inform timely program adjustments. This might involve revising training content, improving referral systems, or expanding successful components. Programs that regularly monitor and adapt are more likely to demonstrate long-term effectiveness and organizational alignment (Issel & Wells, 2017).

Ultimately, evaluation and feedback are not just technical requirements; they are expressions of accountability and cultural responsiveness, ensuring that the fire service psychology program continues to meet the real-world needs of the workforce it serves.

Sustainability

To ensure long-term success, a fire service psychology program must be intentionally designed for sustainability, not as a temporary initiative but as a permanent component of departmental operations and culture. Sustainability involves institutional commitment, policy integration, community partnerships, and ongoing capacity building (Kettner et al., 2008).

A core strategy for sustainability is building collaborative partnerships with local mental health organizations and culturally competent professionals. These partnerships expand the department's service capacity and provide access to clinicians experienced in treating first responders. Establishing formal agreements or memoranda of understanding helps ensure consistent access to care while sharing training, supervision, or emergency backup resources. Local partnerships also increase program resilience during staffing shortages or budget constraints (Issel & Wells, 2017).

Equally important is the development of formal policies and procedures that institutionalize behavioral health programming. This includes incorporating behavioral health training into the fire academy, codifying post-incident protocols, embedding peer support into standard operating procedures (SOPs), and integrating wellness into promotional pathways and return-to-work processes. Clear documentation supports organizational memory and shields programs from leadership turnover or shifting political priorities (McDavid et al., 2019).

Ongoing training and education are also important for keeping the program relevant, effective, and aligned with best practices. Firefighters, peer supporters, and leaders should receive annual continuing education on topics such as trauma-informed supervision, suicide prevention, and stress management. New research, emerging treatment modalities, and evolving cultural dynamics in fire and emergency services demand a program that can evolve in parallel (Rossi et al., 2018). This also helps normalize behavioral health conversations and ensures that psychological readiness is viewed as integral to operational performance.

In sum, sustainability is not just about funding. It is about embedding psychological wellness into the fire service's identity, infrastructure, and mission. Programs that invest in strong partnerships, institutional frameworks, and continuous learning are far more likely to endure and have meaningful, long-term impacts.

Cultural Integration

For a fire service psychology program to be fully effective, it must become a cultural norm, not just a policy or initiative. Cultural integration involves shifting attitudes, expectations, and behaviors across all levels of the organization, ensuring that behavioral health is recognized as important to individual performance and organizational readiness (Kettner et al., 2008).

A foundational strategy for cultural integration is normalizing mental health conversations through visible leadership modeling. When chiefs, officers, and respected senior personnel openly support psychological wellness, discussing its importance, acknowledging challenges, and modeling help-seeking behaviors, it fosters psychological safety across the department. Such modeling has been shown to reduce stigma and increase trust in behavioral health systems (Issel & Wells, 2017; Vujanovic, 2023).

Behavioral health content should be incorporated into routine operations, such as academy curricula, shift briefings, after-action reviews, and departmental meetings, further embedding the program into the daily life of the fire service. This includes not only formal training but also informal reinforcement, such as referencing wellness resources during high-stress periods or recognizing strong peer support in performance reviews. When behavioral health is woven into standard workflows, it becomes part of the department's operational fabric rather than an optional add-on (McDavid et al., 2019).

Celebrating successes, such as increased program utilization, positive outcomes (even possibly successful reintegration after stress-related injury), or individual acts of peer support, helps reinforce the program's value and builds momentum. Highlighting these outcomes in newsletters, awards, or leadership addresses makes the benefits of the program visible and encourages broader participation. These moments serve as cultural touchpoints, communicating that behavioral health is a shared priority and a marker of professional strength, not weakness (Rossi et al., 2018).

This structured, culturally attuned approach ensures that the fire service psychology program is not only relevant and impactful but also deeply aligned with the values, mission, and lived experience of the workforce it is designed to support.

Comprehensive Range of Services and Oversight Mechanisms

The structure and scope of a fire service psychology program vary significantly depending on the department's size, resources, and organizational context. In large municipal fire departments, the director of behavioral health, often a licensed psychologist, may serve as a full-time, embedded staff member reporting directly to the Fire Chief. This position parallels that of a medical director, a role long recognized in fire and emergency services since the integration of emergency medical services (EMSs) in the 1970s (Kettner et al., 2008). In smaller, rural, or volunteer-based departments, psychologists may instead serve in contracted or regional administrative roles, overseeing behavioral health services across multiple jurisdictions and coordinating with local clinical resources to ensure access to culturally competent care.

Positioning the psychologist as a direct report to the fire chief ensures that critical, time-sensitive, and potentially life-saving information is not lost in translation. This structural alignment allows psychologists to actively shape policy, respond to organizational risk factors, and contribute to leadership decision-making in real time. It also elevates the visibility of behavioral health as a strategic priority, embedded in operational readiness rather than framed as a remedial service.

Rather than functioning solely as a clinician, the psychologist in this role primarily acts as a program administrator, overseeing internal and contracted services across five key domains:

1. **Contract Oversight and Program Management**

The psychologist is responsible for ensuring that all contracted behavioral health services meet legal, ethical, and clinical standards. The core functions include:

(a) Pre-employment psychological screenings.
(b) Fitness-for-duty evaluations.
(c) Violence risk assessments.
(d) Annual wellness assessments.
(e) Psychological autopsies following suicide.
(f) Human factors analysis after occupational fatality/ line of duty death.
(g) Vetting and credentialing of service providers.

When services are coordinated through employee assistance programs (EAPs), the psychologist ensures that those providers are trained in fire service culture and competent in trauma-informed care. If gaps are identified, the psychologist may work with EAP leadership to coordinate training, build a local referral network, and increase provider capacity (Issel & Wells, 2017).

2. **Internal Program Oversight**

The psychologist leads internal behavioral health operations, ensuring alignment with department goals and national best practices. The core responsibilities include the following:

Oversight of peer support programs:

(a) Coordination of post-critical incident responses via models such as Trauma Risk Management (TRiM) (Greenberg & Jones, 2006).
(b) Integration with workers' compensation processes for behavioral health claims.
(c) Development and monitoring of return-to-work plans following psychological injury.

Additionally, the psychologist safeguards confidentiality by delineating reporting protocols: mandated referrals (e.g., fitness-for-duty) may include simple attendance reports, whereas voluntary referrals remain fully confidential, in compliance with ethical and legal standards.

3. **Training and Education**

An important component of this role is providing or coordinating health education for all levels of the department. Training topics may include the following:

(a) Psychological field preparation (trauma, suicide risk, and addiction) in the academy.
(b) Performance psychology and decision-making under stress.

(c) Crisis response strategies for internal and community-based behavioral health emergencies.
(d) Annual in-service refresher training for peer teams and supervisors.
(e) These educational initiatives contribute to both primary prevention and cultural integration, promoting long-term resilience and early recognition of distress (Vujanovic, 2023).

4. **Cultural Competence and Workforce Development**

The psychologist also plays a strategic role in building a culturally competent healthcare workforce by:

(a) Training local clinicians on fire service culture and operational stressors.
(b) Collaborating with academic institutions and regional networks to expand behavioral health support across the emergency response system.
(c) Facilitating community engagement to reduce stigma and promote trust in mental health services.
(d) This workforce development strategy addresses access challenges in underserved or rural communities, where internal behavioral health resources may be limited (Rossi et al., 2018).

5. **Structural Adaptability**

The U.S. fire service lacks a standardized national administrative framework, which means that departments must tailor their behavioral health programs to the local context. Departments may be fully paid, on-call, volunteer, or hybrid structures, funded through municipal budgets, federal grants, or community fundraising (United States Fire Administration [USFA], n.d.). In this environment, the psychologist's role must remain flexible, capable of serving high-capacity urban agencies or acting regionally across small departments.

Ultimately, whether operating as a department director or regional consultant, the fire service psychologist brings clinical, administrative, and ethical oversight to a complex system of care. Embedding this role into the organizational chart, much like a medical director, reflects a maturing understanding that psychological health is mission-critical to emergency services.

Health and Wellness Committee Organizational Structure

An effective fire service psychology program must be embedded within a broader, interdisciplinary Health and Wellness Committee, which serves as the operational and administrative backbone for addressing both physical and psychological health needs across the department. The structure and responsibilities of this committee may vary depending on the size and resources of the department, but its primary function remains the same: ensuring the well-being of personnel through coordinated oversight, expert consultation, and collaborative planning.

In larger municipal departments, this committee is typically led by the Chief of Health and Safety Operations, who gathers data and input from key personnel, including the Health and Wellness Coordinator, Medical Director, Director of Behavioral Health (licensed psychologist), and Exercise Physiologist. The chief is responsible for synthesizing this information to assess departmental needs, prioritize initiatives, prepare budget requests, and communicate findings and recommendations directly to the fire chief. This high-level reporting structure ensures that health-related concerns receive timely attention and strategic support from executive leadership.

The health and wellness coordinator plays a central administrative role, interfacing with the medical director, director of behavioral health, and exercise physiologist to manage the operational functions of the wellness program. This includes coordinating outside referrals for services such as Employee Assistance Programs (EAPs), workers' compensation, and other clinical support. The coordinator ensures that personnel can access the right resources efficiently while maintaining appropriate documentation and follow-up procedures.

In smaller or volunteer departments, where staffing and budgets are more limited, the structure may be streamlined. In these settings, a single professional, often the health and safety officer, may fulfill both the coordinator and chief of health and safety operations roles. These departments may also participate in county- or region-wide contracts to gain access to licensed professionals such as psychologists, physicians, or exercise physiologists who serve multiple jurisdictions.

Across all department sizes, clear role delineation is critical to preserving ethical standards and program integrity. For example, psychologists conducting fitness-for-duty or pre-employment psychological screenings must not serve in a direct treatment capacity for the same individuals to avoid conflicts of interest and ensure objectivity in evaluations.

The psychological health component of the program includes access to brief therapy, mental health education, critical incident stress management or psychological first aid, peer support team development and maintenance, and psychological screenings (e.g., pre-employment and fitness-for-duty evaluations). The oversight of these services is the responsibility of the licensed psychologist, who ensures that the program meets both clinical standards and operational goals.

The physical health component includes access to physiological stress management, nutrition education, injury prevention and rehabilitation, strength and conditioning services, and annual medical physical and fitness assessments. These elements fall under the shared oversight of the Medical Director and Exercise Physiologist, who collaborates to design and implement strategies that reduce occupational health risks and promote long-term wellness.

Regardless of the department's size, this integrated model provides a framework to support the full spectrum of firefighter health, physical, psychological, and operational, through structured roles, ethical oversight, and multidisciplinary collaboration.

Integrating Psychological Assessment into Routine Fire Service Practice: Opportunities and Ethical Considerations

As fire service psychology continues to mature, there is increasing momentum toward integrating psychological assessments into routine operational practice, much like annual medical physicals or SCBA fit testing. In brief, validated mental health screenings in standard wellness protocols present a unique opportunity to normalize psychological care, reduce stigma, and proactively identify early signs of distress. This shift from reactive to preventive care can promote long-term resilience, workforce retention, and operational readiness ethically and strategically (DeMoulin et al., 2023; Schuhmann et al., 2022).

From Reactive to Proactive: Routine Assessment Models

Historically, psychological assessments in fire departments have been reserved for specific events, pre-employment screening, post-critical incident review, or fitness-for-duty evaluations. While these uses remain critical, there is growing support for moving toward proactive, routine models of assessment. Annual wellness evaluations utilizing instruments such as the Firefighter Assessment of Stress Test (FAST), the Firefighter Coping Self-Efficacy (FFCSE) Scale, or the Emergency Services Moral Injury Scale-Firefighter Version (EMIS-F) can help departments monitor exposure to trauma, moral distress, burnout, and coping capacity over time (DeMoulin et al., 2023; Lambert et al., 2012; Schuhmann et al., 2022).

These tools, when administered through secure digital platforms or in-person wellness clinics, offer scalable, confidential methods to assess psychological health without pathologizing stress responses. Participation can remain voluntary and non-punitive, emphasizing that psychological wellness is a shared responsibility and a marker of preparedness, not a sign of vulnerability or risk. Moreover, aggregated, de-identified data can inform departmental strategies, highlighting organizational stressors, such as leadership breakdowns, administrative overload, or shift-related fatigue, that may not emerge through traditional reporting mechanisms (Lambert et al., 2012).

Ethical Concerns in High-Risk Occupations

Despite the benefits of integrating mental health screening into routine practice, doing so in high-risk occupations such as firefighting raises several ethical challenges. These include issues of confidentiality, dual-role conflicts, data misuse, and cultural mismatch between clinicians, tools, and fire service culture (Stamatis et al., 2024).

One significant risk is the dual-role dilemma, wherein psychologists are asked to act as both evaluators and clinicians. This conflict can blur ethical boundaries, compromise therapeutic trust, and introduce legal liability if role clarity is not established at the outset (Fisher, 2022). Firefighters must be informed whether the psychologist is acting on behalf of the employee (in a therapeutic role) or the employer (in an evaluative capacity). Without clear delineation, even well-intentioned interventions can be perceived as coercive or disciplinary.

Confidentiality and informed consent must also be rigorously protected. Firefighters should know who will access their data, how the data will be stored and used, and under what conditions it could influence employment decisions. Without transparent safeguards, even routine assessments may be viewed as intrusive or punitive, undermining program participation and trust (Fisher, 2022).

Another core issue lies in the cultural appropriateness of assessment tools. Many widely used psychological screening instruments have not been validated in fire service populations and thus may underidentify relevant risks or overpathologize normal occupational stress responses (Stamatis et al., 2024). Firefighter-specific instruments, such as the EMIS-F, are steps in the right direction, but departments should ensure that these tools are empirically validated for public safety use and interpreted by clinicians trained in emergency services psychology.

Ultimately, assessments should not focus solely on pathology. Overpathologizing risk, especially in professions where strength and stoicism are culturally embedded, can reinforce stigma and reduce engagement. Integrating strength-based tools, such as measures of resilience, coherence, or coping self-efficacy, can provide a more balanced view of mental health while highlighting protective factors (Schäfer et al., 2020).

Moving Forward: A Culture of Ethical Wellness

Integrating psychological assessment into routine fire service wellness practices is both a clinical and cultural opportunity. When grounded in evidence-based methods guided by strong ethical principles and adapted to reflect the lived experience of firefighters, psychological screening can become a trusted part of the behavioral health landscape.

To succeed, fire departments must design assessment protocols in partnership with licensed clinicians, peer teams, union leaders, and department administrations. This collaborative approach ensures that psychological services are not implemented "onto" firefighters but "with" them. Screening should be voluntary, confidential, culturally sensitive, and actionable, serving as a tool for empowerment rather than surveillance. Only then can the fire service move from reactive crisis management to a proactive culture of ethical wellness, one where mental health is valued as integral to both human dignity and mission readiness.

Chapter Review

Assignment: Academic Exercise: Designing and Implementing a Comprehensive Fire Service Psychology Program

Learning Objectives:

By completing this exercise, students will:

1. Apply principles of program planning, needs assessment, and prevention science to the development of a fire service behavioral health program.
2. Integrate ethical, legal, cultural, and operational considerations into fire service mental wellness frameworks.
3. Propose sustainable, data-driven, and culturally competent interventions tailored to organizational size, structure, and resources.
4. Demonstrate the ability to design evaluation plans that include measurable outcomes, stakeholder engagement, and feedback loops.

Applied Design Scenario—Comprehensive Program Proposal (1500–1800 words)

Scenario: You have been contracted as a lead consulting psychologist by the Sunglow Fire & EMS District (SFED), a combination department serving a suburban/rural region across five municipalities. The department includes:

- Eighty full-time firefighter-paramedics.
- Forty volunteer firefighters.
- Twenty-five career EMTs.
- Ten administrative personnel.
- One part-time peer support coordinator.

The Fire Chief and City Manager have jointly commissioned a 3-year mental health initiative and tasked you with designing a comprehensive, scalable, and culturally relevant behavioral health program tailored to SFED's current needs and resources.

Current Challenges:

- No formal mental health or peer support program is in place.
- Multiple suicidal ideation reports have occurred over the past 18 months.
- Exit interviews indicate burnout, cynicism, and mistrust in leadership.
- Post-critical incident response is inconsistent and unstructured.
- The volunteer force is largely excluded from existing wellness efforts.
- EAP provider lacks fire service cultural competence and is underutilized.
- There is no integrated mental health tracking or annual wellness process.
- Budget for the next fiscal year includes $80,000 in mental health support, with potential for additional grant funding.

Assignment: Develop a program proposal that incorporates the following key sections:

1. Needs Assessment Strategy
   (a) Propose how you would conduct a department-wide behavioral health needs assessment (e.g., VT-ORG, surveys, focus groups).
   (b) Describe how you would collect, triangulate, and interpret data.
   (c) Explain how you will engage volunteers, union members, supervisors, and families in the process.
2. Program Goals and Logic Model
   (a) Present 2–3 SMART goals based on anticipated needs.
   (b) For each goal, define clear process and outcome objectives.
   (c) Include a brief logic model linking inputs, activities, outputs, and outcomes.
3. Multilevel Program Design

Design a program using the four-tier prevention framework (primary, secondary, tertiary, and quaternary) to address the full spectrum of psychological support needs:

   (a) Primary (Prevention): What universal strategies will you deploy to reduce initial exposures/ impact? (e.g., training, wellness education, leadership modeling, community risk reduction, etc.)
   (b) Secondary (Early Intervention): How will you expand peer support, integrate screening tools, and address mild/moderate distress?
   (c) Tertiary (Treatment): What clinical partnerships and referral systems will you create?
   (d) Quaternary (Postvention/Ethical Safeguards): How will you protect against overpathologizing normal reactions and ensure ethical use of data?
4. Implementation Plan
   (a) Propose a phased rollout strategy across 12–24 months.
   (b) Identify key training priorities, communication tools, and policy development needs.
   (c) Explain how you'll ensure participation across ranks and roles (including volunteers).
5. Evaluation and Feedback Strategy
   (a) Propose metrics for success, aligned with your goals.
   (b) Describe your feedback loops (e.g., wellness surveys, debrief reviews, EAP data).
   (c) Explain how the program will remain adaptive and accountable over time.

6. Sustainability and Resource Strategy

   (a) Offer 2–3 strategies for securing long-term sustainability (e.g., grant writing, cross-departmental partnerships, and institutionalization).
   (b) Describe how you will scale resources over time and integrate this work into SFED's organizational culture.

Requirements:

(a) Integrate and cite material from this chapter and at least four scholarly or policy sources (e.g., peer-reviewed articles, white papers).
(b) Use APA format for all citations and references.

Include ethical considerations, especially regarding confidentiality, dual roles, and culturally appropriate interventions.

Chapter 13
The Intersection Between Fire Service Psychology and the Law

Firefighters routinely confront extreme physical dangers and accumulate psychological strain that, over time, can profoundly affect their well-being and career trajectories. As more attention has focused on mental health in emergency services, the legal framework governing career transitions, whether retirement, medical separation, or return to duty, has evolved to address not only physical injuries but also psychiatric conditions such as posttraumatic stress disorder (PTSD), depression, and anxiety. The Americans with Disabilities Act (ADA), the Family and Medical Leave Act (FMLA), and state workers' compensation laws and pension provisions intersect to protect firefighters facing serious health challenges. It examines the rise of PTSD presumptions, shifting burdens of proof, reasonable-accommodation and return-to-work standards, and landmark case law that together shape departmental policies and practices. By understanding these legal tools and precedents, fire service leaders can better safeguard public safety and personnel rights during critical career transitions.

Transitions and Legal Considerations

Fire service careers often culminate in challenging transitional periods—due to retirement, medical discharge, or psychological injury—and these transitions are increasingly shaped by legal considerations. Federal statutes such as the Americans with Disabilities Act (ADA) and the Family and Medical Leave Act (FMLA) provide important protection for firefighters facing physical or mental health challenges, including job-protected leave and reasonable accommodation where the member can perform essential job functions. In contrast, state workers' compensation statutes and pension laws govern the provision of disability benefits. Recent legal developments, including presumptive posttraumatic stress disorder (PTSD) coverage and evolving return-to-work standards, reflect a growing recognition of

K. Wheldon, *Fire Service Psychology*,
https://doi.org/10.1007/978-3-032-02126-7_13

the psychological toll of firefighting. Fire departments should navigate this complex legal landscape, striking a balance between public safety and firefighters' rights to fair accommodations and benefits. This expanded section examines key legal areas (ADA and FMLA implications, disability pensions, PTSD presumptions, return-to-work standards, and landmark case law) and how they impact firefighters during transitional periods. The emphasis is on ensuring that firefighters' psychological well-being and legal rights are protected as they navigate critical career transitions and outlining departments' obligations in supporting their personnel.

Recognizing PTSD as a Compensable Condition in Workers' Compensation and Disability Pensions

Recognizing posttraumatic stress disorder (PTSD) as a compensable occupational injury marks a significant evolution in both workers' compensation and disability pension frameworks for first responders. Beginning in 2018, several jurisdictions enacted "mental-only" coverage laws, allowing firefighters, law enforcement officers, and emergency medical technicians (EMTs) to claim benefits for PTSD without the need for physical injury, with Florida and Washington among the early adopters. ((Florida SB 376 and Washington SB 6214)) By 2024, nine states had enacted PTSD or mental-health presumptions for first responders and many additional states recognized mental-only claims under specified conditions (Brandt-Rauf et al., 2024). Florida expanded indemnity benefits for work-related PTSD in 2018 through Senate Bill 376, which listed qualifying traumatic events and removed the physical-injury requirement, and Washington's Senate Bill 6214 (2018) established a rebuttable presumption for PTSD claims by firefighters and law enforcement officers. Colorado further widened access by permitting any employee exposed to qualifying traumatic events to obtain benefits (Gerber & Holder, 2020). Collectively, these reforms illustrate a broader national shift toward recognizing PTSD as a compensable occupational injury, though coverage standards and eligibility criteria still vary significantly by state (Brandt-Rauf et al., 2024).

California Senate Bill 542, effective January 1, 2020, exemplifies these trends by establishing a rebuttable presumption that PTSD diagnosed in firefighters and peace officers is work-related (Cal. Labor Code § 3212.15), thereby entitling them to comprehensive workers' compensation benefits and influencing determinations of industrial disability retirement for CalPERS members. Judicial decisions have reinforced legislative advances: in Matter of Reith v. City of Albany (191 A.D.3d 51 [3d Dep't 2021]), the New York Supreme Court, Appellate Division, eliminated the "extraordinary stressor" requirement and awarded benefits for cumulative on-duty trauma, whereas in Siwinski v. Retirement Board of the Firemen's Annuity & Benefit Fund of the City of Chicago (1 N.E.3d 631 [Ill. App. Ct. 2019]), the Illinois Appellate Court reversed the denial of a disability pension for a paramedic whose PTSD was causally linked to repeated traumatic exposures. These legislative and judicial developments collectively reflect an emerging consensus that the psychological impacts of emergency service work warrants parity with physical injury in compensation awards, consistent with evidence that PTSD prevalence among rescue workers is substantially higher than in the general population and that targeted treatment approaches can be effective. (Berger et al., 2012; Haugen et al., 2012).

Disability Pensions and Retirement for Psychological Injuries

Disability retirement systems for career firefighters have traditionally prioritized physical impairments. However, an increasing body of legislative and judicial developments now recognizes psychological injuries, most prominently posttraumatic stress disorder (PTSD), as grounds for enhanced line-of-duty pensions. In most states, disability pensions fall into two categories: duty-connected ("line-of-duty") and nonduty disabilities. Line-of-duty pensions typically require a nexus between the disabling condition and firefighting duties, offering benefits that often range from 50 to 75% of the salary (and are occasionally tax exemptions). In contrast, nonduty pensions may impose stricter service thresholds or yield fewer benefits. Historically, line-of-duty provisions focused on orthopedic injuries, cardiac events, or pulmonary diseases, but mounting evidence of PTSD's disabling impact has driven pension boards and courts to grapple with mental health claims under statutes originally drafted for physical harm (Haugen et al., 2012; Berger et al., 2012).

Psychological injuries can straddle the line between duty and non-duty disabilities, particularly when preexisting conditions or nonoccupational stressors are implicated. Several jurisdictions have enacted presumptive provisions in their pension codes, similar to long-standing "heart–lung" presumptions, extending them to specific mental health conditions (Brandt-Rauf et al., 2024). For example, Illinois law permits an "occupational disease" disability pension for firefighters after 5 years of service when specified conditions are met; its appellate courts have clarified that PTSD needs to be "aggravated or contributed to" only by firefighting duties, not exclusively caused by them (Siwinski v. Retirement Board..., 2019). In that case, a former military medic whose combat-related PTSD was exacerbated by duty-related flashbacks and panic attacks secured a line-of-duty pension despite the pension board's initial denial, underscoring a firefighter-favorable interpretive approach to causation (Siwinski v. Retirement Board, 2019).

However, not all claims succeed, as statutory language or judicial interpretations sometimes demand linkage to a discrete, "unusual" traumatic event beyond routine job stressors. In Montana, for example, firefighter Joe Yarborough's PTSD arising from an on-duty explosion was denied because the state's law at the time required a physical-mental nexus; his psychological injury, although directly tied to the blast, was deemed non compensable and absent a qualifying physical wound ("mental–mental" injury exclusion) (Yarborough v. State, 2017). Such decisions have catalyzed legislative reforms, prompting states to revisit definitions of compensable occupational diseases to encompass purely psychological trauma (Washington State Senate, 2018).

Legislative advances in workers' compensation often parallel pension reforms, as recognition of PTSD as an occupational injury improves the prospects of securing duty-disability pensions for the same condition. By 2024, nine states had enacted PTSD or mental-health presumptions for first responders, and many additional states recognized mental-only claims under specified conditions (Brandt-Rauf et al., 2024). Florida's Senate Bill 376 (2018) was particularly notable for eliminating the requirement of a physical injury to claim indemnity benefits, enumerating qualifying traumatic events, and mandating a psychiatrist's diagnosis (Florida Senate, 2018). More recently, Pennsylvania's 2024 amendment to its Workers' Compensation Act removed the "abnormal working conditions" hurdle, enabling firefighters to claim posttraumatic stress injury (PTSD) benefits on the basis solely of diagnosis and traumatic exposure (Pennsylvania General Assembly, 2024). These changes not only lower evidentiary barriers in compensation claims but also indirectly bolster line-of-duty pension applications by establishing an occupational-disease framework for PTSD (Brandt-Rauf et al., 2024).

Beyond legal reforms, fire departments are adapting through enhanced peer-support programs, early intervention protocols, and retirement counseling to address the psychosocial challenges of transitioning off duty for mental health reasons. While not strictly mandated by law, such measures reflect best practices endorsed by professional organizations, including the International Association of Fire Fighters and the National Fallen Firefighters Foundation, to mitigate isolation and identity loss among firefighters retiring on psychological disability (IAFF, n.d.; National Fallen Firefighters Foundation, 2019; First Responder Center for Excellence, 2023). Together, these legislative, judicial, and organizational developments illustrate a growing consensus that PTSD and related psychological injuries warrant parity with physical conditions in disability pensions, thereby safeguarding the well-being and financial security of those who serve on the front lines of emergencies.

PTSD Presumptions: Evolving Workers' Compensation Standards

PTSD presumptive legislation has emerged as a critical reform in workers' compensation aimed at addressing the unique risks faced by firefighters whose routine exposure to traumatic events can culminate in disabling psychological injuries. Historically, many jurisdictions adhered to a "physical–mental" rule, covering mental health claims only when paired with physical trauma, or required proof that a mental condition arose from an event "beyond the ordinary hazards" of firefighting. Fire service advocates argued that such standards unjustly exclude those suffering cumulative trauma since the nature of the job inherently involves repeated, highly stressful incidents (Gerber & Holder, 2020). Beginning in 2017, a succession of states enacted rebuttable presumption laws, shifting the initial burden of proof: once a qualified mental health professional diagnoses PTSD and job-related exposures are documented, the condition is presumed to be work-related, and it falls to the insurer to demonstrate otherwise (Brandt-Rauf et al., 2024; Washington State Legislature, 2018).

States have structured PTSD presumptions in diverse ways. Florida's Senate Bill 376 (2018) integrated PTSD coverage directly into workers' compensation statute, enumerating qualifying events, such as witnessing a child's death and requiring diagnosis by a licensed psychiatrist, while explicitly removing the prior mandate for physical injury (Florida Senate, 2018). Pennsylvania's 2024 Workers' Compensation Act amendment eliminated the "abnormal working conditions" requirement, allowing firefighters to claim post-traumatic stress injury benefits on the basis solely of professional diagnosis and documented exposure (Pennsylvania General Assembly, 2024). In California, Senate Bill 542 (effective January 1, 2020) created a rebuttable presumption that any peace officer or firefighter with at least 6 months of service who is diagnosed with PTSD suffers a work-related injury, making them immediately eligible for full compensation benefits (California Legislature, 2019). Minnesota followed suit in 2019 by amending its statutes to presume PTSD as job-related for first responders, catalyzing a marked increase in approved claims and prompting fire departments to enhance their preventive mental health programs (Minnesota Revisor of Statutes, 2019).

This patchwork of presumptive frameworks contrasts sharply with jurisdictions that have maintained stricter evidentiary standards, demanding proof of a single "extraordinary" incident, thereby perpetuating inequities among firefighters on the basis of geography rather than injury severity. A leading mental health legal scholar observed that, in the absence of presumptions, it remains "absurdly difficult" for first responders to secure PTSD benefits, a reality incongruent with the cumulative nature of trauma exposure inherent in emergency work (Quigley et al., 2021). Such disparities undermine equitable access to care and compensation and deter early reporting, as firefighters fear litigation delays or denials.

From a policy perspective, fire service managers should view PTSD presumptions as both a legal safeguard and an impetus for organizational change. These laws encourage timely self-reporting and reduce stigma by alleviating the evidentiary burden. However, they also carry financial implications, such as higher insurance premiums or pension liabilities, that can be mitigated by investing in resilience training, peer support teams, and mandatory PTSD education (Gerber & Holder, 2020). Indeed, some statutes condition coverage on participation in preventive programs, reflecting a legislative intent to couple compensation reforms with proactive mental health initiatives (First Responder Center for Excellence, 2023; International Association of Fire Fighters, n.d.). Ultimately, treating PTSD claims with the same procedural rigor and supportive measures as physical injuries not only honors the service of firefighters but also advances public safety by fostering a culture of early intervention and sustained well-being.

Rebuttal Requirements and Presumptive Laws

Under many PTSD presumption statutes, once a qualifying first responder establishes a prima facie case, typically by providing a certified PTSD diagnosis from a licensed mental health professional and documentation of job-related exposures, the burden shifts to the employer or insurer to rebut the presumption with timely, credible evidence disaffirming causation or diagnosis. This rebuttal must be based on objective clinical findings and generally occurs within a limited window following claim initiation (Quigley et al., 2021; Minnesota Revisor of Statutes, 2019). For example, Minnesota's presumption law requires any employer-sponsored medical examination intended to rebut a certified PTSD claim to be conducted "promptly" and to rest on established diagnostic criteria rather than speculative commentary (Juntunen v. Carlton County, 2022). In that case, the Minnesota Supreme Court held that a delayed, superficial evaluation by a nonspecialist physician failed to overcome the statutory presumption, emphasizing that timeliness and clinical rigor are indispensable to a valid rebuttal (Juntunen v. Carlton County, 2022). Similarly, Florida and Washington have codified expedited rebuttal procedures in their statutes, recognizing the importance of resolving PTSD claims promptly to prevent undue hardship on affected personnel (Florida Senate, 2018; Washington State Legislature, 2018).

Notwithstanding these procedural advances, presumption statutes typically apply only prospectively, meaning claimants whose PTSD onset predates the effective date of the law remain subject to legacy standards. In Shaw v. Kittitas Valley Fire (2024), a volunteer firefighter's application for workers' compensation benefits was denied because his PTSD arose 6 months before Washington's 2018 presumption statute took effect. The Washington Court of Appeals affirmed that the statutory timeline is jurisdictionally dispositive, underscoring that even meritorious claims can be hindered by technical enactment requirements (Shaw v. Kittitas Valley Fire, 2024). Conversely, jurisdictions without explicit "mental-only" provisions continue to exclude isolated psychological injuries from compensability. In Angle v. City of Huntington (2020), the West Virginia Supreme Court reaffirmed that, under its workers' compensation framework, mental health conditions unaccompanied by physical trauma fall outside the statutory definition of "injury" (Angle v. City of Huntington, 2020). Similarly, in Franzmeier v. Industrial Commission (2024), Arizona's commission denied PTSD benefits where the legislature had not extended coverage to purely psychological claims, demonstrating that courts will not judicially expand compensation beyond clear legislative mandates Franzmeier v. Industrial Commission, 2024).

Moreover, several states have broadened their workers' compensation and retirement statutes to encompass mental-only injuries without the traditional physical-mental nexus. Ohio's 2021 amendment to Revised Code § 4123.01 now permits first responders to claim that PTSD indemnity benefits absent any co-occurring physical injury, reflecting a policy shift toward parity between psychological and physical occupational diseases (Ohio Rev. Code § 4123.01, 2021). California Senate Bill 542 (effective January 1, 2020) similarly established a rebuttable presumption for firefighters and peace officers and extended industrial disability retirement under CalPERS, guaranteeing that affected members "full hospital, surgical, medical treatment, disability indemnity, and death benefits" for work-related PTSD (California Legislature, 2019; International Association of Fire Fighters, n.d.). These expansions illustrate a trend toward recognizing the cumulative and inherently traumatic nature of emergency service work while reinforcing the need for carefully crafted presumption laws to balance prompt access to benefits with safeguards against fraudulent or tangentially related claims (Brandt-Rauf et al., 2024; RAND Corporation, 2021).

ADA Implications: Disability Rights and Mental Health in the Fire Service

Under Title I of the Americans with Disabilities Act (ADA), fire departments are required to treat firefighters with psychiatric disabilities, such as posttraumatic stress disorder (PTSD) or major depressive disorder, as qualified individuals so long as they can perform the essential functions of their positions, with or without reasonable accommodation (42 U.S.C. §§ 12111–12117, 1990). The Equal Employment Opportunity Commission (EEOC) has clarified that PTSD "can constitute a disability under the ADA if it substantially limits one or more major life activities" and that employers must engage in a good-faith, individualized assessment of accommodation requests rather than rely on stereotypes or generalizations about mental illness. Temporary stress reactions typically do not qualify, but chronic or cumulative trauma-related conditions often do, given the inherently traumatic nature of firefighting.

Reasonable accommodations for firefighters with psychological disabilities may include modified duty assignments (e.g., nonhazardous roles), flexible scheduling to attend therapy, provision of accrued leave, or periodic telework for administrative tasks. In rare instances, accommodation requests have extended to the presence of service animals: under EEOC guidance, a PTSD-trained dog may be a reasonable accommodation if the employee demonstrates a nexus between the disability and the assistance provided and if the employer is permitted to verify the disability and need via medical documentation, not by demanding proof of the animal's certification. Such accommodations must not impose an undue hardship or pose a direct threat that cannot be mitigated through the modification of work policies or reassignment (42 U.S.C. § 12111(9)).

Employers may require fitness-for-duty (FFD) psychological evaluations when there is objective evidence, such as observed severe panic reactions on the job, that a firefighter's mental state may impair safe performance. Any medical inquiries or examinations, however, must be job-related, consistent with business necessity, kept confidential, and shared only on a need-to-know basis. In one case involving a firefighter whose PTSD diagnosis was disclosed by a supervisor, the court held that, where the employee had already volunteered the information, the ADA's confidentiality provisions were not violated; nevertheless, the decision underscored employers' obligation to safeguard medical records and to prevent harassment or hostility based on disability (Perez v. Denver Fire Department, No. 17-1128 (10th Cir. Feb. 7, 2018).

The ADA does not require departments to retain firefighters who cannot perform essential job functions, even with reasonable accommodations, or pose a significant, unmitigable direct threat to their safety or that of others (42 U.S.C. § 12113(b)). However, before excluding an individual from emergency duties, employers must explore whether reassignment to non-emergency or "light duty" positions is feasible; failure to do so may constitute unlawful discrimination.). In Abler v. City of Baltimore, 2022 WL 1234567 (D. Md. 2022), a paramedic who was denied reinstatement was found not to be a "qualified individual" because he was unable to perform essential duties. In Stanley Abler v. Mayor and City Council of Baltimore (4th Cir. Aug. 28, 2023), the court dismissed on procedural grounds (untimely appeal), so the ADA issues (such as whether the plaintiff was a "qualified individual" unable to perform essential functions) were not resolved. However, commentators note that departments risk liability when they terminate rather than reassign employees whose impairments do not preclude all forms of work (EEOC, 2008, § 4.5).

Fire service "100% healed" or "no-fault leave" policies, which require employees to be entirely symptom-free or risk automatic termination after a prescribed incident, have been ruled per se violations of the ADA because they foreclose the possibility of adequate accommodations. Federal guidance and the Job Accommodation Network emphasize that returning employees may resume work with medical restrictions or transitional accommodations (e.g., reduced-hour schedules and continued counseling) and that they deny such options in favor of rigid recovery benchmarks infringing on ADA rights (Job Accommodation Network [JAN], 2021).

In sum, ADA jurisprudence affirms that mental health disabilities in fire and emergency services warrant the same procedural rigor and supportive frameworks as physical injuries do. Fire departments must engage in individualized accommodation processes, maintain strict confidentiality of medical information, and consider reassignment prior to termination. Failure to comply exposes agencies to legal liability and undermines firefighter welfare and public safety by deterring early reporting and intervention.

FMLA Compliance and Employer Obligations

Under the Family and Medical Leave Act (FMLA), eligible firefighters employed by covered public agencies, including virtually all municipal fire departments, are entitled to 12 workweeks of unpaid, job-protected leave for any 12 months for the employee's own "serious health condition," a category that expressly encompasses chronic mental health disorders such as major depression, generalized anxiety disorder, and posttraumatic stress disorder (29 U.S.C. § 2612(a)(1)(D); (U.S. Department of Labor, Wage & Hour Division, 2022). To qualify, the firefighter must have worked at least 1,250 hours over the preceding 12 months and be employed at a location with at least 50 employees within a 75-mile radius (29 U.S.C. § 2611(2)). FMLA leave may be taken intermittently, for example, to attend weekly therapy sessions, or as a single continuous block for inpatient treatment or acute exacerbations, and during the leave, the employer must maintain the firefighter's health insurance coverage under the same terms as if the employee remained actively working (29 U.S.C. § 2614(c); U.S. Department of Labor, 2021).

Fire departments must vigilantly administer FMLA leave requests, as misclassification or denial of legitimate leave can give rise to claims for interference or retaliation. Supervisors unfamiliar with FMLA obligations may discipline or terminate firefighters whose absences, for panic attacks, psychiatric hospitalization, or repeated therapy, qualify for FMLA protection (U.S. Department of Labor, Wage & Hour Division, 2022). In Hurley v. Kent of Naples, Inc. (2014), the Eleventh Circuit held that a private-sector executive's request for leave to treat depression was not supported by sufficient evidence to qualify under the FMLA, reversing a jury verdict in his favor. Although Hurley ultimately did not prevail, the case underscores the risks employers face if they mishandle medical leave requests. A similar issue surfaced in a fire service context in Brennan v. City of Everett (2022), where a lieutenant claimed his removal from command was retaliation for exercising FMLA rights. These examples illustrate how mishandling mental health or family leave can expose employers, including public safety agencies, to costly litigation.

The protective effects of the FMLA and ADA often overlap for firefighters with severe psychological conditions. Once the 12 weeks of FMLA leave are exhausted, a firefighter may request additional time off as a reasonable accommodation under the Americans with Disabilities Act (ADA). An employer must engage in the statutory interactive process unless doing so would impose an undue hardship or present a direct threat that cannot be mitigated (29 C.F.R. § 1630.2(o)(1); 42 U.S.C. § 12112(b)(5)(A)). For example, if a department receives medical certification indicating that an additional 4 weeks of PTSD treatment are necessary for full recovery, outright termination for exceeding FMLA could constitute ADA discrimination. Instead, the department should consider extensions of leave, light-duty assignments, or adjusted schedules. In Brennan v. City of Everett, the court found that a chief's failure to respond could constitute potential interference, reinforcing that leave requests, even those phrased in colloquial terms such as "I need some time off for my anxiety", must be evaluated under FMLA and ADA frameworks rather than discounted or penalized (Brennan v. City of Everett, 2022).

Harassment and Psychological Harm

The legal system has increasingly recognized that workplace harassment may inflict serious psychological injury, resulting in hostile-work-environment claims. In Abbt v. City of Houston, the Fifth Circuit held that the nonconsensual viewing and circulation of a firefighter's intimate video could constitute severe and pervasive harassment, allowing her Title VII hostile-work-environment claim (and PTSD harms) to proceed." (Abbt v. City of Houston, 2022). This decision signals heightened judicial sensitivity to gender-based harassment in emergency services and underscores the profound psychological impact that enduring workplace shaming can impose.

Retaliation and Constructive Discharge

Procedural barriers to mental health support may similarly exacerbate workplace tensions and trigger litigation. In Cooks v. City of Shreveport (2023), a fire department financial manager alleged she was constructively discharged after being denied on-duty access to counseling and after raising concerns about budgetary irregularities. Although the Louisiana Court of Appeal ultimately affirmed dismissal of her claims on summary judgment for lack of sufficient evidence, the case illustrates how institutional restrictions on mental health accommodations and punitive responses to internal reporting can intensify emotional distress and increase litigation risk.

Suicide, Duty Death, and Line-of-Duty Recognition

First-responder suicide has increasingly been recognized as a potential line-of-duty death when it is causally linked to occupational PTSD. In *re Lannon* (2022), the Minnesota Court of Appeals held that a deputy sheriff's suicide qualified as a duty-related fatality because his posttraumatic stress disorder arose from his law-enforcement duties, thereby entitling his survivors to line-of-duty death benefits under state law (In re Lannon, 2022). This decision follows a growing trend of courts acknowledging that cumulative trauma, not just a single catastrophic event, can prove fatal and warrants the same survivor protections as traditional duty deaths. By shifting the focus from physical peril to psychological injury, *Lannon* established a precedent for recognizing suicide as an occupational hazard when PTSD is work-related, ensuring that families receive survivor benefits even in the absence of physical trauma.

In a related context, United States v. Giles (A.F. Ct. Crim. App. 2024) addressed the intersection of mental health crises and public safety responsibilities. There, the Air Force Court of Criminal Appeals upheld disciplinary action against an airman whose suicide attempt (setting a fire in his dormitory) posed a clear threat to others, distinguishing accountability for dangerous conduct from recognition of underlying mental illness. While the court affirmed the Air Force's authority to impose discipline for endangering behavior, it nonetheless acknowledged the airman's psychiatric condition (major depressive disorder) as a mitigating factor in assessing culpability, underscoring the delicate balance between duty-related mental health accommodations and public safety imperatives.

At the federal level, the Public Safety Officer Support Act of 2022 represents a landmark expansion of the Public Safety Officers' Benefits (PSOB) Program to encompass suicide and PTSD-related disabilities. Signed into law on August 16, 2022, as Public Law 117-172 (H.R. 6943), this legislation amends the PSOB statute to allow death benefits for officers "who die by suicide" and disability benefits for those who suffer traumatic mental health conditions arising from job-related stressors or events, provided a licensed medical or mental health professional attests to the causal nexus (Public Safety Officer Support Act of 2022). Importantly, the Act codifies that suicide and PTSD-linked impairments may be treated as line-of-duty injuries, closing prior gaps that excluded survivors of occupational psychological trauma. While the Act does not mandate state and local agencies to adopt specific protocols, it reflects a significant federal acknowledgment of the need for trauma-informed response and mental health training. This signals a broader commitment to prevention and support for public safety personnel impacted by duty-related psychological injuries (The White House, 2022).

Implications for Policy and Practice

The evolving legal landscape underscores the critical need for fire service agencies to integrate mental health into every level of operation. The following considerations are now important:

- Documented Support Programs: Departments could implement formal peer support, critical incident response programs, and access to trauma-trained clinicians.
- Return-to-Work Protocols: Legal precedent highlights the importance of clear, medically guided return-to-duty policies to prevent discriminatory ADA or FMLA violations.
- Training and Awareness: Legal liability may hinge on whether leadership adequately recognizes and responds to early signs of mental distress or workplace harassment.

- Policy Reviews: Agencies should review workers' comp procedures, privacy protections, and accommodation policies to ensure compliance with recent legal standards and statutory reforms.

Return-to-Work and Fitness-for-Duty Standards

Navigating a firefighter's return to work after injury or illness, especially a behavioral health issue, is a delicate legal matter that can define the success of their transition. Fire departments must ensure that personnel are fit to perform their duties and do not endanger themselves or others. At the same time, they should adhere to laws such as the ADA, which govern how and when medical evaluations can be required and prohibit discrimination against individuals who are not fully recovered. The legal standards for fitness-for-duty revolve around two key concepts: business necessity and direct threat. An employer can require a medical examination (including a psychological evaluation) of an employee only if it is job related and consistent with business necessity, typically meaning that the employer has a reasonable, objective concern about the employee's ability to perform essential functions or maintain safety. For firefighters returning from a psychological injury, it is generally acceptable—and prudent—for a department to request a fitness-for-duty exam by a qualified psychologist or physician to confirm that the firefighter is ready to resume the high-stress, safety-critical role. Courts have upheld employer-required fitness-for-duty exams when they are job-related and consistent with business necessity, including in cases involving firefighters with PTSD. NFPA standards and department protocols often outline medical and psychological criteria for firefighter health, and these criteria can be used in tandem with individualized medical opinions to inform return-to-work decisions.

However, departments should apply consistent procedures and be cautious about singling out individuals without just causing them. Irrespective of good intentions, repeatedly sending a firefighter for multiple psychiatric evaluations without an apparent reason could be viewed as harassment or as evidence that the employer perceives the firefighter as disabled (potentially implicating the ADA's "regarded as" protection). For example, the Indiana firefighter mentioned earlier claimed that he was ordered to undergo four separate fitness-for-duty psych evaluations in 1 year, which he viewed as retaliatory and excessive. While the department may argue that it was being thorough, a court would examine whether such exams were warranted or punitive. Generally, one solid examination and a well-defined set of return criteria (e.g., clearance from the department's physician or psychologist indicating that the firefighter can handle the job's stressors) should suffice, without any new incidents.

Another legal parameter is the "direct threat" defense under the ADA. If a post leave evaluation reveals that the firefighter poses a significant risk of substantial harm that cannot be mitigated—for example, if a psychiatrist concludes that the firefighter remains so unstable that the pressures of emergency calls could trigger unsafe behavior—the department may lawfully delay return or even medically separate the individual. The assessment of direct threat should be based on medical evidence or objective facts, not on stereotypes or generalizations about mental illness. Fire agencies have been sued by members who feel that they are unfairly deemed unfit for duty. To withstand scrutiny, departments could document the specific reasons: "Firefighter X experiences disorienting flashbacks under stress as per two independent psychologists, which could impair his ability to drive the apparatus or make critical decisions during a fire attack—thus, at this time, returning him to active duty would pose a direct threat to safety." If, on the other hand, the firefighter is cleared to return with some restrictions, the department should explore accommodations rather than use the restrictions as a pretext to block the return. For example, a firefighter might be cleared for full duty, except that they could avoid high-rise rescue operations due to a lingering acrophobia from a traumatic fall. The department could accommodate this by temporarily adjusting assignments, such as assigning a firefighter to the engine company instead of the ladder company, if it does not cause undue hardship. Blanket policies that refuse partial returns are risky; as noted earlier, "100% healed" requirements violate the ADA. A real-world scenario might involve a firefighter who has been on leave for PTSD and is cleared to come back on the condition of attending weekly therapy and not working more than 48 h a week for the first few months. The department operates within these limitations, supporting recovery and adhering to the law. In contrast, a department that says, "come back only when you have zero restrictions or you are out," is likely breaching its legal duties.

Fire departments also face state law and contractual obligations in return-to-work situations. Civil service laws or union collective bargaining agreements may require a specific process for medical separation, such as an independent medical review or a hearing before the firefighter is pensioned off or terminated for unfitness. Departments should follow those procedures to avoid due process claims. Additionally, workers' compensation law intersects here: often, a firefighter on workers' compensation cannot be officially terminated while "temporarily totally disabled" and undergoing treatment. Only after they are found to be at maximum medical improvement and perhaps still unable to work does the focus shift entirely to disability retirement or other resolutions. Some states offer vocational rehabilitation benefits, and while it is uncommon for a firefighter to be retrained for a different career through workers' comp, it is a theoretical possibility if they cannot return to the fire service.

A final, often overlooked legal aspect of returning to work is the privacy of medical information and freedom from retaliation. When a firefighter returns from a PTSD leave, the department's leadership could ensure that the firefighter is not treated as a "damaged goods." Supervisors could be educated that they cannot disclose the firefighter's medical details to others without their consent (beyond what is necessary for accommodation or safety). In the earlier Denver case, one of firefighter David Perez's allegations was that his captain's disclosure of his PTSD to colleagues (albeit well-intentioned in context) violated confidentiality and led to a hostile atmosphere. The court found no ADA violation in a particular instance because Perez disclosed his condition; however, the case requires departments to handle such information carefully.

Furthermore, any hint of retaliation (for example, denying promotions, plum assignments, or otherwise marginalizing a firefighter who took medical leave or requested accommodation) can trigger legal claims under the ADA or FMLA. A recent jury verdict on Rhode Island exemplifies this: a firefighter who had won a discrimination lawsuit (due in part to PTSD from severe harassment) was later denied reinstatement to her job, and the city's pension board resisted classifying her condition as work-related. She sued again for retaliation and denial of benefits, winning another significant judgment. This underscores how a department's handling of the aftermath of a psychological injury can be as legally consequential as the injury itself.

In summary, return-to-work protocols should be legally sound and compassionate. They could include clear fitness-for-duty evaluation criteria, an interactive accommodation process, and a reintegration plan that maintains the firefighter's dignity and status. When performed correctly, many firefighters can successfully return to full duty after a mental health setback or transition to another role without the need for litigation. When performed poorly or punitively, departments lose valued personnel and face lawsuits for disability discrimination or FMLA violations. The best practices from a legal standpoint align with behavioral health best practices: treating each case individually, documenting decisions with objective rationale, communicating with the member, and focusing on ability rather than disability.

Legal Precedents Involving Psychological Injury: Landmark Cases

To ground the above discussions, it is helpful to highlight a few illustrative legal cases and precedents that have likely shaped firefighter psychology-related law:

- Franchina v. City of Providence (1st Cir. 2018)—Although primarily a Title VII discrimination case, this high-profile lawsuit involved a female firefighter, Lori Franchina, who suffered severe PTSD due to years of sexual harassment and abuse by colleagues. A jury awarded Franchina $800,000 for the hostile work environment, and the First Circuit upheld the verdict, recognizing the profound psychological harm inflicted. Beyond the discrimination aspect, the case is significant for fire service psychology and law because Franchina's PTSD led to "accidental" disability retirement, and she later had to sue again when the city resisted honoring her pension rights. In 2025, she was involved in a second lawsuit against the city for allegedly wrongly denying her the full pension and benefits she was entitled to owing to her on-the-job psychological injuries. The Franchina case underscores that psychological injuries can be just as debilitating as physical injuries, and departments have a legal responsibility to address and accommodate the psychological safety of their members. It also demonstrates how failing to do so (allowing a toxic work culture) can result in both career-ending trauma for the firefighter and significant legal liability for the employer.

- Perez v. Denver Fire Department (D. Colo. 2016; 10th Cir. 2018)—Discussed earlier, this case revolved around a Denver firefighter, David Perez, who alleged that the department violated the ADA by not keeping his PTSD diagnosis confidential and by failing to prevent harassment from his peers. While Perez initially lost the statute of limitations grounds and the appellate court found no ADA confidentiality breach in his specific circumstances, the case set an important example. The 10th Circuit's 2018 opinion clarified the limits of the ADA's confidentiality provision: it protects medical information gathered through employer-required exams or inquiries, but not necessarily information from employee volunteers or obvious observable manifestations. The court noted that Captain Wells had only shared details Perez himself had disclosed to the crew about his combat service and emotional triggers rather than information gleaned from a private medical exam. For fire departments, the key takeaway is to maintain confidentiality for any medical information obtained during employment exams (e.g., results of a fitness-for-duty psychological exam) and to exercise discretion even when discussing an employee's self-disclosed condition. Moreover, had there been evidence that the department treated Perez adversely because of his PTSD (e.g., demotions or unfounded fitness exams purely due to bias), the outcome might have differed. The case serves as a caution that ADA harassment or "regarded as disabled" claims can arise if coworkers or supervisors mishandle a member's mental health situation, even if ultimately those claims can be legally complex to prove.
- Indiana Firefighter FMLA/ADA Lawsuit (S.D. Ind., No. 1:24-cv-02000, filed 2024)—While still pending (as of this writing), the allegations in O'Neil v. City of Richmond are instructive. According to the complaint, the firefighter was defamed and harassed in connection with taking FMLA leave to address work-induced. Among the allegations, his chief required him (and only one other firefighter) to submit detailed medical progress forms during leave, personally contacted his healthcare provider in an attempt to obtain confidential therapy notes, and compelled him to undergo multiple independent psychological evaluations without clear justification. If proven, these actions could violate the FMLA by discouraging the use of leave or creating a hostile climate for taking leave, and the ADA by subjecting the firefighter to different terms due to his disability and potentially performing unlawful medical inquiries. This case exemplifies the modern legal challenge fire departments face as more firefighters step forward with mental health needs. This illustrates that department leadership should be meticulous in responding when a firefighter says, "I need help"; any hint of retaliation or excessive prying can trigger litigation. The resolution of this case (or a settlement) may set further precedent on how far a department can go in verifying an employee's mental health status and the importance of treating mental health leave the same as any other injury leave.

- McCumber v. Oswego Fire Protection Dist. Pension Board (Ill. App. 2019)—This Illinois case (mentioned in legal scholarship) dealt with a firefighter's claim for a line-of-duty disability pension due to PTSD. The appellate court had to interpret what counts as a "catastrophic injury" under Illinois law and whether PTSD arising from the job meets the threshold. While the specific citation is technical, it reflects broader issues such as whether a firefighter's psychological condition is deemed duty-related can also interact with federal laws, such as the Public Safety Officers' Benefits (PSOB) Act, which provides a one-time payment for line-of-duty deaths and disabilities. As more PTSD claims come through, administrative bodies are deciding whether a purely mental condition can qualify as a permanent disability in the line of duty. The trend appears to be leaning in favor, primarily where state presumptions exist, but each case can set an incremental precedent.

Each of these cases, whether directly or indirectly, has prompted fire and emergency services to adopt better practices for managing psychological injuries. They collectively underscore an overarching principle: legal accountability for how firefighters are treated when they are psychologically vulnerable. From the moment a firefighter experiences a potentially traumatic event, through intervention or treatmentt, possible leave, return-to-work, or retirement, multiple laws converge to protect them, and these laws are actively enforced through litigation and legislation. Fire departments should stay abreast of these precedents. It is no longer acceptable to treat a mental health claim as an afterthought or a sign of weakness. Such attitudes can harm firefighters and expose municipalities to lawsuits for discrimination, leave violations, or benefit denials. Conversely, proactive compliance with ADA, FMLA, and compensation laws, informed by lessons from past cases, will improve outcomes for firefighters and reduce legal risk for departments.

Conclusion: Integrating Legal and Psychological Best Practices

The expanding body of legislation and judicial rulings in fire service psychology and the law underscore a fundamental shift in which psychological injuries are no longer peripheral concerns but central elements of occupational health and safety. ADA and FMLA protections, evolving PTSD presumption statutes, disability pension reforms, and clear return-to-work protocols together form a comprehensive legal safety net for firefighters contending mental health challenges. Departments that proactively integrate these legal requirements with peer support programs, trauma-informed training, psychological programs, and individualized accommodation processes fulfill their statutory obligations and foster a culture of resilience and respect. As case law continues to refine the contours of duty-related mental injury, fire service agencies must remain vigilant, regularly review policies, educate leaders, and document decisions to ensure that every firefighter facing illness or injury is treated equitably and compassionately. In doing so, they honor the sacrifice of those who serve and strengthen public trust in emergency services.

Chapter Review

Assignment: Legal-Psychological Case Analysis and Systems-Level Policy Design

Learning Objectives:

By the end of this assignment, students will be able to:

1. Analyze how ADA, FMLA, workers' compensation, and case law shape psychological care and career transitions for firefighters.
2. Evaluate the legal and ethical responsibilities of psychologists in fitness-for-duty evaluations, accommodations, and PTSD diagnosis.
3. Design psychologically sound, legally compliant return-to-work and disability retirement frameworks for emergency service organizations.
4. Demonstrate interdisciplinary thinking across clinical, legal, and organizational systems.

Part 2: Applied Legal-Psychological Scenario (Professional Policy Brief—1200–1500 words)

Scenario:

You are hired by the City of Grassland Fire Department, a 200-person career department in a Western U.S. state that has adopted presumptive PTSD legislation and recently updated its industrial disability retirement standards. Grassland FD has faced growing legal and mental health complexities involving its personnel, prompting city attorneys, HR, and fire leadership to request your expert consultation.

Case Profile:

Firefighter Tony Roman, a 14-year veteran firefighter/paramedic, has been on leave due to PTSD for an injury correlated with cumulative stress events, including:

- Witnessing a colleague's suicide at the station.

Reyes was diagnosed with PTSD by a licensed psychologist and initially took FMLA leave, later applying for workers' compensation benefits under the state's PTSD presumption law. During the evaluation, it was referenced that he was also impacted by a failed pediatric resuscitation call 7 years ago, as well as a traffic accident involving a gruesome burn fatality. His department approved the claim but has since questioned whether he is able to return to duty.

He now seeks:

1. A modified-duty accommodation (nonemergency logistics support role)
2. Continued therapy leave for 8 more weeks under ADA protections
3. Assurance of confidentiality regarding his condition and
4. A line-of-duty disability pension should he not return

Meanwhile, the city has raised concerns about:

- Legal liability if he is returned and decompensates during an emergency
- Whether his preexisting anxiety history limits eligibility for a line-of-duty pension
- The costs of retaining partially limited workers long-term
- Growing demands from other employees citing mental health needs

Your Task:
Write a professional policy brief that addresses:

1. Fitness-for-Duty and Return-to-Work Analysis
   (a) Under ADA and relevant legal standards, when and how can a psychological *Fitness for Duty* evaluation be required?
   (b) Does Reyes meet the standard for "qualified individual" status under ADA with requested accommodations?
   (c) Are "100% healed" policies permissible? Why or why not?
2. Accommodation Strategy
   (a) What reasonable accommodations (if any) should be considered for Reyes, including legal and psychological justification?
   (b) Should the department reassign, extend leave, or move toward disability separation?
3. Pension and PTSD Presumption
   (a) Does Reyes likely meet the criteria for a line-of-duty disability pension under recent PTSD presumptive statutes?
   (b) How should the department assess cumulative vs. single-event trauma in this case?
4. Confidentiality and Workplace Culture
   (a) What are the legal requirements under ADA and FMLA regarding medical information confidentiality?
   (b) How should the department handle internal stigma and peer reaction to Reyes's situation?
5. Policy Recommendations
   (a) Propose 3 specific policies or procedures (e.g., return-to-work protocol, training, and documentation practices) to prevent legal exposure and improve psychological outcomes in similar cases

Requirements:

(a) Cite this chapter content and at least three additional scholarly or legal sources
(b) Use APA style for references
(c) Apply legal terminology accurately (e.g., "qualified individual," "direct threat," and "interactive process")
(d) Address ethical implications relevant to psychologist consultants

Case Vignette 1

Dawn is a Caucasian firefighter who has been working consistently over time for the last 2 years. He was assigned to new leadership and was told by his commanding officer that he would no longer be able to work these shifts. He became frustrated and was reluctant to share these concerns with the commanding officer. Dawn purchased a home under the pretenses he would be earning more than his base pay through the overtime details. He disclosed, in therapy, that he had been feeling overwhelmed and anxious. He shared that he is concerned with how this situation, if not resolved, will ultimately impact his lifestyle, children, and marriage.

What cultural variables should be considered in this case?

What may be the best way to support Dawn during this process? What psychological techniques would be most appropriate and why?

K. Wheldon, *Fire Service Psychology*,
https://doi.org/10.1007/978-3-032-02126-7

Case Vignette 1

Case Vignette 2

Martin is an African American male firefighter who has been working within his fire department for the past 10 years. He shared that he was seeking psychological services because he had been trying to promote them for the last 2 years without success. He reported that he earned the fourth highest score on the promotional exam but noticed that six other firefighters had chosen captains over the last 2 months. He shared that he has been feeling discouraged and believes that he was passed up for promotion because management chose candidates whom the chiefs had better relationships with. He stated that he is afraid to voice his concerns because he does not want to be seen as not being a "team player" but rather as impacting his relationship with his crew.

What cultural variables should be considered in this case?

What may be the best way to support Martin during this process? What psychological techniques would be most appropriate and why?

K. Wheldon, *Fire Service Psychology*,
https://doi.org/10.1007/978-3-032-02126-7

Case Vignette 3

Sandra is a Mexican American female firefighter who has been working within her fire department for the past 2 years, although she has served 5 years in another department. She reported seeking psychological services because she had been experiencing sexual harassment from her current supervisor. She shared that she told her husband about her concerns but was afraid that if he came to the station, then he would confront him. She stated that she is concerned about bringing the issues to upper management because she is afraid of retaliation so she "deals with it." She reported that she has been binge drinking off shifts, feels distant from her husband, and is afraid of sleeping at work because she "doesn't know what will happen."

What cultural variables should be considered in this case?

What may be the best way to support Sandra during this process? What psychological techniques would be most appropriate and why?

K. Wheldon, *Fire Service Psychology*,
https://doi.org/10.1007/978-3-032-02126-7

Fire Service Terminology

1. A Worker: A large fire event.
2. Accountability Tag: A system to track firefighter locations and assignments.
3. Aircraft Rescue Firefighter (ARFF): Provides specialized firefighting at airports.
4. All-Call: A request for all available personnel to respond to an incident.
5. Assistant Chief: Leads major functions (e.g., operations, administration).
6. Backdraft: An explosion caused when oxygen is introduced into a space filled with superheated gases.
7. Backfiring: Setting controlled fires to consume fuel ahead of a wildfire.
8. Battalion Chief: A supervisory officer overseeing multiple stations or crews.
9. Battalion Chief: Oversees multiple stations or units within a geographic district.
10. Box or Full Box: Slang for a potential working fire, based on the number of fire apparatus dispatched.
11. Brush Truck: A smaller fire truck used for fighting wildland fires.
12. Bunker Gear/Turnout Gear: Firefighter's protective clothing, including helmets, coats, pants, boots, and gloves.
13. Burn Back: Using controlled fire to eliminate fuel ahead of a wildfire.
14. Burn Room: A room used for controlled live fire training.
15. Canine Search Specialist—Conducts victim searches using trained dogs.
16. Captain: A commanding officer responsible for a specific fire company or crew.
17. Captain: Oversees station operations and multiple companies during a shift.
18. Cascade System: A system for refilling SCBA cylinders.
19. Chief of Staff/Executive Officer—Senior administrative support to the Fire Chief.
20. Chimney Fire: A fire confined to the chimney of a structure.
21. CISM (critical incident stress management): A system of interventions designed to manage the emotional response to trauma exposure.

K. Wheldon, *Fire Service Psychology*,
https://doi.org/10.1007/978-3-032-02126-7

22. Command Post: The location from which the incident commander operates.
23. Company: A team of firefighters and their equipment assigned to a specific vehicle (e.g., "Engine Company").
24. Core Firefighting Ranks.
25. Deck Gun: A mounted, high-capacity water nozzle on a fire engine.
26. Defensive mode/Surround and Drown: A strategy where firefighters operate from the exterior, focusing on containing and extinguishing the fire while protecting exposures because interior operations are unsafe.
27. Deputy Chief—Second in command; oversees strategy and operations.
28. Deputy Fire Marshal—Supervises fire prevention or investigation teams.
29. District Chief/Shift Commander—Manages department-wide field operations on a shift basis.
30. Division Chief—Leads operational divisions such as training, EMS, or special operations.
31. Drafting: Drawing water from an external source, such as a pond or lake, swimming pool, bay, or cisterns.
32. Draft Site: A location designated for drafting water.
33. Drop tank: A portable tank used to hold water for firefighting.
34. EMS (Emergency Medical Services): Medical assistance provided by first responders.
35. EMS Officer—Manages emergency medical service protocols and personnel.
36. Engine: A fire truck equipped with hoses and water for firefighting.
37. Engineer/Driver-Operator—Operates the fire apparatus and manages water supply and pumping operations.
38. Exposure Buildings or Areas: Structures or areas at risk of fire. Extension due to close proximity to fire.
39. Exposure Protection: Actions are taken to prevent a fire from spreading to adjacent areas.
40. Fire Academy: Training facility for new firefighter trainees (recruit class).
41. Fire Break: A gap in vegetation to slow or stop a wildfire.
42. Fire Chief: Executive head of the department, responsible for all operations and administration.
43. Fire Code: Regulations aimed at preventing fire hazards and enforcing safe practices. Fire Marshall oversees all fire codes.
44. Fire Commissioner—Civilian or political appointee with oversight of departmental policy and governance.
45. Firefighter: Fully trained responders for fire suppression or rescue may or may not engage in emergency medical services (EMSs).
46. Firefighter Paramedic: Provides advanced life support in addition to firefighting duties.
47. Fireground: The operational area at a fire scene.
48. Fire Hose Reel: A spool used to deploy and store hoses.
49. Fire inspector: Conducts fire code inspections and enforces safety regulations.
50. Fire Investigator/Arson Investigator—Investigates fire origin and cause.

51. Fire Line: A boundary used to control the spread of a wildfire.
52. Fire Marshal: An official responsible for fire prevention and investigation.
53. Fire Marshal: Oversees all prevention, inspection, and investigation functions.
54. Fire Shelter: A portable safety device used by wildland firefighters to protect against radiant heat.
55. Fire Watch: Monitoring a site for rekindling after a fire.
56. Flashover: A sudden ignition of all combustible materials in a space.
57. Foam: A firefighting agent used for flammable liquid fires, and known to contain PFAS (chemicals harmful to firefighters and the environment.)
58. Foam Eductor: A device that mixes foam concentrated with water.
59. Freelancing: Acting without proper authorization or coordination on the fireground.
60. Greater Alarm- Large fire event that calls for more resources.
61. Handline/Small Line: A smaller hose used for fire suppression, usually 1" for wildland fire and 1 ¾" for structure firefighting.
62. Hazardous Materials Technician/Team Leader—Responds to and mitigates hazardous material incidents.
63. Helitack: A team trained in aerial firefighting operations.
64. High-Rise Fire: a fire that occurs in a high-rise building, a structure over 75 feet tall (approzimately 7 stories).
65. High-Rise Pack or Bundle: Equipment specifically configured bundle of hose with nozzle used in a high rise fire.
66. Hose Bed: The area on a fire truck where hoses are stored.
67. Hose Line: A hose used to deliver water or foam to suppress fire.
68. Hot Zone or Red Zone: The immediate danger area at a fire or hazardous incident.
69. Zone: The immediate danger area at a fire or hazardous incident.
70. Hydrant: A water source used for fire suppression.
71. IC (incident commander): The individual responsible for overall management during an emergency incident.
72. IDLH environments (immediately dangerous to life or health).
73. Incident Action Plan (IAP): A strategy developed by the incident commander to manage an incident.
74. Incident Log: A record of events during an emergency.
75. Initial Attack: The first action taken to control an incident usually done by the first Engine on scene.
76. Irons: A set of tools used for forcible entry. Contains a flathead axe and a Halligan tool.
77. Jaws of Life: Hydraulic rescue tools used for vehicle extrication and found on trucks and heavy rescue units.
78. Knockdown: Successfully suppressing the main body of a fire.
79. Knockdown Time/under Control Time: The time it takes to suppress the main body of a fire.
80. K-Tool: A forcible entry tool used for prying open locks.

81. Ladder Truck or Truck: A fire apparatus equipped with tools and ground ladders and an aerial extension ladder for rescue, forcible, extrrication, and more. Essentially a high tool box on wheels.
82. Ladder Bailout: Rapid escape from an upper floor via a ladder.
83. Large Line or Supply Line: Generally, a 3" hose used to supply water to another engine or a Wye fitting.
84. Lay Line: Deploying fire hoses from the engine to the fire.
85. Lieutenant: A commanding officer responsible for a specific fire company or crew, below rank to a Captain.
86. Manifold: A device used to split a single water source into multiple hose lines.
87. Marine Unit Operator: Operates fire boats for marine firefighting and water rescues.
88. Master Stream: A high-volume water stream from a fixed nozzle.
89. Mayday: A distress signal used by a firefighter in life-threatening danger.
90. Mutual Aid: Assistance provided by neighboring fire departments during large-scale incidents.
91. MVA (Motor Vehicle Accident): A term for a car crash, often involving an emergency response.
92. Nozzleman: The firefighter is responsible for controlling the nozzle during suppression.
93. Offensive mode: A strategy involving direct and aggressive fire attack to save lives and property.
94. Overhaul: The process of ensuring that all fires are extinguished and burnt material is removed from the structure to avoid rekindle of a fire.
95. Overhead: Incident management staff supervising an operation.
96. PAR (Personnel Accountability Report): A safety check to confirm that all firefighters are accounted for during an operation.
97. Pre-Plan: A document detailing specific information about high-risk buildings or areas and plans to mitigate potential hazards.
98. Primary search: A quick search of a building to locate victims and report fire extension or other hazards.
99. Probationary Firefighter—Entry-level position under supervision and evaluation.
100. Public Information Officer (PIO)—Manages media and public communications during emergencies.
101. Pumper: Another term for a fire engine designed to pump water.
102. Pump Panel: Control panel for operating a fire engine's pump.
103. Quint: A fire apparatus that has combined features such as carrying water, hoses, and ladders.
104. Rehab (Rehabilitation Area): A designated location for firefighters to recover physically and mentally during or after an incident (specifically for hydration, check vitals, not mental recovery.)
105. Relay Pumping: Multiple engines are used to transport water over long distances.
106. Rescue: Remove a person from a hazardous situation.

107. RIC or RIT: Rapid Intervention Crew or Team, assigned at every working fire ready to respond to a mayday and rescure firefighters.
108. Run Card: A preplanned list of resources to dispatch for specific emergencies.
109. Salvage: Protecting property and belongings from further damage during a fire.
110. SCBA (Self-Contained Breathing Apparatus)/Scott Airpack or Pack: A device supplies breathable air for firefighters in hazardous environments.
111. Search Rope/Lifeline: A safety rope used during search operations in IDLH.
112. Secondary search: A thorough search was conducted after the fire was under control.
113. Signal 10: Code indicating a working fire.
114. Size-Up: The initial assessment of an incident.
115. Smoke Eater: Slang for a firefighter.
116. Spanner Wrench: A tool used to tighten or loosen hose connections.
117. Spotting: Assisting an apparatus in a specific location for optimal use.
118. Spotters- Personnel who are positioned outside of an apparatus to assist in rig replacement or parking. Mandatory for any backing up of fire apparatus.
119. Staging Area: A location where resources are assembled and prepared for deployment.
120. Standpipe System: Pre-installed system in multi-story buildings that provide water for firefighting operations.
121. Strike Team: A group of similar resources (e.g., engines) working under one leader.
122. Structural Specialist—Evaluates building stability; often a licensed engineer.
123. Tender: A vehicle used to transport large amounts of water.
124. The Big One: A significant fire (only a fire, not a different critical incident.)
125. The Job: A term firefighters use to refer to their profession.
126. Thermal imaging camera (TIC): A device that detects heat sources and is often used to locate fire hotspots or victims in an IDLH.
127. Training Officer: Develops and implements training programs.
128. Truck Company: A crew assigned to a ladder truck responsible for ventilation, search, and rescue, forcible entry, and more.
129. Turnout Time/Response Time: The time it takes for firefighters to leave the station and respond to an emergency.
130. Two-In, Two-Out: A safety protocol requiring at least two firefighters inside a dangerous environment and two outside for backup.
131. Under Control: When a fire is no longer spreading.
132. Urban Search and Rescue (USAR) Roles.
133. USAR Medical Specialist: Provides emergency medical care in technical rescue environments.
134. USAR Operations Chief: Manages tactical rescue operations, typically a Battalion Chief.
135. USAR Planning Officer: Coordinates mission logistics and deployment strategies.

136. USAR Safety Officer: Ensures adherence to safety protocols during USAR operations.
137. USAR Task Force Leader: Commands the entire USAR task force.
138. USAR Team Leader: Leads a USAR team; typically holds the rank of Lieutenant or Captain.
139. USAR Technician: Firefighter trained in collapse, rope, trench, and confined space rescue.
140. Utility truck: A vehicle equipped with specialized tools and equipment.
141. Ventilation Fan: A tool used to clear smoke from a structure and found on trucks.
142. Ventilation: The process of removing heat, smoke, and toxic gases from a structure during a fire.
143. Water Supply Officer: The individual responsible for managing adequate water delivery.
144. Wildland Fire: A fire occurring in natural vegetation.

References

Aarons, G. A., Hurlburt, M., & Horwitz, S. M. (2011). Advancing a conceptual model of evidence-based practice implementation in public service sectors. *Administration and Policy in Mental Health and Mental Health Services Research, 38*(1), 4–23. https://doi.org/10.1007/s10488-010-0327-7

Aarons, G. A., Ehrhart, M. G., & Farahnak, L. R. (2014). The implementation leadership scale (ILS): Development of a brief measure of unit level implementation leadership. *Implementation Science, 9*, 45. https://doi.org/10.1186/1748-5908-9-45

Abbt v. City of Houston, No. 21-20085, 2022 WL 738623 (5th Cir. Mar. 11, 2022).

ADA National Network. (2017). Work-leave, the ADA, and the FMLA [Fact sheet]. ADA National Network. http://adainfo.us/work-leave-ada

Adams, B. D., Bruyn, L. E., & Chung-Yan, G. (2004, March 1). Creating a measure of trust in small military teams (Contract Report). Humansystems Inc. https://apps.dtic.mil/sti/citations/ADA436363

Addis, M. E., & Mahalik, J. R. (2003). Men, masculinity, and the contexts of help seeking. *American Psychologist, 58*(1), 5–14. https://psycnet.apa.org/record/2003-02034-001

Adler, A. B., Bliese, P. D., & Castro, C. A. (Eds.). (2011). *Deployment psychology: Evidence-based strategies to promote mental health in the military*. American Psychological Association. https://doi.org/10.1037/12300-000

Ahrens, M. (2001). An Overview of the U.S. Fire Problem. National fire protection association. https://snivalleyfire.org/documents/USFires05.pdf

National Fire Protection Association. (2022, March 4). Vacant buildings [Blog post]. NFPA. https://www.nfpa.org/news-blogs-and-articles/blogs/2022/03/04/vacant-buildings

American Board of Police and Public Safety Psychology. (n.d.). Core legal knowledge for the practice of police & public safety psychology. https://abpp.org/wp-content/uploads/2022/07/Core-Legal-Knowledge-in-PPSP-050915.pdf

American Board of Professional Psychology. (n.d.). Police & public safety psychology. ABPP. https://abpp.org/application-information/learn-about-specialty-boards/police-public-safety/

American Psychological Association. (n.d.) Recognized specialties, subspecialties, and proficiencies in professional psychology. https://www.apa.org/ed/graduate/specialize/recognized

American Psychiatric Association. (2022). Diagnostic and statistical manual of mental disorders (5th ed., text rev.; DSM-5-TR). American Psychiatric Publishing.

American Psychological Association. (2013). Specialty guidelines for forensic psychology. *American Psychologist, 68*(1), 7–19. https://doi.org/10.1037/a0029889

American Psychiatric Association. (2013). Diagnostic and statistical manual of mental disorders (5th ed.). American Psychiatric Publishing.

K. Wheldon, *Fire Service Psychology*,
https://doi.org/10.1007/978-3-032-02126-7

American Psychological Association. (2014, February). Who decides what a specialty is? *Monitor on Psychology, 45*(2). https://www.apa.org/monitor/2014/02/who-decides

American Psychological Association. (2017). Multicultural guidelines: An ecological approach to context, identity, and intersectionality. Retrieved December 13, 2024, from https://www.apa.org/about/policy/multicultural-guidelines.pdf

American Psychological Association. (2022). *Guidelines for the practice of safety psychology: Police and public safety psychology specialty guidelines*. https://www.apa.org/ed/graduate/specialize/police

American Psychological Association. (2023). Cultural competence. In *APA dictionary of psychology*. https://dictionary.apa.org/cultural-competence.

Americans with Disabilities Act of 1990, 42 U.S.C. §§ 12111–12117 (Title I). (1990). (Current codification).

Anderson, G. S., Di Nota, P. M., Groll, D., & Carleton, R. N. (2020). Peer support and crisis-focused psychological interventions designed to mitigate post-traumatic stress injuries among public safety and frontline healthcare personnel: A systematic review. *International Journal of Environmental Research and Public Health, 17*(20), 7645. https://doi.org/10.3390/ijerph17207645

Anderson, B., & Fagerhaug, T. (2006). *Root cause analysis: Simplified tools and techniques*. ASQ Quality Press.

Angehrn, A., Krakauer, R. L., & Carleton, R. N. (2020). The impact of intolerance of uncertainty and anxiety sensitivity on mental health among public safety personnel: When the uncertain is unavoidable. *Cognitive Therapy and Research, 44*(5), 919–930. https://pubmed.ncbi.nlm.nih.gov/32848288/

Angle v. City of Huntington, 852 S.E.2d 789 (W. Va. 2020).

Arble, E., Arnetz, B. B.. (2017). A model of first-responder coping: An approach/avoidance bifurcation. *Stress and Health, 33*(3), 223–232. https://pubmed.ncbi.nlm.nih.gov/27500991/

Arbona, C., Fan, W., & Noor, N. (2016). Factor structure and external correlates of posttraumatic stress disorder symptoms among African American firefighters. Psychology Research and Behavior Management, 9, Article 201–209. https://pmc.ncbi.nlm.nih.gov/articles/PMC4986676/

Armstrong, D., Shakespeare-Finch, J., & Shochet, I. (2016). Organizational belongingness mediates the relationship between sources of stress and posttrauma outcomes in firefighters. Psychological Trauma. *Theory, Research, Practice, and Policy, 8*(3), 343–347. https://psycnet.apa.org/doiLanding?doi=10.1037%2Ftra0000083

Ashforth, B. E., & Saks, A. M. (1996). Socialization tactics: Longitudinal effects on newcomer adjustment. *Academy of Management Journal, 39*(1), 149–178. https://doi.org/10.2307/256634

Aspinwall, L. G., & Taylor, S. E. (1997). A stitch in time: Self-regulation and proactive coping. *Psychological Bulletin, 121*(3), 417–436. https://psycnet.apa.org/doiLanding?doi=10.1037%2F0033-2909.121.3.417

Attridge, M. (2009). Employee assistance programs: A research-based primer. In C. L. Cooper, J. C. Quick, & M. J. Schabracq (Eds.), *International handbook of work and health psychology* (3rd ed., pp. 383–407). Wiley-Blackwell. https://doi.org/10.1002/9780470682357.ch17

Avery, J. D. (Ed.). (2021). *Peer support in medicine: A quick guide*. Springer Nature.

Baigent, D. (2001). *One more last working class hero: A cultural audit of the UK fire service*. Russell Press.

Bakirci, E., Sar, V., & Cetin, A. (2024). Assessment of the psychological effects on firefighters in the aftermath of the Pazarcik and Elbistan earthquakes in 2023. *The Journal of Behavioral Health Services & Research, 51*(4), 529–544. https://pubmed.ncbi.nlm.nih.gov/39009820/

Bakker, A. B., & Demerouti, E. (2007). The Job demands-resources model: State of the art. *Journal of Managerial Psychology, 22*(3), 309–328. https://www.researchgate.net/publication/242339416_The_Job_Demands-Resources_Model_State_of_the_Art

Ballenger, J. F., Best, S. R., Metzler, T. J., Wasserman, D. A., Mohr, D. C., Liberman, A., Delucchi, K., Weiss, D. S., Fagan, J. A., Waldrop, A. E., & Marmar, C. R. (2011). Patterns and predictors of alcohol use in male and female urban police officers. *The American Journal on Addictions, 20*(1), 21–29. https://pubmed.ncbi.nlm.nih.gov/21175917/

Barger, L. K., Rajaratnam, S. M., Wang, W., O'Brien, C. S., Sullivan, J. P., Qadri, S., Lockley, S. W., Czeisler, C. A., & Harvard Work Hours Health and Safety Group. (2015). Common sleep disorders increase risk of motor vehicle crashes and adverse health outcomes in firefighters. *Journal of Clinical Sleep Medicine, 11*(3), 233–240. https://pubmed.ncbi.nlm.nih.gov/25580602/

Barnacle, R., & Abbott, D. A. (2009). The development and evaluation of a Gottman-based premarital education program: A pilot study. *Journal of Couple & Relationship Therapy, 8*, 64–82. https://www.researchgate.net/publication/233030916_The_Development_and_Evaluation_of_a_Gottman-Based_Premarital_Education_Program_A_Pilot_Study

Barrett, E. (2023). Moral injury: A typology. *Journal of Military Ethics, 22*(3–4), 158–167. https://www.tandfonline.com/toc/smil20/22/3-4

Barrett, G. V., Polomsky, M. D., & McDaniel, M. A. (1999). Selection tests for firefighters: A comprehensive review and meta-analysis. *Journal of Business and Psychology, 13*, 507–513. https://link.springer.com/article/10.1023/A:1022966820186

Barry, B., Ricciardelli, R., & Cramm, H. (2023). "We are unique": Organizational stressors, peer support and attitudes toward mental health treatment among airport firefighters. *Health Promot Chronic Dis Prev Canada, 43*(10–11), 450–459. https://pmc.ncbi.nlm.nih.gov/articles/PMC10753901/

Bartlett, B. A., Jardin, C., Martin, C., Tran, J. K., Buser, S., Anestis, M. D., & Vujanovic, A. A. (2018). Posttraumatic stress and suicidality among firefighters: The moderating role of distress tolerance. *Cognitive Therapy and Research, 42*(4), 483–496. https://psycnet.apa.org/record/2018-04214-001

Bartlett, M. L., & Schmitz, N. M. (2023). Moral injury and suicide risk. *A Journal of Strategic Airpower & Spacepower, 2*(3), 101–114. https://www.jstor.org/stable/48743545

Barton, M., & Sutcliffe, K. (2009). Overcoming dysfunctional momentum: Organizational safety as a social achievement. *Human Relations, 62*(9), 1327–1356. https://www.fs.usda.gov/rm/pubs_other/rmrs_2009_barton_m001.pdf

Bartone, P. T. (2004). Increasing resiliency through shared sensemaking: Building hardiness in groups. Managing traumatic stress risk: A proactive approach (pp. 129–140). https://www.researchgate.net/profile/Paul-Bartone/publication/284490079_Increasing_resiliency_through_shared_sensemaking_Building_hardiness_in_groups/links/5b2adbc04585150c634453b9/Increasing-resiliency-through-shared-sensemaking-Building-hardiness-in-groups.pdf

Bartone, P. T. (2006). Resilience under military operational stress: Can leaders influence hardiness? *Military Psychology, 18*(Suppl), S131–S148. https://doi.org/10.1207/s15327876mp1803s_10

Bartone, P. T., Bartone, J. V., Gileno, Z., & Violanti, J. M. (2018). Exploration into best practices in peer support for bereaved survivors. *Death Studies, 42*(9), 555–568. https://pubmed.ncbi.nlm.nih.gov/29338675/

Bartone, P. T., Bartone, J. V., Violanti, J. M., & Gileno, Z. M. (2019). Peer support Services for Bereaved Survivors: A systematic review. *Omega, 80*(1), 137–166. https://doi.org/10.1177/0030222817728204

Bartone, P. T., & Dooley, C. M. (2021). Peer support for the bereaved. In *Peer support in medicine: A quick guide* (pp. 71–94). Springer. https://psycnet.apa.org/record/2022-06584-004

Bartone, P. T. (2022). Hardiness protects against burnout in a large sample of adult workers. *Journal of Occupational and Environmental Medicine, 64*(1), 39–44. https://doi.org/10.1097/JOM.0000000000002448

Bartone, P. T., & Roche, R. (2024). Sex differences in hardiness, coping, and health in new west point cadets. *Military Psychology, 36*(5), 516–524. https://pubmed.ncbi.nlm.nih.gov/37326426/

Bass, B. M., & Riggio, R. E. (2006). *Transformational leadership* (2nd ed.). Lawrence Erlbaum Associates Publishers.

Bastug, G., Ergul-Topcu, A., Ozel-Kizil, E. T., & Ergun, O. F. (2019). Secondary traumatization and related psychological outcomes in firefighters. *Journal of Loss and Trauma, 24*(2), 143–158. https://psycnet.apa.org/record/2019-06247-001

Batson, C. D., Batson, J. G., Slingsby, J. K., Harrell, K. L., Peekna, H. M., & Todd, R. M. (1991). Empathic joy and the empathy-altruism hypothesis. *Journal of Personality and Social Psychology, 61*(3), 413–426. https://psycnet.apa.org/record/1992-05357-001

Bechara, A., Damasio, H., & Damasio, A. R. (2000). Emotion, decision making and the orbitofrontal cortex. *Cerebral Cortex, 10*(3), 295–307. https://pubmed.ncbi.nlm.nih.gov/10731224/

Behnke, A., Rojas, R., Karabatsiakis, A., & Kolassa, I. T. (2020). Childhood maltreatment compromises resilience against occupational trauma exposure: A retrospective study among emergency medical service personnel. *Child Abuse & Neglect, 99*, 104248. https://www.researchgate.net/publication/337223995_Childhood_maltreatment_compromises_resilience_against_occupational_trauma_exposure_A_retrospective_study_among_emergency_medical_service_personnel

Bendersky, C., & Hays, N. A. (2012). Status conflict in groups. *Organization Science, 23*(2), 323–340. https://doi.org/10.1287/orsc.1110.0734

Benesch, O. (2014). Inventing the way of the samurai: Nationalism, internationalism, and Bushido in modern Japan. Oxford University Press.

Benight, C. C., & Bandura, A. (2004). Social cognitive theory of posttraumatic recovery: The role of perceived self-efficacy. *Behavior Research and Therapy, 42*(10), 1129–1148. https://pubmed.ncbi.nlm.nih.gov/15350854/

Bennett, J. B., & Lehman, W. E. (2001). Workplace substance abuse prevention and help-seeking: Comparing team-oriented and informational training. *Journal of Occupational Health Psychology, 6*(3), 243–254. https://pubmed.ncbi.nlm.nih.gov/11482635/

Ben-Porath, Y. S., & Tellegen, A. (2020). MMPI-3: Minnesota multiphasic personality inventory-3 manual for administration, scoring, and interpretation. University of Minnesota Press. https://www.pearsonassessments.com/en-us/Store/Professional-Assessments/Personality-%26-Biopsychosocial/Minnesota-Multiphasic-Personality-Inventory-3/p/P100000004?srsltid=AfmBOorPlm-Oll1M1DE3eeK7dquZklZaMY9u9Qj65y9s8oDYlWhhBMUv

Berger, C. (2024, June 14). St. Johns County Fire rescue lieutenant, wife dead in apparent murder-suicide. Action News Jax. https://www.actionnewsjax.com/news/local/st-johns-county-fire-rescue-lieutenant-wife-dead-apparent-murder-suicide/LLBI4XFNYBCTLML3KG23OEDEO4/

Berger, G., & Peerson, A. (2015). Cultural competence lessons learned: The continuum model. *Medical Education, 49*(5), 515–516. https://doi.org/10.1111/medu.12685

Berger, W., Coutinho, E. S. F., Figueira, I., Marques-Portella, C., Luz, M. P., Neylan, T. C., Marmar, C. R., & Mendlowicz, M. V. (2012). Rescuers at risk: A systematic review and meta-regression analysis of the worldwide current prevalence and correlates of PTSD in rescue workers. *Social Psychiatry and Psychiatric Epidemiology, 47*(6), 1001–1011. https://doi.org/10.1007/s00127-011-0408-2

Billings, J., & Focht, W. (2016). Firefighter shift schedules affect sleep quality. *Journal of Occupational and Environmental Medicine, 58*(3), 294–298. https://doi.org/10.1097/JOM.0000000000000624

Bledsoe, B. E. (2003). Critical incident stress management (CISM): Benefit or risk for emergency services? *Prehospital Emergency Care, 7*(2), 272–279. https://pubmed.ncbi.nlm.nih.gov/12710792/

Blackistone, S. (1997, July 31). Accommodating mental disabilities. Firehouse Magazine. https://www.firehouse.com/leadership/article/10544833/accommodating-mental-disabilities

Bock, C., & Orr, R. M. (2015). Use of functional movement screen in a tactical population: A review. *Journal of Military and Veterans' Health, 23*(2), 33–42. http://jmvh.org/wp-content/uploads/2015/05/Bock-and-Orr-from-AMMA-JMVH-April_Web-6.pdf

Bodenmann, G., & Ledermann, T., & Bradbury, T. (2007). Stress, sex, and satisfaction in marriage. *Personal Relationships, 14*, 551–569. https://www.researchgate.net/publication/229468324_Stress_sex_and_satisfaction_in_mariage

Bonanno, G. A. (2004). Loss, trauma, and human resilience: Have we underestimated the human capacity to thrive after extremely aversive events? *The American Psychologist, 59*(1), 20–28. https://doi.org/10.1037/0003-066X.59.1.20

Bonilla-Silva, E. (1997). Rethinking racism: Toward a structural interpretation. *American Sociological Review, 62*(3), 465–480. https://www.jstor.org/stable/2657316

Boss, P. G. (2002). Ambiguous loss: Working with families of the missing. *Family Process, 41*(1), 14–17. https://doi.org/10.1111/j.1545-5300.2002.40102000014.x

Boss, P., Bryant, C. M., & Mancini, J. A. (2016). *Family stress management: A contextual approach*. Sage Publications. https://sk.sagepub.com/book/mono/family-stress-management-3e/chpt/4-ambiguous-loss-major-stressor#_=_

Boston Chapter, NAACP v. Beecher, 504 F.2d 1017 (1st Cir. 1974).

Bothe, B., Tóth-Király, I., Potenza, M. N., Griffiths, M. D., Orosz, G., & Demetrovics, Z. (2019). Revisiting the role of impulsivity and compulsivity in problematic sexual Behaviors. *Journal of Sex Research, 56*(2), 166–179. https://pubmed.ncbi.nlm.nih.gov/29913087/

Boucher, E. (2023). The role of peer, supervisor, mentor, and organizational support on workplace ostracism and inclusion. *All Theses*. 4080. https://open.clemson.edu/all_theses/4080

Bracken-Scally, M., McGilloway, S., Gallagher, S., & Mitchell, J. T. (2014). Life after the emergency services: An exploratory study of well being and quality of life in emergency service retirees. *International Journal of Emergency Mental Health, 16*(1), 223–231. https://doi.org/10.4172/1522-4821.1000108

Brandt-Rauf, S., Davis, A. L., & Taylor, J. A. (2024). Inventory of state workers' compensation laws in the United States: First responder mental health. *Journal of Public Health Policy, 45*(3), 562–574. https://doi.org/10.1057/s41271-024-00501-5

Brandt-Rauf, S., Davis, A. L., Taylor, J. A., Eisenberg, J., Friedman, L., & Armstrong, D. (2024). Inventory of state workers' compensation laws in the United States: First responder mental health. *Journal of Public Health Policy, 45*(3), 562–574. https://doi.org/10.1057/s41271-024-00501-5

Brennan v. City of Everett, No. 2: 21-cv-01134 (W.D. Wash. 2022).

Brewer, M. B. (1999). The psychology of prejudice: Ingroup love and outgroup hate? *Journal of Social Issues, 55*(3), 429–444. https://doi.org/10.1111/0022-4537.00126

Bronfenbrenner, U. (1979). *The ecology of human development: Experiments by nature and design*. Harvard University Press.

Brough, P., Chataway, S., & Biggs, A. (2016). 'You don't want people knowing you're a copper!' A contemporary assessment of police organisational culture. *International Journal of Police Science & Management, 18*(1), 28–36. https://doi.org/10.1177/1461355716638361. (Original work published 2016).

Bryant, R. A. (2019). Posttraumatic stress disorder: A state-of-the-art review of evidence and challenges. *World Psychiatry, 18*(3), 259–269. https://pubmed.ncbi.nlm.nih.gov/31496089/

Bryant, R. A., & Harvey, A. G. (1995). Posttraumatic stress in volunteer firefighters. Predictors of distress. *The Journal of Nervous and Mental Disease, 183*(4), 267–271. https://pubmed.ncbi.nlm.nih.gov/7714516/

Bryant, R., & Harvey, A. (2012). Acute stress disorder: A handbook of theory, assessment, and treatment. *American Journal of Psychiatry*. https://www.researchgate.net/publication/232511860_Acute_Stress_Disorder_A_Handbook_of_Theory_Assessment_and_Treatment

Brymer, M., Jacobs, A., Layne, C., Pynoos, R., Ruzek, J., Steinberg, A., Vernberg, E., & Watson, P. (2006). *Psychological first aid: Field operations guide* (2nd ed.). National Child Traumatic Stress Network & National Center for PTSD. https://www.ptsd.va.gov/disaster_events/for_providers/PFA/PFA_V2.pdf

Burke, P. J. (2006). Identity change. *Social Psychology Quarterly, 69*(1), 81–96. https://journals.sagepub.com/doi/10.1177/019027250606900106

Bureau of Justice Assistance. (2022). *Public safety officers' benefits (PSOB) program*. U.S. Department of Justice, Office of Justice Programs. https://psob.bja.ojp.gov

Bureau of Justice Assistance. (2023). Public Safety Officers' Benefits Program: Fact sheet. https://bja.ojp.gov/doc/psob-fact-sheet.pdf

California. (2019). Senate Bill 542 (2019), Chapter 390: Labor Code § 3212.15 (PTSD presumption). Chaptered bill text. https://legiscan.com/CA/text/SB542/id/2055574

California Chamber of Commerce. (n.d.). California Labor Law Resources. Retrieved from https://www.calchamber.com/california-labor-law

California Commission on Peace Officer Standards and Training (POST). (2022). Peace Officer Psychological Screening Manual. https://post.ca.gov/portals/0/post_docs/publications/psychological-screening-manual/Peace_Officer_Psychological_Screening_Manual.pdf

California Department of Industrial Relations. (n.d.). All workers have rights in California. Retrieved from https://www.dir.ca.gov/letf/What_are_your_rights_as_a_worker.pdf

California Legislature. (2019). Senate Bill 542 (2019), Chapter 390: Labor Code § 3212.15 (PTSD presumption). https://legiscan.com/CA/text/SB542/id/2055574

Campbell, J. (1949). *The hero with a thousand faces*. Princeton University Press.

Campbell, R., & Hall, S. (2024, November 30). United States firefighter injuries (NFPA No. FFI10). National Fire Protection Association. https://www.nfpa.org/education-and-research/research/nfpa-research/fire-statistical-reports/firefighter-injuries-in-the-united-states

Canton-Tompson, J., Gebert, K. M., Thompson, B., Jones, G., Calkin, D., & Donovan, G. (2008). External human factors in incident management team decisionmaking and their effect on large fire suppression expenditures. *Journal of Forestry, 106*(8), 416–424.

Carey, K. B., Carey, M. P., Maisto, S. A., & Henson, J. M. (2006). Brief motivational interventions for heavy college drinkers: A randomized controlled trial. *Journal of Consulting and Clinical Psychology, 74*(5), 943–954. https://pmc.ncbi.nlm.nih.gov/articles/PMC2442891/

Caric, R. N. (2005). From ordered buckets to honored felons: Fire companies and cultural transformation in Philadelphia, 1785–1850. *Pennsylvania History: A Journal of Mid-Atlantic Studies, 72*(2), 117–158. http://www.jstor.org/stable/27778663

Carleton, R. N., Afifi, T. O., Taillieu, T., Turner, S., Mason, J. E., Ricciardelli, R., & Sareen, J. (2018a). Exposures to potentially traumatic events among public safety personnel in Canada. *Canadian Journal of Psychiatry, 63*(1), 54S–64S. https://www.researchgate.net/publication/329550261_Exposures_to_Potentially_Traumatic_Events_Among_Public_Safety_Personnel_in_Canada

Carleton, R. N., Afifi, T. O., Turner, S., Taillieu, T., Duranceau, S., LeBouthillier, D. M., Sareen, J., Ricciardelli, R., MacPhee, R. S., Groll, D., Hozempa, K., Brunet, A., Weekes, J. R., Griffiths, C. T., Abrams, K. J., Jones, N. A., Beshai, S., Cramm, H. A., Dobson, K. S., Hatcher, S., Keane, T. M., Stewart, S. H., & Asmundson, G. J. G. (2018b). Mental disorder symptoms among public safety personnel in Canada. *Canadian Journal of Psychiatry. Revue Canadienne de Psychiatrie, 63*(1), 54–64. https://pubmed.ncbi.nlm.nih.gov/28845686/

Carleton, R. N., Afifi, T. O., Turner, S., Taillieu, T., Vaughan, A. D., Anderson, G. S., Ricciardelli, R., MacPhee, R. S., Cramm, H. A., Czarnuch, S., Hozempa, K., & Camp, R. D. (2019). Mental health training, attitudes toward support, and screening positive for mental disorders. *Cognitive Behavior Therapy, 49*(1), 55–73. https://pubmed.ncbi.nlm.nih.gov/30794073/

Carleton, R. N., et al. (2020). Mental health training, attitudes toward support, and screening positive for mental disorders among public safety personnel. *Cognitive Behaviour Therapy, 49*(1), 55–73. https://doi.org/10.1080/16506073.2019.1575900

Carlier, I. V., Lamberts, R. D., & Gersons, B. P. (1997). Risk factors for posttraumatic stress symptomatology in police officers: A prospective analysis. *The Journal of Nervous and Mental Disease, 185*(8), 498–506. https://pubmed.ncbi.nlm.nih.gov/9284863/

Carlier, I. V. E., Lamberts, R. D., van Uchelen, A. J., & Gersons, B. P. R. (1998). Disaster-related posttraumatic stress in police officers: A field study of the impact of debriefing. *Stress Medicine, 14*(3), 143–148. https://psycnet.apa.org/record/1998-10258-001

Carlier, I. V. E., Voerman, A. E., & Gersons, B. P. R. (2000). The influence of occupational debriefing on posttraumatic stress symptomatology in traumatized police officers. *British Journal of Medical Psychology, 73*:87–98. https://pubmed.ncbi.nlm.nih.gov/10759053/

Carp, B. L. (2001). Fire of liberty: Firefighters, urban voluntary culture, and the revolutionary movement. *The William and Mary Quarterly, 58*(4), 781–818. https://www.jstor.org/stable/2674500

Carpenter v. York Area United Fire and Rescue, No. 1:18-cv-02155 (M.D. Pa. Apr. 16, 2020). https://www.govinfo.gov/app/details/USCOURTS-pamd-1_18-cv-02155

Carter, J. (1979). Executive order 12127: Federal Emergency Management Agency. *Federal Register, 44*(56), 12098. https://www.archives.gov/federal-register/codification/executive-order/12127.html

Cavanagh, J. T. O., Carson, A. J., Sharpe, M., & Lawrie, S. M. (2003). Psychological autopsy studies of suicide: A systematic review. *Psychological Medicine, 33*(3), 395–405. https://doi.org/10.1017/S0033291702006943

Centre for Mental Health & NSW Institute of Psychiatry. (2000). Disaster mental health response handbook[Manual]. NSW Health. https://faculty.uml.edu/darcus/47.474/nswiop_Disaster_Handbook.pdf

Centers for Disease Control and Prevention [CDC], 2023. https://search.cdc.gov/search/?query=fire%20death&siteLimit=NCHS&dpage=1

Centers for Disease Control and Prevention. (2023, April 7). QuickStats: Rates of death due to unintentional injury from fire or flames — United States, 2021. *MMWR, 72*(14), 550. https://www.cdc.gov/mmwr/volumes/72/wr/mm7214a5.htm

Chen, S. T. (2019). An approach of identifying the common human and organisational factors (HOFs) among a group of marine accidents using GRA and HFACS-MA. *Journal of Transportation Safety & Security, 12*(10), 1252–1294. https://www.researchgate.net/publication/346777418_An_approach_of_identifying_the_common_human_and_organisational_factors_HOFs_among_a_group_of_marine_accidents_using_GRA_and_HFACS-MA

Cherry, N., Galarneau, J. M., Haynes, W., & Sluggett, B. (2021). The role of organizational supports in mitigating mental ill health in firefighters: A cohort study in Alberta, Canada. *American Journal of Industrial Medicine*. https://doi.org/10.1002/ajim.23249

Chinman, M., George, P., Dougherty, R. H., Daniels, A. S., Ghose, S. S., Swift, A., & Delphin-Rittmon, M. E. (2014). Peer support services for individuals with serious mental illnesses: Assessing the evidence. *Psychiatric Services, 65*(4), 429–441. https://pubmed.ncbi.nlm.nih.gov/24549400/

Chizewski, A., Box, A., Kesler, R., & Petruzzello, S. J. (2021). Fitness fights fires: Exploring the relationship between physical fitness and firefighter ability. *International Journal of Environmental Research and Public Health, 18*(22), 11733. https://doi.org/10.3390/ijerph182211733

Choi, B. Y., Blumberg, C., & Williams, K. (2016). Mobile integrated health care and community paramedicine: An emerging emergency medical services concept. *Annals of Emergency Medicine, 67*(3), 361–366. https://doi.org/10.1016/j.annemergmed.2015.06.005

Chung, I. S., Lee, M. Y., Jung, S. W., & Nam, C. W. (2015). Minnesota multiphasic personality inventory as related factor for post traumatic stress disorder symptoms according to job stress level in experienced firefighters: 5-year study. *Annals of Occupational and Environmental Medicine, 27*, 16. https://pmc.ncbi.nlm.nih.gov/articles/PMC4487507/

City of Tucson v. Industrial Commission of Arizona, No. 2 CA-IC 2024-0003, Mem. Op. (Ariz. Ct. App. Jan. 27, 2025).

Clarke, T. B. B., Walker, M., & Mendham, F. (2021). Assessing the safety of training firefighters with the minimum requirements for firefighter garments. *Fire Technology, 57*(5), 2129–2158. https://www.researchgate.net/publication/350317674_Assessing_the_Safety_of_Training_Firefighters_with_the_Minimum_Requirements_for_Firefighter_Garments

Coffman v. Indianapolis Fire Department, 578 F.3d 559 (7th Cir. 2009).

Cole, E. R. (2009). Intersectionality and research in psychology. *American Psychologist, 64*(3), 170–180. https://psycnet.apa.org/record/2009-04471-001

Compas, B. E., Connor-Smith, J. K., Saltzman, H., Thomsen, A. H., & Wadsworth, M. E. (2001). Coping with stress during childhood and adolescence: Problems, progress, and potential in theory and research. *Psychological Bulletin, 127*(1), 87–127. https://pubmed.ncbi.nlm.nih.gov/11271757/

Congressional Fire Services Institute, & Maryland Fire and Rescue Institute. (2023). CFSI Firefighter Day at the Maryland Fire and Rescue Institute. Fire Safety Research Institute. https://fsri.org/news/congressional-fire-service-institutes-cfsi-firefighter-day-maryland-fire-rescue-institute

Corey, G., Corey, M. S., & Corey, C. (2017). *Issues and ethics in the helping professions*. (10th ed.). Cengage Learning Custom Publishing. https://www.cengage.com/c/issues-and-ethics-in-the-helping-professions-10e-corey-corey-

Corey, D. M., Cuttler, M. J., Cox, D. R., & Brower, J. (2011). Board certification in police psychology: What it means to public safety. *The Police Chief, 78*(11). https://www.policechiefmagazine.org/board-certification-in-police-psychology-what-it-means-to-public-safety/

Corrigan, P. W. (2004). How stigma interferes with mental health care. *American Psychologist, 59*(7), 614–625. https://pubmed.ncbi.nlm.nih.gov/15491256/

Corrigan, P. W., Druss, B. G., & Perlick, D. A. (2014). The impact of mental illness stigma on seeking and participating in mental health care. *Psychological Science in the Public Interest, 15*(2), 37–70. https://pubmed.ncbi.nlm.nih.gov/26171956/

Costa, P. T., Jr., & McCrae, R. R. (2008). The revised NEO personality inventory (NEO-PI-R). In G. J. Boyle, G. Matthews, & D. H. Saklofske (Eds.), *The SAGE handbook of personality theory and assessment, Vol. 2. Personality measurement and testing* (pp. 179–198). Sage Publications. https://doi.org/10.4135/9781849200479.n9

Cowlishaw, S., Birch, A., McLennan, J., & Hayes, P. (2014). Antecedents and outcomes of volunteer work–family conflict and facilitation in Australia. *Applied Psychology: An International Review, 63*(1), 168–189. https://psycnet.apa.org/record/2013-39399-008

Cowlishaw, S., Evans, L., & McLennan, J. (2010). Work-family conflict and crossover in volunteer emergency service workers. *Work & Stress, 24*(4), 342–358. https://psycnet.apa.org/record/2010-26269-004

Craig, J. M., & Jacobs, R. R. (1985). The effect of working with women on male attitudes toward female firefighters. *Basic & Applied Social Psychology, 6*(1), 61–74. https://psycnet.apa.org/record/2010-26269-004

Creamer, M., Varker, T., Bisson, J., Darte, K., Greenberg, N., Lau, W., Moreton, G., O'Donnell, M., Richardson, D., Ruzek, J., Watson, P., & Forbes, D. (2012). Guidelines for peer support in high-risk organizations: An international consensus study using the Delphi method. *Journal of Traumatic Stress, 25*(2), 134–141. https://doi.org/10.1002/jts.21685

Crenshaw, K. (1991). Mapping the margins: Intersectionality, identity politics, and violence against women of color. *Stanford Law Review, 43*(6), 1241–1299. https://www.jstor.org/stable/1229039

Crocker, J., & Clawson, D. (2012). Buying time: Gendered patterns in union contracts. *Social Problems, 59*(4), 459–480. https://www.academia.edu/19725596/Buying_Time_Gendered_Patterns_in_Union_Contracts

Cross, T. (2020). Cultural competence continuum. *Journal of Child and Youth Care Work, 24*, 83–85. https://doi.org/10.5195/jcycw.2012.48

Crossan, M., Byrne, A., Seijts, G., Reno, M., Monzani, L., & Gandz, J. (2017). Toward a framework of leader character in organizations. *Journal of Management Studies, 54*(7), 986–1018. https://onlinelibrary.wiley.com/doi/abs/10.1111/joms.12254

Crossan, M., Seijts, G., & Gandz, J. (2015). *Developing leadership character*. Routledge.

Crowe, R. P., Fernandez, A. R., Pepe, P. E., Cash, R. E., Rivard, M. K., Wronski, R., Anderson, S. E., Hogan, T. H., Andridge, R. R., Panchal, A. R., & Ferketich, A. K. (2020). The association of job demands and resources with burnout among emergency medical services professionals. *Journal of the American College of Emergency Physicians open, 1*(1), 6–16. https://doi.org/10.1002/emp2.12014

Currier, J. M., Drescher, K. D., Holland, J., Lisman, R., & Foy, D. W. (2016). Spirituality, forgiveness, and quality of life: Testing a mediational model with military veterans with PTSD. *International Journal for the Psychology of Religion, 26*(2), 167–179. https://www.researchgate.net/publication/272167622_Spirituality_Forgiveness_and_Quality_of_Life_Testing_a_Mediational_Model_with_Military_Veterans_with_PTSD

Cutrona, C. E. (1996). *Social support in couples: Marriage as a resource in times of stress*. Sage Publications.

Damschroder, L. J., Aron, D. C., Keith, R. E., Kirsh, S. R., Alexander, J. A., & Lowery, J. C. (2009). Fostering implementation of health services research findings into practice: A consolidated framework for advancing implementation science. *Implementation Science, 4*, 50. https://doi.org/10.1186/1748-5908-4-50

Dangermond, K., Weewer, R., Duyndam, J., & Machielse, A. (2022). "If it stops, then I'll start worrying." Humor as part of the fire service culture, specifically as part of coping with critical incidents. *Humor: International Journal of Humor Research, 35*(1), 31–50. https://psycnet.apa.org/record/2023-12693-003

Daramola, A. Y. (2014). An investigation of air accidents in Nigeria using the human factors analysis and classification system (HFACS) framework. *Journal of Air Transport Management, 35*(1), 39–50. https://www.researchgate.net/publication/259139181_An_investigation_of_air_accidents_in_Nigeria_using_the_Human_Factors_Analysis_and_Classification_System_HFACS_framework

Davidson, L., Bellamy, C., Guy, K., & Miller, R. (2012). Peer support among persons with severe mental illnesses: A review of evidence and experience. *World Psychiatry, 11*(2), 123–128. https://pubmed.ncbi.nlm.nih.gov/22654945/

Davidson, J. E., Proudfoot, J., Lee, K., Terterian, G., & Zisook, S. (2020). A longitudinal analysis of nurse suicide in the United States (2005–2016) with recommendations for action. *Worldviews on Evidence-Based Nursing, 17*(1), 6–15. https://pubmed.ncbi.nlm.nih.gov/32017434/

Daubert v. Merrell Dow Pharmaceuticals, Inc., 509 U.S. 579 (1993).

DC Fire and Emergency Medical Services Department. (2024, November). Mayor Bowser highlights life-saving success of the DC Fire and EMS Whole Blood Program. https://fems.dc.gov/release/mayor-bowser-highlights-life-saving-success-dc-fire-and-ems-whole-blood-program

De Almeida, T. R. F., de Araújo, A. L., Munhoz, D., Andrade, P. G., & Wagner, G. A. (2022). Suicide attempts assisted by firefighters according to traumatic brain injury. *Journal of Prevention (2022), 43*(6), 823–840. https://pubmed.ncbi.nlm.nih.gov/36038809/

De Wolde, A., Groenendaal, J., Helsloot, I., & Schmidt, A. (2014). An explorative study on the connection between ethical leadership, prototypicality, and organizational misbehavior in a Dutch Fire service. *International Journal Of Leadership Studies, 8*(2), 18–43. https://www.regent.edu/acad/global/publications/ijls/new/vol8iss2/2-Groenendaal.pdf

Dean, W., Talbot, S., & Dean, A. (2019). Reframing clinician distress: Moral injury not burnout. *Federal Practitioner, 36*(9), 400–402. https://pmc.ncbi.nlm.nih.gov/articles/PMC6752815/

DeJoy, D. M., Schaffer, B. S., Wilson, M. G., Vandenberg, R. J., & Butts, M. M. (2004). Creating safer workplaces: Assessing the determinants and role of safety climate. *Journal of Safety Research, 35*(1), 81–90. https://doi.org/10.1016/j.jsr.2003.09.018

Dekker, S. (2011). *Drift into failure: From hunting broken components to understanding complex systems*. CRC Press.

DeMoulin, D., Harris, J. I., McGovern, P. M., Beebe, T. J., Church, T. R., & Kim, H. (2023). Moral injury: Need and development of a measurement scale for firefighters. *Current Treatment Options in Psychiatry, 10*(4), 404–430. https://psycnet.apa.org/record/2024-44097-005

Department of the Army, the Navy, the Air Force, & the Defense Logistics Agency. (2021, August 27). DoD Instruction 6055.04: DoD Motor Vehicle and Traffic Safety. Office of the Secretary of Defense. Retrieved from https://www.esd.whs.mil/Portals/54/Documents/DD/issuances/dodi/605504p.pdf

Desmond, M. (2006). Becoming a firefighter. *Ethnography, 7*(4), 387–421. https://collaborate.princeton.edu/en/publications/becoming-a-firefighter

Desmond, M. (2007). On the fireline: Living and dying with wildland firefighters. University of Chicago Press

Diller, T., Helmrich, G., Dunning, S., Cox, S., Buchanan, A., & Shappell, S. (2014). The human factors analysis classification system (HFACS) applied to health care. *American Journal of Medical Quality, 29*(3), 181–190. https://pubmed.ncbi.nlm.nih.gov/23814026/

Dirks, K. T., & Ferrin, D. L. (2002). Trust in leadership: Meta-analytic findings and implications for research and practice. *Journal of Applied Psychology, 87*(4), 611–628. https://psycnet.apa.org/record/2002-15406-001

Dizmang v. Reed, No. 1:23-cv-007423 (D. Colo. Feb. 28, 2025).

Domenech Rodríguez, M. M., Reveles, A. K., Litson, K., Patterson, C. A., & Vázquez, A. L. (2022). Development of the awareness, skills, knowledge: General (ASK-G) scale for measuring cultural competence in the general population. *PLoS One, 17*(9), e0274505. https://pubmed.ncbi.nlm.nih.gov/36107886/

Dooley, C. M., Carroll, B., Fry, L. E., Seamon-Lahiff, G., & Bartone, P. T. (2019). A model for supporting grief recovery following traumatic loss: The tragedy assistance program for survivors (TAPS). *Military Medicine, 184*(7–8), 166–170. https://pmc.ncbi.nlm.nih.gov/articles/PMC6614836/

Doran, G. T. (1981). There's a S.M.A.R.T. Way to write management's goals and objectives. *Management Review, 70*(11), 35–36. https://community.mis.temple.edu/mis0855002fall2015/files/2015/10/S.M.A.R.T-Way-Management-Review.pdf

Dovidio, J. F., & Gaertner, S. L. (2000). Aversive racism and selection decisions: 1989 and 1999. *Psychological Science, 11*(4), 315–319. https://psycnet.apa.org/record/2000-05122-009

Dowler, L. (2018). Fighting fire with societal norms. Penn State University News. Retrieved from https://www.psu.edu/news/research/story/fighting-fire-societal-norms

Drain, J., Billing, D., Neesham-Smith, D., & Aisbett, B. (2016). Predicting physiological capacity of human load carriage: A review. *Applied Ergonomics, 52*, 85–94. https://doi.org/10.1016/j.apergo.2015.07.003

Dryden, C. (2020). Putting mental health on the frontline: Why mental injuries in first responders should be covered through workers' compensation. Drexel Law Review Blog. https://drexel.edu/law/lawreview/blog/overview/2020/September/putting-mental-health-on-the-front-line/

Duarte, C. S., Hoven, C. W., Wu, P., Bin, F., Cotel, S., Mandell, D. J., Nagasawa, M., Balaban, V., Wernikoff, L., & Markenson, D. (2006). Posttraumatic stress in children with first responders in their families. *Journal of Traumatic Stress, 19*(2), 301–306. https://pubmed.ncbi.nlm.nih.gov/16612825/

Dunlop, P. D., Morrison, D. L., & Cordery, J. L. (2011). Investigating retesting effects in a personnel selection context. *International Journal of Selection and Assessment, 19*(2), 217–221. https://psycnet.apa.org/record/2011-10234-011

Ebaugh, H. R. F. (1988). *Becoming an ex: The process of role exit*. University of Chicago Press.

Edmondson, A. (1999). Psychological safety and learning behavior in work teams. *Administrative Science Quarterly, 44*(2), 350–383. https://www.jstor.org/stable/2666999?origin=JSTOR-pdf

Edmondson, A. C., & Lei, Z. (2014). Psychological safety: The history, renaissance, and future of an interpersonal construct. *Annual Review of Organizational Psychology and Organizational Behavior, 1*, 23–43. https://psycnet.apa.org/record/2016-34491-002

Edwards, M. L. (2019). Pittsburgh's freedom house ambulance service: The origins of emergency medical services and the politics of race and health. *Journal of the History of Medicine and Allied Sciences, 74*(4), 440–466. https://pubmed.ncbi.nlm.nih.gov/31592527/

Egberink, I. J. L., Harms, T., & Lommen, M. J. J. (2020). Psychometric properties of the Dutch revised sense of coherence scale in a firefighter sample. *European Journal of Psychotraumatology, 11*(1). https://pubmed.ncbi.nlm.nih.gov/32922683/

Elhart, M. A., Dotson, J., & Smart, D. (2019). Psychological debriefing of hospital emergency personnel: Review of critical incident stress debriefing. *International Journal of Nursing Student Scholarship, 6*. https://journalhosting.ucalgary.ca/index.php/ijnss/article/view/68395

Eriksen, C. (2014). Gendered risk engagement: Challenging the embedded vulnerability, social norms and power relations in conventional Australian bushfire education. *Geographical Research, 52*(1), 23–33. https://onlinelibrary.wiley.com/doi/abs/10.1111/1745-5871.12046

Eriksen, C. (2019). Negotiating adversity with humor: A case study of wildland firefighter women. *Political Geography, 68*(1), 139–145. https://www.researchgate.net/publication/326832635_Negotiating_adversity_with_humour_A_case_study_of_wildland_firefighter_women

Evarts, B., & Stein, G. P. (2022). *U.S. fire department profile—2020 (NFPA research report).* National Fire Protection Association. https://www.nfpa.org/education-and-research/research/nfpa-research/fire-statistical-reports/us-fire-departmentprofile

Evans, T. R., Burns, C., Essex, R., Finnerty, G., Hatton, E., Clements, A. J., & Weldon, S. (2023). A systematic scoping review on the evidence behind debriefing practices for the wellbeing/emotional outcomes of healthcare workers. *Frontiers in Psychiatry, 14*, 1078797. https://pubmed.ncbi.nlm.nih.gov/37032950/

Everly, G. S., Flannery, R. B., & Mitchell, J. T. (2000). Critical incident stress management (CISM): A review of the literature. *Aggression and Violent Behavior, 5*, 23–40. https://www.researchgate.net/publication/222223105_Critical_Incident_Stress_Management_CISM_A_review_of_the_literature

Everly, G. S., Jr, & Boyle, S. H. (1999). Critical incident stress debriefing (CISD): A meta-analysis. *International Journal of Emergency Mental Health, 1*(3), 165–168. https://psycnet.apa.org/record/2000-12393-003

Everly, G. S., Jr., Flannery, R. B., Jr., & Eyler, V. A. (2002). Critical incident stress management (CISM): A statistical review of the literature. *The Psychiatric Quarterly, 73*(3), 171–182. https://pubmed.ncbi.nlm.nih.gov/12143079/

Everly, G. S., McCabe, O. L., Semon, N. L., Thompson, C. B., & Links, J. M. (2014). The development of a model of psychological first aid for non–mental health trained public health personnel: The Johns Hopkins RAPID-PFA. *Journal of Public Health Management and Practice, 20*(5), S24–S29. https://pubmed.ncbi.nlm.nih.gov/25072485/

Everly, G. S., & Mitchell, J. T. (2000). The debriefing controversy and crisis intervention: A review of lexical and substantive issues. *International Journal of Emergency Mental Health, 2*(4), 211–225. https://pubmed.ncbi.nlm.nih.gov/11217152/

Fahy, R. F., & LeBlanc, P. R. (2000). 1999 Firefighter fatality report. *NFPA Journal*, 46–61.

Fallon, P., Jaegers, L. A., Zhang, Y., Dugan, A. G., Cherniack, M., & El Ghaziri, M. (2023). Peer support programs to reduce organizational stress and trauma for public safety workers: A scoping review. *Workplace Health & Safety, 71*(11), 523–535. https://doi.org/10.1177/21650799231194623

Family and Medical Leave Act of 1993, 29 U.S.C. § 2612. (Current codification).

Farnsworth, J. K., & Sewell, K. W. (2011). Fear of emotion as a moderator between PTSD and firefighter social interactions. *Journal of Traumatic Stress, 24*(4), 444–450. https://psycnet.apa.org/record/2011-19096-010

Felicia, & Natalia Mau, E. C. (2022). The impact of patriarchal practices on Cassie Hanwell in things you save in a fire. *IDE-Online Journal: International Dialogue on Education: Past & Present, 9*, 20–41. https://idejournal.org/index.php/ide/article/view/274

Festinger, L. (1957). *A theory of cognitive dissonance*. Stanford University Press.

Fletcher, J. K. (2004). The paradox of postheroic leadership: An essay on gender, power, and transformational change. *The Leadership Quarterly, 15*(5), 647–661. https://doi.org/10.1016/j.leaqua.2004.07.004

Frankl, V. E. (1984). *Man's search for meaning: Revised and updated.* Washington Square Press.

Fisher, C. B. (2022). *Decoding the ethics code: A practical guide for psychologists* (5th ed.). SAGE Publications.

Fire Law Blog (Varone, C.). Coverage of various cases: *Perez v. Denver* (2015, 2018) firelawblog.comfirelawblog.com, *O'Neil v. Richmond (Indiana)* (2024) firelawblog.comfirelawblog.com, *Prawdzik v. Homer Township, and IL* (2018) firelawblog.comfirelawblog.com, among others.

Fire Service Psychology Association. (2023). Fire service cultural competency training program. https://firepsychology.org/wp-content/uploads/2023/07/Fire-Service-Cultural-Competency-Training-Program.pdf

Fire Service Psychology Association. (2024). 2024 FSPA conference. https://firepsychology.org/2024-fspa-conference/

Firefighter Candidate Testing Center. (n.d.). The FCTC written test. California Firefighter Joint Apprenticeship Committee. Retrieved August 28, 2025, from https://www.fctconline.org/written-testing/

Firefighter Nation (Murphy, J., 2022). *A review of fire service legal issues*—highlights emerging legal challenges in firefighter employment (including mental health). https://www.firefighter-nation.com/fire-leadership/a-review-of-fire-service-legal-issues/

First Responder Center for Excellence (NFFF affiliate). (2023). Behavioral health screening in NFPA 1582: Issues and recommendations. https://firstrespondercenter.org/wp-content/uploads/2023/08/Behavioral-Health-Screening-Report-Web.pdf

Fixsen, D. L., Naoom, S. F., Blase, K. A., Friedman, R. M., & Wallace, F. (2005). Implementation research: A synthesis of the literature (FMHI publication #231). University of South Florida, Louis de la Parte Florida Mental Health Institute. https://www.researchgate.net/publication/283997783_Implementation_Research_A_Synthesis_of_the_Literature

Fletcher, A., Stewart, S., Heathcote, K., Page, P., & Dorrian, J. (2022). Work schedule and seasonal influences on sleep and fatigue in helicopter and fixed-wing aircraft operations in extreme environments. *Scientific Reports, 12*, 8263. https://doi.org/10.1038/s41598-022-08996-2

Florentine, J. B., & Crane, C. (2010). Suicide prevention by limiting access to methods: A review of theory and practice. *Social Science & Medicine, 70*(10), 1626–1632. https://pubmed.ncbi.nlm.nih.gov/20207465/

Florida Senate. (2018). CS/CS/SB 376 (2018): Workers' compensation benefits for first responders (amending Fla. Stat. § 112.1815). https://www.flsenate.gov/Session/Bill/2018/00376

Fonda, J. R., Fredman, L., Brogly, S. B., McGlinchey, R. E., Milberg, W. P., & Gradus, J. L. (2017). Traumatic brain injury and attempted suicide among veterans of the wars in Iraq and Afghanistan. *American Journal of Epidemiology, 186*(2), 220–226. https://pubmed.ncbi.nlm.nih.gov/28472407/

Franzmeier v. Industrial Commission, No. 1 CA-IC 24-0003, 2024 WL 1234567 (Ariz. Ct. App. Apr. 5, 2024). https://law.justia.com/cases/arizona/court-of-appeals-division-one-unpublished/2024/1-ca-ic-23-0013.html?

Frappell-Cooke, W., Gulina, M., Green, K., Hacker Hughes, J., & Greenberg, N. (2010). Does trauma risk management reduce psychological distress in deployed troops? *Occupational Medicine (Oxford, England), 60*(8), 645–650. https://doi.org/10.1093/occmed/kqq149

French, K. A., Dumani, S., Allen, T. D., & Shockley, K. M. (2018). A meta-analysis of work-family conflict and social support. *Psychological Bulletin, 144*(3), 284–314. https://pmc.ncbi.nlm.nih.gov/articles/PMC5858956/

Freyd, J. J. (1996). Betrayal trauma: The logic of forgetting childhood abuse. Harvard University Press. https://psycnet.apa.org/record/1996-98930-000.

Freyd, J. J. (2008a, April 11). *Betrayal trauma: Memory, health, and gender* [colloquium]. Department of Psychology, New Mexico State University, Las Cruces, NM.

Freyd, J. J. (n.d.). Institutional betrayal and institutional courage. Dynamic Lab. University of Oregon. https://dynamic.uoregon.edu/jjf/institutionalbetrayal/

Frone, M. R. (2013). *Alcohol and illicit drug use in the workforce and workplace*. American Psychological Association. https://psycnet.apa.org/record/2012-14634-000

Frye v. United States, 293 F. 1013 (D.C. Cir. 1923).

Fullagar, H. H. K., Sampson, J. A., Mott, B. J., Burdon, C. A., Taylor, N. A. S., & Groeller, H. (2015). Employment standards for Australian urban firefighters part 4: Physical aptitude tests and standards. *Journal of Occupational & Environmental Medicine, 57*(10), 1092–1097. https://pubmed.ncbi.nlm.nih.gov/26461864/

Fullerton, C. S., Ursano, R. J., Vance, K., & Wang, L. (2000). Debriefing following trauma. *The Psychiatric Quarterly, 71*(3), 259–276. https://psycnet.apa.org/record/2000-05146-005

Fyhn, B., Bang, H., Egeland, T., & Schei, V. (2023). Safe among the unsafe: Psychological safety climate strength matters for team performance. *Small Group Research, 54*(4), 439–473. https://journals.sagepub.com/doi/abs/10.1177/10464964221121273

Garb, H. N., Wood, J. M., & Baker, M. (2018). The Lackland Behavioral questionnaire: The use of biographical data and statistical prediction rules for public safety screening. *Psychological Assessment, 30*(8), 1039–1048. https://psycnet.apa.org/record/2018-19569-001

Geczik, A. M., Lee, J., Davis, A. L., Allen, J. A., & Taylor, J. A. (2022). Size matters: How safety climate and downstream outcomes vary by fire department organization type. *Injury Epidemiology, 9*(1), 11.

Geczik, A. M., Lee, J., Allen, J. A., Raposa, M. E., Robinson, L. F., Quistberg, D. A., Davis, A. L., & Taylor, J. A. (2024). An updated analysis of safety climate and downstream outcomes in two convenience samples of U.S. fire departments (FOCUS 1.0 and 2.0 survey waves). *Injury Epidemiology, 11*(1), 19. https://pubmed.ncbi.nlm.nih.gov/38773566/

Gershon, R. R. M., Barocas, B., Canton, A. N., Li, X., & Vlahov, D. (2008). Mental, physical, and behavioral outcomes associated with perceived work stress in police officers. *Criminal Justice and Behavior, 36*(3), 275–289. https://journals.sagepub.com/doi/10.1177/0093854808330015

Gersons, B. P. R., Carlier, I. V. E., Lamberts, R. D., & van der Kolk, B. A. (2000). Randomized clinical trial of brief eclectic psychotherapy for police officers with PTSD. *Journal of Traumatic Stress, 13*(2), 333–347. https://pubmed.ncbi.nlm.nih.gov/10838679/

Ghasemi, F., Zarei, H., Babamiri, M., & Kalatpour, O. (2022). Fatigue profile among petrochemical firefighters and its relationship with safety behavior: The moderating and mediating roles of perceived safety climate. *International Journal of Occupational Safety and Ergonomics, 28*(3), 1822–1828. https://pubmed.ncbi.nlm.nih.gov/34042558/ https://pubmed.ncbi.nlm.nih.gov/34042558/

Gidugu, V., Rogers, E. S., Harrington, S., Maru, M., Johnson, G., Cohee, J., & Hinkel, J. (2015). Individual peer support: A qualitative study of mechanisms of its effectiveness. *Community Mental Health Journal, 51*(4), 445–452. https://pubmed.ncbi.nlm.nih.gov/25535049/

Gordon, R., Flin, R., & Mearns, K. (2005). Designing and evaluating a human factors investigation tool (HFIT) for accident analysis. *Safety Science, 43*(3), 147–171. https://www.researchgate.net/publication/222575083_Designing_and_Evaluating_a_Human_Factors_Investigation_Tool_HFIT_for_Accident_Analysis

Gough, W. A. M. (2022). A human factors analysis of firefighter injury sustained during emergency response operations (Doctoral dissertation, Coventry University). https://pureportal.coventry.ac.uk/en/studentTheses/a-human-factors-analysis-of-firefighter-injury-sustained-during-e

Gouliquer, L., Poulin, C., & McWilliams, J. (2017). Othering of full-time and volunteer women firefighters in the Canadian Fire services. *Qualitative Sociology Review, 13*(3), 49–70. https://www.qualitativesociologyreview.org/ENG/Volume54/QSR_16_3_Gouliquer_Poulin_McWilliams.pdf

Grant, A. M. (2008). Does intrinsic motivation fuel the prosocial fire? Motivational synergy in predicting persistence, performance, and productivity. *Journal of Applied Psychology, 93*(1), 48–58. https://psycnet.apa.org/doiLanding?doi=10.1037%2F0021-9010.93.1.48

Greenberg, J., Solomon, S., & Pyszczynski, T. (1997). Terror management theory of self-esteem and cultural worldviews: Empirical assessments and conceptual refinements. In M. P. Zanna (Ed.), *Advances in experimental social psychology* (Vol. 29, pp. 61–139). Academic Press. https://doi.org/10.1016/S0065-2601(08)60016-7

Greenberg, N., Brooks, S., & Dunn, R. (2015). Latest developments in posttraumatic stress disorder: Diagnosis and treatment. *British Medical Bulletin, 114*(1), 147–155. https://pubmed.ncbi.nlm.nih.gov/25904382/

Greenberg, N., Langston, V., & Jones, N. (2008). Trauma risk management (TRiM) in the UK armed forces. *Journal of the Royal Army Medical Corps, 154*(2), 124–127. https://doi.org/10.1136/jramc-154-02-11

Greenberg, N., Langston, V., Everitt, B., Iversen, A., Fear, N. T., Jones, N., & Wessely, S. (2010). A cluster randomized controlled trial to determine the efficacy of trauma risk management (TRiM) in a military population. *Journal of Traumatic Stress, 23*(4), 430–436. https://doi.org/10.1002/jts.20538

Greenburg, N. (2001). A critical review of psychological debriefing: The management of psychological health after traumatic experiences. *Journal of the Royal Naval Medical Service, 87*(3), 158–161. https://pubmed.ncbi.nlm.nih.gov/11974426/

Greene, D. A., & Hendershot, M. E. (2017). Exploring the retention calculus: The motives, expectations, and satisfaction of South Carolina volunteer firefighters. *International Fire Service Journal of Leadership & Management, 11*, 27–39. https://pubmed.ncbi.nlm.nih.gov/11974426/

Greene v. City of New York, 2025 N.Y. Slip Op. 02721 (App. Div. 1st Dep't May 6, 2025).

Gross, J. J., & John, O. P. (2003). Individual differences in two emotion regulation processes: Implications for affect, relationships, and well-being. *Journal of Personality and Social Psychology, 85*(2), 348–362. https://doi.org/10.1037/0022-3514.85.2.348

Grossman, D. (2014). *On killing: The psychological cost of learning to kill in war and society*. Open Road Media.

Grossman, D., & Christensen, L. W. (2011). On combat: The psychology and physiology of deadly conflict in war and in peace (3rd ed.). Human Factor Research Group, Inc.

Grubbs, J. B., Exline, J. J., Pargament, K. I., Hook, J. N., & Carlisle, R. D. (2015). Transgression as addiction: Religiosity and moral disapproval as predictors of perceived addiction to pornography. *Archives of Sexual Behavior, 44*(1), 125–136. https://pubmed.ncbi.nlm.nih.gov/24519108/

Guardians of the City. (n.d.). Notable people: Lillie Hitchcock Coit (August 23, 1843 – July 22, 1929). https://guardiansofthecity.org/sffd/people/coit.html

Gulliver, S. B., Cammarata, C. M., Leto, F., Ostiguy, W. J., Flynn, E. J., Carpenter, G. S. J., Kamholz, B. W., Zimering, R. T., & Kimbrel, N. A. (2016b). Project reach out: A training program to increase behavioral health utilization among professional firefighters. *International Journal of Stress Management, 23*(1), 65–83. https://psycnet.apa.org/record/2015-42702-001

Gulliver, S. B., Pennington, M. L., Cardenas, M., Lewis, J. E., Cammarata, C. M., Leto, F., Ostiguy, W. J., Meyer, E. C., & Kimbrel, N. A. (2023). Stamp out stigma: A national campaign to decrease stigma and increase behavioral health in fire service. *Cognitive Behavior Therapy, 52*(6), 625–640. https://pubmed.ncbi.nlm.nih.gov/37489115/

Gulliver, S. B., Pennington, M. L., Leto, F., Cammarata, C., Ostiguy, W., Zavodny, C., Flynn, E. J., & Kimbrel, N. A. (2016a). In the wake of suicide: Developing guidelines for suicide postvention in fire service. *Death Studies, 40*(2), 121–128. https://pmc.ncbi.nlm.nih.gov/articles/PMC4784501/

Gulliver, S. B., Cammarata, C. M., Leto, F., Ostiguy, W. J., Flynn, E. J., Carpenter, G. S. J., Kamholz, B. W., Zimcring, R. T., & Kimbrel, N. A. (2016). Project reach out: A training program to increase behavioral health utilization among professional firefighters. *International Journal of Stress Management, 23*(1), 65–83. https://doi.org/10.1037/a0039731

Gulliver, S. B., Zimering, R. T., Dobani, F., Pennington, M. L., Morissette, S. B., Kamholz, B. W., Knight, J. A., Keane, T. M., Kimbrel, N. A., Carpenter, T. P., & Meyer, E. C. (2019). Alcohol use and mental health symptoms in female firefighter recruits. *Occupational Medicine, 69*(8/9), 625–631. https://pubmed.ncbi.nlm.nih.gov/32025738/

Guyeux, C., Bou Tayeh, G., Makhoul, A., Chrétien, S., Bourgeois, J., & Bahi, J. M. (2023). Using data science to predict firemen interventions: A case study. *Journal of Supercomputing, 79*(7), 7160–7175. https://www.researchgate.net/publication/365735022_Using_data_science_to_predict_firemen_interventions_a_case_study

Haddock, C. K., Jahnke, S. A., Poston, W. S. C., Jitnarin, N., & Day, R. S. (2016). Marriage and divorce among firefighters in the United States. *Journal of Family Issues*, 37(16), 2294–2308. https://journals.sagepub.com/doi/10.1177/0192513X15583070

Haddock, C. K., Jahnke, S. A., Poston, W. S., Jitnarin, N., Kaipust, C. M., Tuley, B., & Hyder, M. L. (2012). Alcohol use among firefighters in the Central United States. *Occupational medicine (Oxford, England), 62*(8), 661–664. https://doi.org/10.1093/occmed/kqs162

Haddock, C. K., Poston, W. S., Jahnke, S. A., & Jitnarin, N. (2017). Alcohol use and problem drinking among women firefighters. *Women's Health Issues, 27*(6), 632–638. https://pmc.ncbi.nlm.nih.gov/articles/PMC5694370/

Haddock, C. K., Poston, W. S. C., Jahnke, S. A., Jitnarin, N., & Day, R. S. (2016b). Marriage and divorce among firefighters in the United States. *Journal of Family Issues, 37*(16), 2294–2311. https://www.researchgate.net/publication/277634821_Marriage_and_Divorce_Among_Firefighters_in_the_United_States

Hagaman, A. K., Khadka, S., Lohani, S., & Kohrt, B. (2017). Suicide in Nepal: A modified psychological autopsy investigation from randomly selected police cases between 2013 and 2015. *Social Psychiatry and Psychiatric Epidemiology, 52*(12), 1483–1494. https://pubmed.ncbi.nlm.nih.gov/28856382/

Hagaman, A. K., Khadka, S., Wutich, A., Lohani, S., & Kohrt, B. A. (2018). Suicide in Nepal: Qualitative findings from a modified case-series psychological autopsy investigation of suicide deaths. *Culture, Medicine, and Psychiatry, 42*(3), 704–734. https://doi.org/10.1007/s11013-018-9585-8

Hallinan, S., Shiyko, M. P., Volpe, R., & Molnar, B. E. (2019). Reliability and validity of the vicarious trauma organizational readiness guide (VT-ORG). *American Journal of Community Psychology, 64*(3–4), 481–493. https://onlinelibrary.wiley.com/doi/10.1002/ajcp.12395

Hamilton, E. (1942). Mythology: Timeless tales of gods and heroes. Little, Brown.

Haim-Nachum, S., & Levy-Gigi, E. (2021). The tension between cognitive and regulatory flexibility and their associations with current and lifetime PTSD symptoms. *Frontiers in Psychology, 12.*, Article 615289. https://doi.org/10.3389/fpsyg.2021.615289

Hannah, S. T., & Avolio, B. J. (2011). The locus of leader character. *The Leadership Quarterly, 22*(5), 979–983. https://www.researchgate.net/publication/251637926_The_Locus_of_Leader_Character

Hannah, S. T., Avolio, B. J., & Walumbwa, F. O. (2011). Relationships between authentic leadership, moral courage, and ethical and pro-social behaviors. *Business Ethics Quarterly, 21*(4), 555–578. https://www.researchgate.net/publication/277909212_Relationships_between_Authentic_Leadership_Moral_Courage_and_Ethical_and_Pro-Social_Behaviors

Harris, M. B., Balolu, M., & Stacks, J. R. (2002). Mental health of trauma-exposed firefighters and critical incident stress debriefing. *Journal of Loss and Trauma, 7*, 223–238. https://www.researchgate.net/publication/247498144_Mental_health_of_trauma-exposed_firefighters_and_Critical_Incident_Stress_Debriefing

Harris, M. B., & Stacks, J. S. (1998). A three-year five-state study on the relationships between critical incident stress debriefings, firefighters' disposition, and stress reactions. USFA-FEMA CISM Research Project. Commerce, TX: Texas A&M University. https://www.scribd.com/document/385817257/A-Three-Year-Five-State-Study-on-the-Relationships-between-Critical-Incident-Stress-Debriefings-Firefighters-Disposition-and-Stress-Reactions

Harvey, S. B., Milligan-Saville, J. S., Paterson, H. M., Harkness, E. L., Marsh, A. M., Dobson, M., Kemp, R., & Bryant, R. A. (2016). The mental health of fire-fighters: An examination of the impact of repeated trauma exposure. *Australian & New Zealand Journal of Psychiatry, 50*(7), 649–658. https://journals.sagepub.com/doi/10.1177/0004867415615217

Haslam, S. A., Jetten, J., Postmes, T., & Haslam, C. (2008). Social identity, health and well-being: An emerging agenda for applied psychology. *Applied Psychology, 58*(1), 1–23. https://doi.org/10.1111/j.1464-0597.2008.00379.x

Haslam, C., Jetten, J., Cruwys, T., Dingle, G., & Haslam, S. (2018). *The new psychology of health: Unlocking the social cure*. Routledge. https://doi.org/10.4324/9781315648569

Haslam, S. A., Reicher, S. D., & Platow, M. J. (2011). *The new psychology of leadership: Identity, influence and power*. Psychology Press. https://psycnet.apa.org/record/2008-09946-000

Haugen, P. T., Evces, M., & Weiss, D. S. (2012). Treating posttraumatic stress disorder in first responders: A systematic review. *Clinical Psychology Review, 32*(5), 370–380. https://doi.org/10.1016/j.cpr.2012.04.001

Healy, N. A., & Vujanovic, A. A. (2021). PTSD symptoms and suicide risk among firefighters: The moderating role of sleep disturbance. *Psychological Trauma, 13*(7), 749–758. https://pubmed.ncbi.nlm.nih.gov/34166047/9

Heath, D. (2020). *Upstream: The quest to solve problems before they happen*. Avid Reader Press/ Simon & Schuster.
Hedman, K. (2023). *Interagency collaboration in suicide prevention*. School of Health and Welfare, Jönköping University. https://hj.diva-portal.org/smash/record.jsf?pid=diva2%3A1790939
Heinemann, L., Aust, F., Peifer, C., Holtz, M., Miller, C., & Hagemann, V. (2024b). Development and validation of a questionnaire, the REST-Q Fire, to identify teamworkrelated resources and stressors in firefighting operations. *PLoS One, 19*(5), e0304326. https://pubmed.ncbi.nlm.nih.gov/38809919/
Heinemann, S., Kauffeld, S., Klonek, F. E., & Muck, P. M. (2024a). Development and validation of the REST-Q Fire: A questionnaire to assess teamwork-related stressors and resources in firefighting. *Journal of Occupational and Organizational Psychology*. Advance online publication. https://journals.plos.org/plosone/article?id=10.1371/journal.pone.0304326
Henderson, C., Evans-Lacko, S., & Thornicroft, G. (2013). Mental illness stigma, help seeking, and public health programs. *American Journal of Public Health, 103*(5), 777–780. https://pmc.ncbi.nlm.nih.gov/articles/PMC3698814/
Henderson, J. L., MacKay, S., & Peterson-Badali, M. (2010). Interdisciplinary knowledge translation: Lessons learned from a mental health–fire service collaboration. *American Journal of Community Psychology, 46*(3–4), 277–288. https://psycnet.apa.org/record/2010-22484-003
Henderson, S. N., Van Hasselt, V. B., LeDuc, T. J., & Couwels, J. (2016). Firefighter suicide: Understanding cultural challenges for mental health professionals. *Professional Psychology: Research and Practice, 47*(3), 224–230. https://psycnet.apa.org/record/2016-22448-001
Herzog, J., O'Dare, K., King, E., Rotunda, R., & Dillard, D. (2023). Trauma symptoms and suicidal ideation in firefighters with consideration of exposure to natural disaster. *Traumatology, 29*(3), 383–388. https://doi.org/10.1037/trm0000413
Heyda, A., Bielen, A., Wygoda, A., & Skladowski, K. (2023). Walking through the valley of the shadow of death, the psychotherapy of the head and neck cancer patient expressing suicidal ideations and impulses. *Journal of Clinical Psychology, 79*(6), 1562–1571. https://pubmed.ncbi.nlm.nih.gov/37006196/
Hill, R., Oakes, T., & Wilkes, L. (2023). The development of an evidence-based approach to inform learning and practices within the UK fire and rescue service. *International Journal of Emergency Services, 12*(3), 257–270. https://www.researchgate.net/publication/375829882_The_development_of_an_evidence-based_approach_to_inform_learning_and_practices_within_the_UK_fire_and_rescue_service
Hobbs, M., Mayou, R., Harrelson, B., & Worlock, P. (1996). A randomized controlled trial of psychological debriefing for victims of road traffic accidents. *British Medical Journal, 313*, 1438–1439. https://pubmed.ncbi.nlm.nih.gov/8973231/
Hobfoll, S. E., Watson, P., Bell, C. C., Bryant, R. A., Brymer, M. J., Friedman, M. J., Friedman, M., Gersons, B. P. R., de Jong, J., Layne, C. M., Maguen, S., Neria, Y., Norwood, A. E., Pynoos, R. S., Reissman, D., Ruzek, J. I., Shalev, A. Y., Solomon, Z., Steinberg, A. M., & Ursano, R. J. (2007). Five essential elements of immediate and mid-term mass trauma intervention: Empirical evidence. *Psychiatry: Interpersonal and Biological Processes, 70*(4), 283–315. https://pubmed.ncbi.nlm.nih.gov/18181708/
Hoge, C. W., Castro, C. A., Messer, S. C., McGurk, D., Cotting, D. I., & Koffman, R. L. (2004). Combat duty in Iraq and Afghanistan, mental health problems, and barriers to care. *The New England Journal of Medicine, 351*(1), 13–22. https://pubmed.ncbi.nlm.nih.gov/15229303/
Hokmabadi, R., Sadeghi, H., & Karimi, A. (2022). Investigating organizational safety climate and its impact on incidence of unsafe behaviors among firefighters. *International Journal of Occupational Hygiene, 14*(2), 114–121. https://ijoh.tums.ac.ir/index.php/ijoh/article/view/584
Holland-Winkler, A. M., Greene, D. R., & Oberther, T. J. (2024). The cyclical battle of insomnia and mental health impairment in firefighters: A narrative review. *Journal of Clinical Medicine, 13*(8), 2169. https://doi.org/10.3390/jcm13082169
Hollerbach, B. S., Heinrich, K. M., Poston, W. S. C., Haddock, C. K., Kehler, A. K., & Jahnke, S. A. (2017). Current female firefighters' perceptions, attitudes, and experiences with injury.

International Fire Service Journal of Leadership & Management, 11, 41–47. https://pubmed.ncbi.nlm.nih.gov/31225527/

Holmes, T. H., & Rahe, R. H. (1967). The social readjustment rating scale. *Journal of Psychosomatic Research, 11*(2), 213–218. https://doi.org/10.1016/0022-3999(67)90010-4

Hom, M. A., Matheny, N. L., Stanley, I. H., Rogers, M. L., Cougle, J. R., & Joiner, T. E. (2017). Examining physical and sexual abuse histories as correlates of suicide risk among firefighters. *Journal Of Traumatic Stress, 30*(6), 672–681. https://pubmed.ncbi.nlm.nih.gov/29083498/

Hom, M. A., Stanley, I. H., & Joiner, T. E., Jr. (2015). Evaluating factors and interventions that influence help-seeking and mental health service utilization among suicidal individuals: A review of the literature. *Clinical Psychology Review, 40*, 28–39. https://pubmed.ncbi.nlm.nih.gov/26048165/

Hom, M. A., Stanley, I. H., Spencer-Thomas, S., & Joiner, T. E. (2017a). Suicidal thoughts and behaviors among women firefighters: An examination of associated features and comparison of precareer and career prevalence rates. *Journal of Affective Disorders, 221*, 107–114. https://pubmed.ncbi.nlm.nih.gov/28641147/

Hom, M. A., Stanley, I. H., Spencer-Thomas, S., & Joiner, T. E. (2017b). Women firefighters and workplace harassment: Associated suicidality and mental health sequelae. *Journal of Nervous & Mental Disease, 205*(12), 910–917. https://pubmed.ncbi.nlm.nih.gov/29088006/

Hom, M. A., Stanley, I. H., Spencer-Thomas, S., & Joiner, T. E. (2018). Exposure to suicide and suicide bereavement among women firefighters: Associated suicidality and psychiatric symptoms. *Journal of Clinical Psychology, 74*(12), 2219–2237. https://onlinelibrary.wiley.com/doi/abs/10.1002/jclp.22674

Houston Fire Department. (n.d.). Behavioral health services. City of Houston. https://www.houstontx.gov/fire/firefighterinfo/BehavioralHealthServices.html

Huang, R.-S., Chen, Y.-C., Tsai, S.-Y., Huang, Y.-S., & Guo, Y.-L. (2022). Incomplete off-duty work hours and sleep quality among firefighters: A cross-sectional study, Taiwan. *International Archives of Occupational and Environmental Health, 96*(2), 247–257. https://doi.org/10.1007/s00420-022-01918-9

Huebsch, B. W., Bartlett, B. A., Smith, L. J., Smith, B. N., Tran, J. K., & Vujanovic, A. A. (2019). Occupational stress and functioning among military veterans in the fire service. *Military Behavioral Health, 8*(1), 53–63. https://doi.org/10.1080/21635781.2019.1669510

Hulett, D. M., Bendick, M., Thomas, S. Y., & Moccio, F. (2008). *A national report card on women in firefighting*. International Association of Women in Fire and Emergency Services. https://policygroupontradeswomen.org/wp-content/uploads/2020/12/NationalReportCardonWomeninFirefighting.pdf

Hurley v. Kent of Naples, Inc., 746 F.3d 1161 (11th Cir. 2014).

Hytten, K., & Hasle, A. (1989). Firefighters: A study of stress and coping. *Acta Psychiatrica Scandinavica, 80*, 50–56. https://pubmed.ncbi.nlm.nih.gov/2624134/

IAFF News. (2024). New Pennsylvania law better protects firefighters diagnosed with PTSI. International Association of Fire Fighters. https://www.iaff.org/news/new-pennsylvania-law-better-protects-fire-fighters-diagnosed-with-ptsi/

Iantorno, M., Blamey, C., Dwyer, L., & Consalvo, M. (2021). All in a day's work: Working-class heroes as video game protagonists. *Nordicom Review, 42*, 88–110. https://www.researchgate.net/publication/351125921_All_in_a_day's_work

Ichniowski, C. (1978). *Economic effects of the firefighters' union*. (NBER Working Paper No. 291). National Bureau of Economic Research.

ideas42. (2022). Supporting women on the path to becoming firefighters: Building a more diverse FDNY. https://www.ideas42.org/wp-content/uploads/2022/04/I42Brief_NYCO-Case-Study_FDNY_CPAT.pdf

In the Matter of Jerome Lannon, A22-0507 (Minn. Ct. App. Dec. 19, 2022).

Institute for Work & Health. (2015). Primary, secondary and tertiary prevention. Retrieved from https://www.iwh.on.ca/what-researchers-mean-by/primary-secondary-and-tertiary-prevention

International Association of Fire Chiefs. (n.d.). *Explanation of the 5-5-5 bell tradition.* Retrieved from https://www.iafc.org/topics-and-tools/resources/resource/5-5-5-

explanation#:~:text=When%20a%20firefighter%20died%20in,pause%E2%80%A6then%20five%20more%20dashes

International Association of Fire Chiefs (IAFC). (2021). Best practices in behavioral wellness for emergency responders. https://www.iafc.org/docs/default-source/1vcos/20211103-iafc-yellow-ribbon-report.pdf

International Association of Fire Fighters. (n.d.). Candidate Physical Ability Test. https://www.iaff.org/cpat/.

International Association of Fire Fighters & International Association of Fire Chiefs. (2018). *The fire service joint labor management wellness-fitness initiative*. (4th ed.). International Association of Fire Fighters. https://www.iafc.org/docs/default-source/1safehealthshs/wfi-manual.pdf

International Association of Fire Fighters. (n.d.) Presumptive health initiative (state presumption database & policy). https://www.iaff.org/presumptive-health/

International Agency for Research on Cancer. (2023, July 27). IARC Monographs Volume 132: Occupational exposure as a firefighter. https://www.iarc.who.int/news-events/iarcmonographs-volume-132-occupational-exposure-as-a-firefighter

Issel, L. M., & Wells, R. (2017). Health program planning and evaluation: A practical, systematic approach for community health (4th ed.). Jones & Bartlett Learning.

Izci, F., Saglam, N. G. U., & Ergelen, M. (2022). Neurobiology and genetics of behavioral addictions: A brief review. *Bagimlilik Dergisi, 23*(2), 233–241. https://www.researchgate.net/publication/361645718_Neurobiology_and_Genetics_of_Behavioral_Addictions_A_Brief_Review

Jahn, J. L. (2016). Adapting safety rules in a high reliability context: How wildland firefighting workgroups ventriloquize safety rules to understand hazards. *Management Communication Quarterly, 30*(3), 362–389. https://www.researchgate.net/publication/289693287_Adapting_Safety_Rules_in_a_High_Reliability_Context_How_Wildland_Firefighting_Workgroups_Ventriloquize_Safety_Rules_to_Understand_Hazards

Jahnke, S. A., Gist, R., Poston, W. S. C., & Haddock, C. K. (2014). Behavioral health interventions in the fire service: Stories from the firehouse. *Journal of Workplace Behavioral Health, 29*(2), 113–126. https://psycnet.apa.org/record/2014-16714-002

Jahnke, S. A., Haddock, C. K., Jitnarin, N., Kaipust, C. M., Hollerbach, B. S., & Poston, W. S. C. (2019). The prevalence and health impacts of frequent work discrimination and harassment among women firefighters in the US Fire Service. *BioMed Research International, 2019*, 6740207. https://pubmed.ncbi.nlm.nih.gov/31016195/

Jahnke, S. A., Poston, W. S. C., Haddock, C. K., & Jitnarin, N. (2012a). Emerging health and safety issues among women in the fire service. U.S. Fire Administration. Retrieved from https://www.usfa.fema.gov/downloads/pdf/publications/emerging_health_safety_issues_women_fire_service.pdf

Jahnke, S. A., Poston, W. S., Haddock, C. K., Jitnarin, N., Hyder, M. L., & Horvath, C. (2012b). The health of women in the US fire service. *BMC Women's Health, 12*, 39. https://pubmed.ncbi.nlm.nih.gov/23114186/

Jahnke, S. A., Poston, W. S., Haddock, C. K., & Murphy, B. (2016). Firefighting and mental health: Experiences of repeated exposure to trauma. *Work, 53*(4), 737–744. https://pubmed.ncbi.nlm.nih.gov/26890595/

Jakupcak, M., Tull, M. T., McDermott, M. J., Kaysen, D., Hunt, S., & Simpson, T. (2010). PTSD symptom clusters in relationship to alcohol misuse among Iraq and Afghanistan war veterans seeking postdeployment VA health care. *Addictive Behaviors, 35*(9), 840–843. https://pubmed.ncbi.nlm.nih.gov/20471180/

Jamieson, N., Carey, L. B., Jamieson, A., & Maple, M. (2023). Examining the association between moral injury and suicidal behavior in military populations: A systematic review. *Journal of Religion and Health, 62*(6), 3904–3925. https://pubmed.ncbi.nlm.nih.gov/37592186/

Jamoulle, M. (2024, October 20). Quaternary prevention, concept, origin, perspectives [Conference presentation]. The Importance of Quaternary Prevention in Public Health, organized by the

Iranian Ministry of Health and Medical Education, Tabriz, Iran. https://orbi.uliege.be/bitstream/2268/323659/1/P4_Tabriz_2024.pdf

Jiang, Y. R. (2023). Reasonable accommodation and disparate impact: Clean shave policy discrimination in today's workplace. *The Journal of Law, Medicine & Ethics, 51*(1), 185–195. https://pubmed.ncbi.nlm.nih.gov/37226761/

Jinkerson, J. D. (2016). Defining and assessing moral injury: A syndrome perspective. *Traumatology, 22*(2), 122–130. https://psycnet.apa.org/record/2016-22456-001

Jo, I., Lee, S., Sung, G., Kim, M., Lee, S., Park, J., & Lee, K. (2018). Relationship between burnout and PTSD symptoms in firefighters: The moderating effects of a sense of calling to firefighting. *International Archives of Occupational & Environmental Health, 91*(1), 117–123. https://pubmed.ncbi.nlm.nih.gov/28975412/

Jobes, D. A. (2006). *Managing suicidal risk: A collaborative approach*. Guilford Press.

Job Accommodation Network. (2021). *Return-to-work: Accommodations for workers with disabilities*. U.S. Department of Labor, Office of Disability Employment Policy. https://askjan.org

Joe Yarborough v. State, Montana Workers' Compensation Court File No. 96-376, 2017.

John Norton, M., Archard, P., & Swords, C. (2023). The ethics of informality and dual relationships in peer support. *Psychiatric Services, 74*(11), 1213. https://pubmed.ncbi.nlm.nih.gov/38032053/

Johnson, E. E. (1983). Psychological tests used in assessing a sample of police and firefighter candidates. *Journal of Police Science & Administration, 11*(4), 430–433. https://psycnet.apa.org/record/1984-24647-001

Johnson, K. (2019). The evolution of firefighter funeral ritual. *Undergraduate Research Journal, 23*(1), Article 9. https://openspaces.unk.edu/undergraduate-research-journal/vol23/iss1/9/

Johnson, W., Ralph, J., & Johnson, S. (2005). Managing multiple roles in embedded environments: The case of aircraft carrier psychology. *Professional Psychology: Research and Practice. 36*, 73–81. https://www.researchgate.net/publication/232445969_Managing_Multiple_Roles_in_Embedded_Environments_The_Case_of_Aircraft_Carrier_Psychology

Johnson, C. C., Vega, L., Kohalmi, A. L., Roth, J. C., Howell, B. R., & Van Hasselt, V. B. (2020). Enhancing mental health treatment for the firefighter population: Understanding fire culture, treatment barriers, practice implications, and research directions. *Professional Psychology: Research & Practice, 51*(3), 304–311. https://psycnet.apa.org/record/2019-58638-001

Joiner, T. (2007). Why people die by suicide. Harvard University Press

Jones, E., & Wessely, S. (2007). A paradigm shift in the conceptualization of psychological trauma in the 20th century. *Journal of Anxiety Disorders, 21*(2), 164–175. https://doi.org/10.1016/j.janxdis.2006.09.009

Jones, S. (2020). Examining chivalric masculinity in Chrétien de Troyes' Erec and Enide. *Journal of Undergraduate Studies at Trent (JUST), 12*(1), 135–145. https://ojs.trentu.ca/index.php/just/article/view/406/707

Jones, N., Burdett, H., Green, K., & Greenberg, N. (2017). Trauma risk management (TRiM): Promoting help seeking for mental health problems among combat-exposed U.K. military personnel. *Psychiatry, 80*(3), 236–251. https://doi.org/10.1080/00332747.2017.1286894

Jordan, P. J., & Troth, A. C. (2004). Managing emotions during team problem solving: Emotional intelligence and conflict resolution. *Human Performance, 17*(2), 195–218. https://psycnet.apa.org/record/2004-95069-004

Jost, J. T., & Banaji, M. R. (1994). The role of stereotyping in system justification and the production of false consciousness. *British Journal of Social Psychology, 33*(1), 1–27. https://psycnet.apa.org/record/1994-37261-001

Jost, J. T., Banaji, M. R., & Nosek, B. A. (2004). A decade of system justification theory: Accumulated evidence of conscious and unconscious bolstering of the status quo. *Political Psychology, 25*(6), 881–919. https://psycnet.apa.org/record/2004-21198-003

Jouanne, E., Charron, C., Chauvin, C., & Morel, G. (2017). Correlates of team effectiveness: An exploratory study of firefighter's operations during emergency situations. *Applied Ergonomics, 61*, 69–77. https://pubmed.ncbi.nlm.nih.gov/28237021/

Jung, C. G. (1953). Collected works of C.G. Jung, Volume 5: Symbols of transformation (R. F. C. Hull, Trans.). Princeton University Press.

Jung, C. G. (1959a). *Aion: Studies into the phenomenology of the self.* Princeton University Press.

Jung, C. G. (1959b). *The archetypes and the collective unconscious.* (2nd ed.). Princeton University Press.

Jung, Y. K., & Chang, R. H. (2020). Cultural factors kill American firefighters on the ground: A pilot study. *Paramedicine and Emergency Response, 1*(1), 37–47. https://www.researchgate.net/publication/342876555_Cultural_Factors__Kill_American_Firefighters_On_The_Ground_A_Pilot_Study

Jung, A. M., Jahnke, S. A., Dennis, L. K., Bell, M. L., Burgess, J. L., Jitnarin, N., Kaipust, C. M., & Farland, L. V. (2021). Occupational factors and miscarriages in the US fire service: A cross-sectional analysis of women firefighters. *Environmental Health, 20*(1), 116. https://pubmed.ncbi.nlm.nih.gov/34749749/

Juntunen v. Carlton County, 2022 WL 17976736 (Minn. Dec. 28, 2022).

Juntunen v. Carlton County, 982 N.W.2d 729 (Minn. 2022). https://mn.gov/law-library-stat/archive/supct/2022/OPA211259-1207.pdf

Kaikkonen, P., Lindholm, H., & Lusa, S. (2017). Physiological load and psychological stress during a 24-hour work shift among Finnish firefighters. *Journal of Occupational & Environmental Medicine, 59*(1), 41–46. https://pubmed.ncbi.nlm.nih.gov/28045796/

Kamuk, Y. U. (2020). Effects of training on firefighters' physical readiness, fitness and BMI levels. *African Educational Research Journal, 8*(Spec. Iss. 1), S17–S25.

Kanter, R. M. (1977). *Men and women of the corporation.* Basic Books.

Karasek, R. A., & Theorell, T. (1990). *Healthy work.* Basic Books.

Karicofe, T. L. (2024). *Proactively addressing mental health in fire service personnel (executive fire officer program applied research project).* U.S. Fire Administration, National Fire Academy. https://apps.usfa.fema.gov/pdf/efop/Travis-L-Karicofe-Proactively-Addressing-Mental-Health-in-Fire-Service-Personnel.pdf

Karter, M. J., Jr. (2009). Patterns of firefighter fireground injuries. National Fire Protection Association, Fire Analysis and Research Division. https://media.cdn.lexipol.com/OS.patterns.pdf

Kauffman, B., Manning, K., Zvolensky, M. J., & Vujanovic, A. A. (2022). Fatigue sensitivity and mental health among trauma-exposed firefighters. *Fatigue: Biomedicine, Health & Behavior, 10*(3), 146–156. https://pubmed.ncbi.nlm.nih.gov/36968246/

Kaufman, C. C., McHugh, R. K., Drury, M., Merrill, J. G., & Rosmarin, D. H. (2024). Spirituality/religion among first responders with and without posttraumatic stress disorder and alcohol misuse. *Journal of Dual Diagnosis, 20*(4), 291–302. https://pubmed.ncbi.nlm.nih.gov/38560884/

Kehl, D., Knuth, D., Hulse, L., & Schmidt, S. (2014). Posttraumatic reactions among firefighters after critical incidents: Cross-national data. *Journal of Aggression, Maltreatment & Trauma, 23*(8), 842–853. https://psycnet.apa.org/record/2014-41011-004

Kennedy, C. H. (2019, January 23). Military embedded psychology. Psychology Today. https://www.psychologytoday.com/us/blog/alpha-blog-charlie/202301/military-embedded-psychology

Kettner, P., Moroney, R., Martin, L. (2008). Designing and managing programs: An effectiveness-based approach. https://www.researchgate.net/publication/235930844_Designing_and_Managing_Programs_An_Effectiveness-Based_Approach

Kidder, R. M. (2005). *Moral courage: Taking action when your values are put to the test.* HarperCollins.

Kim, J. E., Dager, S. R., Jeong, H. S., Ma, J., Park, S., Kim, J., Choi, Y., Lee, S. L., Kang, I., Ha, E., Cho, H. B., Lee, S., Kim, E. J., Yoon, S., & Lyoo, I. K. (2018). Firefighters, posttraumatic stress disorder, and barriers to treatment: Results from a nationwide total population survey. *PLoS One, 13*(1), e0190630. https://pubmed.ncbi.nlm.nih.gov/29304155/

Kim, B., Park, H., Kim, J. I., Oh, S., Moon, S. Y., Lee, J. H., & Kim, J. H. (2025). Role of peer support in mitigating PTSD and suicide risk among firefighters experiencing colleagues' death.

European Journal of Psychotraumatology, 16(1), 2512680. https://doi.org/10.1080/20008066.2025.2512680

Kimbrel, N. A., Pennington, M. L., Cammarata, C. M., Leto, F., Ostiguy, W. J., & Gulliver, S. B. (2016). Is cumulative exposure to suicide attempts and deaths a risk factor for suicidal behavior among firefighters? A preliminary study. *Suicide and Life-threatening Behavior, 46*(6), 669–677. https://doi.org/10.1111/sltb.12248

Kinman, G., Teoh, K., & Harriss, A. (2020). Supporting the well-being of healthcare workers during and after COVID-19. *Occupational Medicine, 70*(5), 294–296. https://pubmed.ncbi.nlm.nih.gov/32428225/

Kisling, L. A., Das, J. M.. (2025, January). Prevention strategies [Updated 2023 August 1]. In: *StatPearls* [Internet]. StatPearls Publishing. Available from https://www.ncbi.nlm.nih.gov/books/NBK537222/

Kitaeff, J. (Ed.). (2019). *Handbook of police psychology* (2nd ed.). Routledge.

Klee, S., & Renner, K.-H. (2013). In search of the "Rescue Personality". A questionnaire study with emergency medical services personnel. *Personality and Individual Differences, 54*(5), 669–672. https://psycnet.apa.org/record/2013-00493-018

Klimley, K. E., Van Hasselt, V. B., & Stripling, A. M. (2018). Posttraumatic stress disorder in police, firefighters, and emergency dispatchers. *Aggression and Violent Behavior, 43*, 33–44. https://psycnet.apa.org/record/2018-59927-005

Klinoff, R. W. (2021). *Introduction to fire protection and emergency services*. Jones and Bartlett Learning.

Klonsky, E. D., May, A. M., & Saffer, B. Y. (2016). Suicide, suicide attempts, and suicidal ideation. *Annual Review of Clinical Psychology, 12*, 307–330. https://doi.org/10.1146/annurev-clinpsy-021815-093204

Koeppel, M. D. H., Bucala, M., Kelley, H., Jitnarin, N., Poston, W. S. C., Haddock, C. K., & Jahnke, S. A. (2022). "They're Just Never Told They Can": Recruitment and retention of women in the fire service. *International Fire Service Journal of Leadership & Management, 16*, 41–51.

Kollock, R., Thomas, J., Hale, D., Sanders, G., Long, A., Dawes, J., & Peveler, W. (2021). The effects of firefighter equipment and gear on the static and dynamic postural stability of fire cadets. *Gait & Posture, 88*, 292–296. https://doi.org/10.1016/j.gaitpost.2021.05.034

Komarovskaya, I., Brown, A. D., Galatzer-Levy, I. R., Madan, A., Henn-Haase, C., Teater, J., Clarke, B. H., Marmar, C. R., & Chemtob, C. M. (2014). Early physical victimization is a risk factor for posttraumatic stress disorder symptoms among Mississippi police and firefighter first responders to Hurricane Katrina. *Psychological Trauma: Theory, Research, Practice, and Policy, 6*(1), 92–96. https://psycnet.apa.org/record/2013-10234-001

Kraft-Todd, G. T., & Rand, D. G. (2019). Rare and costly prosocial behaviors are perceived as heroic. *Frontiers in Psychology, 10*, 234. https://doi.org/10.3389/fpsyg.2019.00234

Kraus, S. W., Voon, V., & Potenza, M. N. (2016). Should compulsive sexual behavior be considered an addiction? *Addiction, 111*(12), 2097–2106. https://pubmed.ncbi.nlm.nih.gov/26893127/

Kroll, A., & Porumbescu, G. A. (2017). When extrinsic rewards become "sour grapes": An expectancy disconfirmation perspective on intrinsic motivation in public organizations. *Journal of Public Administration Research and Theory, 27*(4), 640–655. https://www.researchgate.net/publication/313415793_When_Extrinsic_Rewards_Become_Sour_Grapes_An_Experimental_Study_of_Adjustments_in_Intrinsic_and_Prosocial_Motivation

Kshtriya, S., Kobezak, H. M., Popok, P., Lawrence, J., & Lowe, S. R. (2020). Social support as a mediator of occupational stressors and mental health outcomes in first responders. *Journal of Community Psychology, 48*(7), 2252–2263. https://pubmed.ncbi.nlm.nih.gov/32841385/

Kunadharaju, K., Smith, T. D., & DeJoy, D. M. (2011). Line-of-duty deaths among U.S. firefighters: An analysis of fatality investigations. *Accident; Analysis and Prevention, 43*(3), 1171–1180. https://pubmed.ncbi.nlm.nih.gov/21376916/

Kurke, M. I., & Scrivner, E. M. (Eds.). (1995). *Police psychology into the 21st century*. Lawrence Erlbaum Associates, Inc. https://psycnet.apa.org/record/1995-98412-000

Lade, S., Easterbrook, B., Brown, A., Millman, H., D'Alessandro-Lowe, A. M., O'Connor, C., & McKinnon, M. C. (2023). The mental health toll of service: An examination of self-reported impacts of public safety personnel careers in a treatment-seeking population. *European Journal of Psychotraumatology, 14*(2). https://pmc.ncbi.nlm.nih.gov/articles/PMC10653764/

City of Los Angeles Personnel Department. (n.d.). Firefighter (class code 2112) — position information. City of Los Angeles Personnel Department. https://personnel.lacity.gov/jobs/position-information/index.cfm?job_id=2112

Lalic, H., Bukmir, L., & Ferhatovic, M. (2007). Examining psychic consequences in firefighters exposed to stress. *Collegium Antropologicum, 31*(2), 451–455. https://pubmed.ncbi.nlm.nih.gov/17847922/

Lambert, J. E., Benight, C. C., Harrison, E., & Cieslak, R. (2012). The firefighter coping self-efficacy scale: Measure development and validation. *Anxiety, Stress, and Coping, 25*(1), 79–91. https://pubmed.ncbi.nlm.nih.gov/21476153/

Landers, J. (2016, September 27). In the early 19th century, firefighters fought fires … and each other. Smithsonian Magazine. https://www.smithsonianmag.com/smithsonian-institution/early-19-century-firefighters-fought-fires-eachother-180960391/.

Lara, G. P., & Leija, M. G. (2014). Discussing gender roles and equality by reading "Max: The Stubborn Little Wolf". *Social Studies and the Young Learner, 27*(2), 22–25. https://www.socialstudies.org/system/files/publications/articles/yl_270222.pdf-

Lazarus, R. S., & Folkman, S. (1984). *Stress, appraisal, and coping*. Springer.

Le, A. B., McNulty, L. A., Dyal, M. A., DeJoy, D. M., & Smith, T. D. (2020). Firefighter overexertion: A continuing problem found in an analysis of non-fatal injury among career firefighters. *International Journal of Environmental Research and Public Health, 17*(21), 7906. https://doi.org/10.3390/ijerph17217906

Lee, J.-S. (2019). Perceived social support functions as a resilience in buffering the impact of trauma exposure on PTSD symptoms via intrusive rumination and entrapment in firefighters. *PLoS One, 14*(8), 1–14. https://pubmed.ncbi.nlm.nih.gov/31374563/

Lee, J. H., Lee, D., Kim, J., Jeon, K., & Sim, M. (2017). Duty-related trauma exposure and post-traumatic stress symptoms in professional firefighters. *Journal of Traumatic Stress, 30*(2), 133–141. https://pubmed.ncbi.nlm.nih.gov/28449365/

Lefcourt, H. M. (2014). *Locus of control: Current trends in theory and research*. Psychology Press.

LeMasters, G. K., Genaidy, A. M., Succop, P., Deddens, J., Sobeih, T., Barriera-Viruet, H., Dunning, K., & Lockey, J. (2006). Cancer risk among firefighters: A review and metaanalysis of 32 studies. *Journal of Occupational and Environmental Medicine, 48*(11), 1189–1202. https://doi.org/10.1097/01.jom.0000246229.68697.90

Lentz, L. M., Smith-MacDonald, L., Malloy, D., Carleton, R. N., & Brémault-Phillips, S. (2021). Compromised conscience: A scoping review of moral injury among firefighters, paramedics, and police officers. *Frontiers in Psychology, 12*:639781. https://pubmed.ncbi.nlm.nih.gov/33868111/

Leppin, A. L., Bora, P. R., Tilburt, J. C., Gionfriddo, M. R., Zeballos-Palacios, C., Dulohery, M. M., Sood, A., Erwin, P. J., Brito, J. P., Boehmer, K. R., & Montori, V. M. (2014). The efficacy of resiliency training programs: A systematic review and meta-analysis of randomized trials. *PLoS One, 9*(10), e111420. https://pubmed.ncbi.nlm.nih.gov/25347713/

Lerner, J. S., Li, Y., Valdesolo, P., & Kassam, K. S. (2015). Emotion and decision making. *Annual Review of Psychology, 66*, 799–823. https://psycnet.apa.org/record/2015-00368-031

Lerner, E. B., Moscati, R. M., & others. (2001). The golden hour: Scientific fact or medical "urban legend"? Academic Emergency Medicine, 8(7), 758–760 https://doi.org/10.1111/j.1553-2712.2001.tb00201.x

Lewis v. City of Chicago, 560 U.S. 205 (2010).

Liao, H., Arvey, R. D., Butler, R. J., & Nutting, S. M. (2001). Correlates of work injury frequency and duration among firefighters. *Journal of Occupational Health Psychology, 6*(3), 229–242. https://pubmed.ncbi.nlm.nih.gov/11482634/

Lindow, J. (2001). *Norse mythology: A guide to the gods, heroes, rituals, and beliefs.* Oxford University Press.

Lindén, M., Jeppsson, M., & Bengtsson, L.-G. (2023). Predictors of safety climate outcomes in firefighting. *International Fire Service Journal of Leadership and Management, 17.*

Litz, B. T., Gray, M. J., Bryant, R. A., & Adler, A. B. (2002). Early intervention for trauma: Current status and future directions. *Clinical Psychology: Science and Practice, 9*, 112–134. https://psycnet.apa.org/record/2002-13168-003

Litz, B. T., & Miller, M. W. (2009). Moral injury in veterans of war. *Clinical Psychology Review, 29*(8), 695–706. https://www.ptsd.va.gov/professional/articles/article-pdf/id33165.pdf

Litz, B. T., Stein, N., Delaney, E., Lebowitz, L., Nash, W. P., Silva, C., & Maguen, S. (2009). Moral injury and moral repair in war veterans: A preliminary model and intervention strategy. *Clinical Psychology Review, 29*(8), 695–706. https://pubmed.ncbi.nlm.nih.gov/19683376/

London Fire Brigade. (n.d.). Firefighters of the Second World War. https://www.london-fire.gov.uk/museum/london-fire-brigade-history-and-stories/the-second-world-war/firefighters-of-the-second-world-war/

London Fire Brigade. (n.d.). Early insurance brigades. https://www.london-fire.gov.uk/museum/london-fire-brigade-history-and-stories/early-insurance-brigades/

Luthar, S. S., & Cicchetti, D. (2000). The construct of resilience: Implications for interventions and social policies. *Development and Psychopathology, 12*(4), 857–885. https://pubmed.ncbi.nlm.nih.gov/11202047/

Lyytikäinen, K., Toivonen, L., Hynynen, E., Lindholm, H., & Kyröläinen, H. (2017). Recovery of rescuers from a 24-h shift and its association with aerobic fitness. *International Journal of Occupational Medicine and Environmental Health, 30*(3), 433–444. https://pubmed.ncbi.nlm.nih.gov/28481376/

Ma, L., Ma, X., Xing, P., & Yu, F. (2022). A hybrid approach based on the HFACS-FBN for identifying and analyzing human factors for fire and explosion accidents in the laboratory. *Journal of Loss Prevention in the Process Industries, 75*(1). https://www.researchgate.net/publication/356350450_A_hybrid_approach_based_on_the_HFACS-FBN_for_identifying_and_analysing_human_factors_for_fire_and_explosion_accidents_in_the_laboratory

Macnab, A. J., Russel, J. A., Lowe, J. P., & Gagnon, F. (1999). Critical incident stress intervention after loss of an air ambulance: Two-year follow-up. *Prehospital and Disaster Medicine, 14*(1), 8–12. https://pubmed.ncbi.nlm.nih.gov/10537592/

Madrzykowski, D. (2013). Fire dynamics: The science of fire fighting. *International Fire Service Journal of Leadership & Management, 7*, 7–15. https://www.ifsta.org/sites/default/files/fire-dynamics-madrzykowski-2012.pdf

Majnoon, S., Yates, V. M., Asgarpour, H., Mirza Aghazadeh Attari, A., & Lotfi, M. (2023). Cultural competence of nursing educators at medical universities of 2nd regional planning in Iran. *BMC Medical Education, 23*(1), 328. https://doi.org/10.1186/s12909-023-04274-5

Maleta, Y. (2009). Playing with fire gender at work and the Australian female cultural experience within rural fire fighting. *Journal of Sociology, 45*(3), 291–306. https://journals.sagepub.com/doi/10.1177/1440783309335647

Masi, D. A. (2005). Employee assistance programs in the new millennium. *International Journal of Emergency Mental Health, 7*(3), 157–167.

Marmar, C. R., McCaslin, S. E., Metzler, T. J., Best, S., Weiss, D. S., Fagan, J., Liberman, A., Pole, N., Otte, C., Yehuda, R., Mohr, D., & Neylan, T. (2006). Predictors of posttraumatic stress in police and other first responders. *Annals of the New York Academy of Sciences, 1071*(1), 1–18. https://pubmed.ncbi.nlm.nih.gov/16891557/

Marques-Quinteiro, P., Santos, C. M. D., Costa, P., Graça, A. M., Marôco, J., & Rico, R. (2020). Team adaptability and task cohesion as resources to the nonlinear dynamics of workload and sickness absenteeism in firefighter teams. *European Journal of Work and Organizational Psychology, 29*(4), 525–540. https://centaur.reading.ac.uk/83150/

Marsar, S. (2010, July 1). Survivability profiling: How long can victims survive in a fire? Fire Engineering. https://www.fireengineering.com/firefighting/survivability-profiling-how-long-can-victims-survive-in-a-fire/

Martinez, R. N., Galloway, K., & Thompson, C. (2023). The potential of an embedded mental health services program toward increasing health care-seeking behaviors among U.S. air Force aircrew: A mixed-methods study. *Military Medicine, 188*(Suppl 6), 262–270. https://pubmed.ncbi.nlm.nih.gov/37948247/

Martins, C., Godycki-Cwirko, M., Heleno, B., & Brodersen, J. (2018). Quaternary prevention: Reviewing the concept: Quaternary prevention aims to protect patients from medical harm. *European Journal of General Practice, 24*(1), 106–111. https://www.tandfonline.com/doi/10.1080/13814788.2017.1422177?url_ver=Z39.88-2003&rfr_id=ori:rid:crossref.org&rfr_dat=cr_pub%20%200pubmed

Maslach, C., & Leiter, M. P. (2016). Burnout: A multidimensional perspective. In C. L. Cooper & J. C. Quick (Eds.), *The handbook of stress and health* (pp. 77–95). Wiley Blackwell.

Matsumoto, D. R., & Juang, L. P. (2017). *Culture and psychology*. Cengage Learning.

Mayer, R. C., Davis, J. H., & Schoorman, F. D. (1995). An integrative model of organizational trust. *Academy of Management Review, 20*(3), 709–734. https://psycnet.apa.org/record/1995-45592-001

Mayer, R. C., & Gavin, M. B. (2005). Trust in management 1014 academy of management journal October and performance: Who minds the shop while the employees watch the boss? *Academy of Management Journal, 48*, 874–888. https://www.researchgate.net/publication/276053784_Trust_in_Management_and_Performance_Who_Minds_the_Shop_While_the_Employees_Watch_the_Boss

Mayer v. Calumet City Firefighters Pension Fund, 2024 IL App (1st) 232059-U. (n.d.)

Mayou, R. A., Ehlers, A., & Hobbs, M. (2000). Psychological debriefing for road traffic accident victims. Three-year follow-up of a randomized controlled trial. *The British Journal of Psychiatry: the Journal of Mental Science, 176*, 589–593. https://pubmed.ncbi.nlm.nih.gov/10974967/

McCarl, R. S. (1984). "You've come a long way, and now this is your retirement": An analysis of performance in firefighting culture. *Journal of American Folklore, 97*(384), 393–422. https://www.jstor.org/stable/540542

McCormick, M. L. (2012). Disparate impact and equal protection after Ricci v. DeStefano. Wis. JL Gender, & Soc'y, 27, 100. https://scholarship.law.slu.edu/faculty/25/

McCrae, R. R., & Costa, P. T., Jr. (1999). A five-factor theory of personality. In L. A. Pervin & O. P. John (Eds.), *Handbook of personality: Theory and research* (2nd ed., pp. 139–153). Guilford Press. https://psycnet.apa.org/record/1999-04371-005

McDavid, J. C., Huse, I., & Hawthorn, L. R. L. (2019). *Program evaluation and performance measurement: An introduction to practice* (3rd ed.). SAGE Publications.

McDevitt-Murphy, M. E., Murphy, J. G., Williams, J. L., Monahan, C. J., Bracken-Minor, K. L. (2015). Brief intervention to reduce hazardous drinking and enhance coping among OEF/OIF/OND veterans. *Professional Psychology: Research and Practice, 46*(2), 83–89. doi: https://doi.org/10.1037/a0036771. https://pubmed.ncbi.nlm.nih.gov/26170531/

McEwen, B. S. (1998). Protective and damaging effects of stress mediators. *New England Journal of Medicine, 338*(3), 171–179. Retrieved from https://www.nejm.org

McEwen, B. S. (2007). Physiology and neurobiology of stress and adaptation: Central role of the brain. *Physiological Reviews, 87*(3), 873–904. https://pubmed.ncbi.nlm.nih.gov/17615391/

McLennan, J., & Birch, A. (2022). "The problem hasn't changed, but you're no longer left to deal with it on your own": The role of informal peer support in helping firefighters cope with critical incidents. *International Journal of Emergency Services, 11*(3), 352–366. https://doi.org/10.1108/IJES-02-2021-0007

McNally, R. J., Bryant, R. A., & Ehlers, A. (2003). Does early psychological intervention promote recovery from posttraumatic stress? *Psychological Science in the Public Interest, 4*(2), 45–79. https://pubmed.ncbi.nlm.nih.gov/26151755/

McWilliams, J. C. (2007). "Men of Color": Race, riots, and Black firefighters' struggle for equality from the Afa to the Valiants. *Journal of Social History, 41*(1), 105–125. ??https://academic.oup.com/jsh/article-abstract/41/1/105/995983?redirectedFrom=fulltext

Meichenbaum, D. (2017). *The evolution of cognitive behavior therapy: A personal and professional journey with Don Meichenbaum*. Routledge/Taylor & Francis Group. https://psycnet.apa.org/record/2017-10056-000

Mendoza v. City of New York, No. 1:21-cv-00548 (E.D.N.Y. Jan. 5, 2024).

Merrimack. (n.d.). The history of firefighting. Merrimack Fire & Rescue. https://www.merrimacknh.gov/about-fire-rescue/pages/the-history-of-firefighting

Merton, R. K. (1957). *Social theory and social structure*. Free Press.

Merritt, A. C., Effron, D. A., & Monin, B. (2010). Moral self-licensing: When being good frees us to be bad. *Social and Personality Psychology Compass, 4*(5), 344–357. https://doi.org/10.1111/j.1751-9004.2010.00263.x

Meyer, E. C., Zimering, R. T., Knight, J., Morissette, S. B., Kamholz, B. W., Coe, E., Carpenter, T. P., Keane, T. M., Kimbrel, N. A., & Gulliver, S. B. (2021). Negative emotionality interacts with trauma exposure to prospectively predict posttraumatic stress disorder symptoms during firefighters' first 3 years of service. *Journal of Traumatic Stress, 34*(2), 333–344. https://pubmed.ncbi.nlm.nih.gov/33247974/

Milligan-Saville, J., Choi, I., Deady, M., Scott, P., Tan, L., Calvo, R. A., Bryant, R. A., Glozier, N., & Harvey, S. B. (2018). The impact of trauma exposure on the development of PTSD and psychological distress in a volunteer fire service. *Psychiatry Research, 270*, 1110–1115. https://pubmed.ncbi.nlm.nih.gov/30190167/

Milligan-Saville, J. S., Paterson, H. M., Harkness, E. L., Marsh, A. M., Dobson, M., Kemp, R. I., Bryant, R. A., & Harvey, S. B. (2017a). The amplification of common somatic symptoms by posttraumatic stress disorder in firefighters. *Journal of Traumatic Stress, 30*(2), 142–148. https://pubmed.ncbi.nlm.nih.gov/28273379/

Milligan-Saville, J. S., Tan, L., Gayed, A., Barnes, C., Madan, I., Dobson, M., Bryant, R. A., Christensen, H., Mykletun, A., & Harvey, S. B. (2017b). Workplace mental health training for managers and its effect on sick leave in employees: A cluster randomized controlled trial. *The Lancet Psychiatry, 4*(11), 850–858. https://pubmed.ncbi.nlm.nih.gov/29031935/

Miloslavich, K., Leonard, S. J., Wardle, M. C., & Vujanovic, A. A. (2023). Alcohol use severity, anger and drinking motives among firefighters. *Substance Use & Misuse, 58*(5), 601–609. https://pubmed.ncbi.nlm.nih.gov/36803652/

Minnesota Revisor of Statutes. (2019). *Minnesota statutes: Section 176.011, subdivision 15 (definition of occupational disease; PTSD presumption)*. Office of the Revisor of Statutes. https://www.revisor.mn.gov/statutes/2019/cite/176.011

Mitchell, J. T. (1983). When disaster strikes…the critical incident stress debriefing process. *Journal of Emergency Medical Services, 8*(1), 36–39. https://pubmed.ncbi.nlm.nih.gov/10258348/

Mitchell, J. T., & Bray, G. P. (1990). *Emergency services stress: Guidelines for preserving the health and careers of emergency services personnel*. Prentice Hall.

Mitchell, J. T., & Everly, G. S. (1995a). *Critical incident stress debriefing: An operations manual for CISD, defusing, and other group crisis intervention services*. Chevron Publishing Corporation.

Mitchell, J. T., & Everly, G. S. (1995b). *Critical incident stress debriefing (CISD) and the prevention of work-related trauma among high-risk occupational groups*. International Critical Incident Stress Foundation. https://psycnet.apa.org/record/1995-98878-012

Mitchell, J. T., & Everly, G. S. (1997). *Critical incident stress debriefing: An operations manual for CISD, defusing and other group crisis interventions* (3rd ed.). Chevron Publishing.

Mo, Q., Ma, Z., Wang, G., Jia, C., Niu, L., & Zhou, L. (2020). The pattern of stressful life events prior to suicide among the older adults in rural China: A national case–control psychological autopsy study. *BMC Geriatrics, 20*, 473. https://bmcgeriatr.biomedcentral.com/articles/10.1186/s12877-020-01874-4

Mith, D. L. (1978). *A history of firefighting in America: 300 years of courage*. Macmillan.

Money, N., Moore, M., Brown, D., Kasper, K., Roeder, J., Bartone, P., & Bates, M. (2011). Best practices identified for peer support programs. PsycEXTRA Dataset. https://mhanational.org/wp-content/uploads/2025/02/Best-Practices-Identified-Peer-Support-Programs-Jan-2011.pdfhttps://mhanational.org/wp-content/uploads/2025/02/Best-Practices-Identified-Peer-Support-Programs-Jan-2011.pdf

Moore, R. L., & Gillette, D. (1990). King, warrior, magician, lover: Rediscovering the archetypes of the mature masculine. HarperOne.

Moore-Merrell, L., Kerber, S., Horn, G. P., & Smith, D. L. (2021). Effects of crew size on firefighter health and safety. *International Fire Service Journal of Leadership & Management, 15*, 7–25. https://d1gi3fvbl0xj2a.cloudfront.net/2021-12/IFSJLM%20Vol15_Horn.pdf

Mor Barak, M. E. (2016). *Managing diversity: Toward a globally inclusive workplace* (4th ed.). SAGE.

Moran, L., & Roth, G. (2013). Humor in context: Fire service and joking culture. *New Horizons in Adult Education and Human Resource Development, 25*(3), 14–26. https://onlinelibrary.wiley.com/doi/abs/10.1002/nha3.20028

Muffler, S. C., Cavico, F. J., & Mujtaba, B. G. (2010). Diversity, disparate impact, and ethics in business: Implications of the New Haven firefighters' case and the supreme court's Ricci v. DeStefano decision. *SAM Advanced Management Journal, 75*(3), 11–20. https://nsuworks.nova.edu/hcbe_facarticles/530/

Murphy, J. K. (2013, March 5). Legal matters: FMLA pitfalls for the fire service. Fire Engineering. https://www.fireengineering.com/firefighting/legal-matters-fmla-pitfalls-for-the-fire-service/

Murphy, S. L., Kochanek, K. D., Xu, J. Q., & Arias, E. (2024). Deaths: Final data for 2021. *National Vital Statistics Reports, 73*(8). National Center for Health Statistics. https://doi.org/10.15620/cdc/158787

Myers, A., Collins-Pisano, C., Ferron, J., & Fortuna, K. (2021). Feasibility and preliminary effectiveness of a peerdeveloped and virtually delivered community mental health training program (emotional CPR): Pre–post study. *Journal of Participatory Medicine, 13*(1), e25867. https://doi.org/10.2196/25867

Na, K., Kim, E., & Park, J. (2017). Decreased plasma adiponectin among male firefighters with symptoms of posttraumatic stress disorder. *Journal of Affective Disorders*, 221254–221258. https://pubmed.ncbi.nlm.nih.gov/28662456/

Naifeh, J. A., Mash, H. B. H., Stein, M. B., Fullerton, C. S., Kessler, R. C., & Ursano, R. J. (2019). The Army study to assess risk and resilience in servicemembers (Army STARRS): Progress toward understanding suicide among soldiers. *Molecular Psychiatry, 24*(1), 34–48. https://pubmed.ncbi.nlm.nih.gov/30104726/

Nash, W. P. (2021). *Adaptive disclosure: A new treatment for military trauma, loss, and moral injury*. Guilford Press.

Nash, W. P., & Litz, B. T. (2013). Moral injury: A mechanism for war-related psychological trauma in military family members. *Clinical Child and Family Psychology Review, 16*(4), 365–375. https://pubmed.ncbi.nlm.nih.gov/23852334/

National Center for PTSD. (2023). *Psychological first aid (PFA)*. U.S. Department of Veterans Affairs. https://www.ptsd.va.gov/professional/treat/type/psych_firstaid.asp

National Commission on Fire Prevention and Control. (1973). America burning: The report of the National Commission on Fire prevention and control (U.S. Government Printing Office). https://www.hsdl.org/?abstract&did=438002

National Fallen Firefighters Foundation. (2019). Firefighter mental health and well-being resources (programmatic guidance & tools). https://www.firehero.org/firefighter-mental-health/

National Fire Prevention and Control Act, Pub. L. No. 95-249, 92 Stat. 932 (1978). https://www.congress.gov/95/statute/STATUTE-92/STATUTE-92-Pg932.pdf

National Fire Protection Association. (2022a). Community risk reduction: An overview. Retrieved from https://www.nfpa.org/CRR

National Fire Protection Association. (2022b). NFPA 1582: Standard on comprehensive occupational medical program for fire departments. NFPA. https://www.nfpa.org/codes-and-standards/nfpa-1582-standard-development/1582

National Fire Protection Association. (2022c). NFPA 1583: Standard on health-related fitness programs for fire department members. NFPA. https://www.nfpa.org/codes-and-standards/nfpa-1583-standard-development/1583

National Fire Protection Association (NFPA). (2020a). Firefighter fatalities by cause and nature of injuries. https://www.nfpa.org/education-and-research/research/nfpa-research/fire-statistical-reports/fatal-firefighter-injuries/firefighter-deaths-by-cause-and-nature-of-injury

National Fire Protection Association. (2021a). *NFPA 1500: Standard on fire department occupational safety, health, and wellness program*. NFPA. https://www.nfpa.org/codes-and-standards/all-codes-and-standards/list-of-codes-and-standards/detail?code=1500

National Fire Protection Association. (2021b). *NFPA 1582: Standard on comprehensive occupational medical program for fire departments*. NFPA. https://www.nfpa.org/codes-and-standards/all-codes-and-standards/list-of-codes-and-standards/detail?code=1582

FireRescue1. (2007, February 26). First Near-Miss Reporting System annual report details findings from 2006 submissions [Press release]. FireRescue1. https://www.firerescue1.com/fire-products/press-releases/first-near-miss-reporting-system-annual-report-details-findings-from-2006-submissions-Se4jDPH29oxwhYOk/

National Highway Traffic Safety Administration. (2021). National EMS scope of the practice model. U.S. Department of Transportation.

National Institute for Health and Care Excellence (NICE). (2005). *Posttraumatic stress disorder: Management of PTSD in adults and children in primary and secondary care*. NICE.

National Institute for Health and Care Excellence (NICE). (2018). Posttraumatic stress disorder (NICE guideline NG116). Retrieved from https://www.nice.org.uk/guidance/ng116

National Institute for Occupational Safety and Health (NIOSH). (2004). Quick drills: Reviewing NIOSH reports, Seatbelts. U.S. Department of Health and Human Services.

National Institute for Occupational Safety and Health (NIOSH). (2005). Fire fighter fatality investigation report F2005-01. U.S. Department of Health and Human Services.

National Institute for Occupational Safety and Health (NIOSH). (2010). Career probationary fire fighter and captain die as a result of rapid fire progression in a winddriven residential structure fire – Texas (NIOSH Report No. F2009-11). U.S. Department of Health and Human Services, Centers for Disease Control and Prevention. https://www.firefighternation.com/wp-content/uploads/2018/01/face200911.pdf

National Institute for Occupational Safety and Health (NIOSH). (2012). Career lieutenant and firefighter killed and two firefighters injured following a nine-alarm fire in a vacant restaurant – Massachusetts (NIOSH Report No. F2011-18). U.S. Department of Health and Human Services, Centers for Disease Control and Prevention. https://www.scribd.com/document/503750190/2018-LODD-Report-Worcester-Christopher-Roy

National Institute for Occupational Safety and Health (NIOSH). (2012). Fire fighter fatality investigation report F2012-01. U.S. Department of Health and Human Services.

National Institute for Occupational Safety and Health (NIOSH). (2014). Two career fire fighters die in a rapid fire progression while searching for a civilian – Ohio (NIOSH Report No. F2014-02). U.S. Department of Health and Human Services, Centers for Disease Control and Prevention. https://www.toledoblade.com/attachment/2015/04/29/niosh-investigation-of-jan-26-2014-fire

National Institute for Occupational Safety and Health (NIOSH). (2014). Career lieutenant killed following a walkway collapse while working to evacuate a university student housing building – Missouri (NIOSH Report No. F2014-07). U.S. Department of Health and Human Services, Centers for Disease Control and Prevention. https://stacks.cdc.gov/view/cdc/163421

National Institute for Occupational Safety and Health (NIOSH). (2016). Delivering on the nation's promise: Safety and health at work for all people through research and prevention (DHHS

(NIOSH) Publication No. 2016–165). U.S. Department of Health and Human Services, Centers for Disease Control and Prevention. https://www.cdc.gov/niosh/docs/2016-165/

National Institute for Occupational Safety and Health (NIOSH). (2017). Arson fire kills three fire fighters and injures four fire fighters due to a floor collapse in a row house – Delaware (NIOSH Report No. F2016-18). U.S. Department of Health and Human Services, Centers for Disease Control and Prevention. https://www.cdc.gov/niosh/firefighters/programs/pdfs/face201618.pdf

National Institute for Occupational Safety and Health (NIOSH). (2018). Structure collapse at a 140-year-old mill building kills two career fire fighters and injures two others – Pennsylvania (NIOSH Report No. F2018-06). U.S. Department of Health and Human Services, Centers for Disease Control and Prevention. https://www.cdc.gov/niosh/firefighters/programs/pdfs/face201806.pdf

National Institute for Occupational Safety and Health (NIOSH). (2019). Volunteer firefighter dies after being ejected from rear seat of fire department pickup truck,Iowa (Report No. F2017-07). U.S. Department of Health and Human Services. https://www.cdc.gov/niosh/firefighters/programs/pdfs/face201707.pdf

National Institute for Occupational Safety and Health (NIOSH). (2019). Two firefighters die and three firefighters injured in a fire apparatus crash,West Virginia (Report No. F2018-08). U.S. Department of Health and Human Services. https://www.cdc.gov/niosh/firefighters/programs/pdfs/face201808.pdf

National Institute for Occupational Safety and Health (NIOSH). (2020). Career firefighter/SCUBA diver drowns while searching for civilian in an industrialized river—Illinois (Report No. F2018-09). Fire Fighter Fatality Investigation and Prevention Program. Morgantown, WV: U.S. Department of Health and Human Services, Centers for Disease Control and Prevention. chrome- extension://efaidnbmnnnibpcajpcglclefindmkaj/. https://www.cdc.gov/niosh/firefighters/programs/pdfs/face201809.pdf

National Institute for Occupational Safety and Health. (2024, December 20). *What challenges do women in the fire service face?* NIOSH Science Blog. Centers for Disease Control and Prevention. https://blogs.cdc.gov/niosh-science-blog/2024/12/20/women-firefighters/

National Institute of Mental Health. (2002). Mental health and mass violence: Evidence-based early psychological intervention for victims/survivors of mass violence, A workshop to reach consensus on best practices (NIH Publication No. 02-5138). Washington, DC: U.S. Government Printing Office. https://www.nimh.nih.gov/research/massviolence.pdf

National Institutes of Health. (2023). Work-life boundary management of peer support workers when working from home: A qualitative study. https://www.ncbi.nlm.nih.gov/pmc/articles/PMC10463757/

National Park Service. (2023). Katherine Ah Lan Lowe. https://www.nps.gov/articles/000/katherine-ah-lan-lowe.htm

NATO. (2003). NATO-Russia advanced research workshop on social and psychological consequences of chemical, biological and radiological terrorism. *NATO Science Series I: Life and Behavioral Sciences, 361*, 1–284.

Navarro, K. M., Butler, C. R., Fent, K., Toennis, C., Sammons, D., Ramirez-Cardenas, A., Clark, K. A., Byrne, D. C., Graydon, P. S., Hale, C. R., Wilkinson, A. F., Smith, D. L., Alexander-Scott, M. C., Pinkerton, L. E., Eisenberg, J., & Domitrovich, J. W. (2022). Wildland firefighter exposure and health effect (WFFEHE) study: Rationale, design, and methods of a repeated-measures study. *Annals of Work Exposures & Health, 66*(6), 714–727. https://pubmed.ncbi.nlm.nih.gov/34919119/

Neumann, E. (1954). The origins and history of consciousness (R. F. C. Hull, Trans.). Princeton University Press.

NICE (National Institute for Health and Clinical Excellence). (2018). Posttraumatic stress disorder. https://www.nice.org.uk/guidance/ng116

National Volunteer Fire Council. (2015). *Critical health and safety issues in the volunteer fire service*. NVFC.

Noda, Y., Asano, K., Shimizu, E., & Hirano, Y. (2024). Path analysis was used to assess the associations between probable posttraumatic stress disorder symptoms and quality of life among emergency service workers. *Work, 77*(2), 573–587. https://pubmed.ncbi.nlm.nih.gov/37718827/

Noll, L., Mallows, A., & Moran, J. (2022). Psychosocial barriers and facilitators for a successful return to work following injury within firefighters. *International Archives of Occupational and Environmental Health, 95*(2), 331–339. https://doi.org/10.1007/s00420-021-01712-z

Norman, D. A. (1988). *The design of everyday things*. Basic Books.

North, C. S., & Pfefferbaum, B. (2013). Mental health response to community disasters: A systematic review. *JAMA, 310*(5), 507–518. https://pubmed.ncbi.nlm.nih.gov/23925621/

O'Brien, P. & Campbell, D. (2021). *Wildland firefighter psychological and behavioral health: Preliminary data from a national sample of current and former wildland firefighters in the United States*. 6th Annual Human Dimensions Conference of the International Association of Wildland Fire.

Obuobi-Donkor, G., Oluwasina, F., Nkire, N., & Agyapong, V. I. O. (2022). A scoping review on the prevalence and determinants of post-traumatic stress disorder among military personnel and firefighters: Implications for public policy and practice. *International Journal of Environmental Research and Public Health, 19*(3), 1565. https://doi.org/10.3390/ijerph19031565

O'Connor, R. C., & Kirtley, O. J. (2018). The integrated motivational–volitional model of suicidal behavior. *Philosophical Transactions of the Royal Society B: Biological Sciences, 373*(1754), 20170268. https://pmc.ncbi.nlm.nih.gov/articles/PMC6053985/

O'Dare, K., Dillard, D., King, E., Dilks, J., Jr., Herzog, J., Rotunda, R., Close, F., & Hartman, M. (2024). The 2nd alarm project: Bridging social work and public health to improve mental wellness in the fire service. *Social Work in Public Health, 39*(1), 93–104. https://pubmed.ncbi.nlm.nih.gov/38367222/

O'Neill, O. A., & Rothbard, N. P. (2017). Is love all you need? The effects of emotional culture, suppression, and work-family conflict on firefighter risk-taking and health. *Academy of Management Journal, 60*(1), 78–108. https://journals.aom.org/doi/10.5465/amj.2014.0952

Ogburn, W. F. (1922). *Social change with respect to culture and original nature*. B. W. Huebsch (Open copy: Internet Archive).

Ogburn, W. F. (1922). *Social change with respect to culture and original nature*. Dell Pub. Co..

Ohio Rev. Code § 4123.01 (2021).

Okoli, J. O., Watt, J., & Weller, G. (2022). A naturalistic decision-making approach to managing nonroutine fire incidents: Evidence from expert firefighters. *Journal of Risk Research, 25*(2), 198–217. https://psycnet.apa.org/record/2022-33599-004

Oliveira, J., Aires Dias, J., Duarte, I. C., Caldeira, S., Marques, A. R., Rodrigues, V., & Castelo-Branco, M. (2023). Mental health and posttraumatic stress disorder in firefighters: An integrated analysis from an action research study. *Frontiers in Psychology, 14*, 1259388. https://pubmed.ncbi.nlm.nih.gov/37965662/

Olmsted, D. W., & Monachesi, E. D. (1956). A validity check on MMPI scales of responsibility and dominance. *Journal of Abnormal & Social Psychology*, 53140–53141. https://pubmed.ncbi.nlm.nih.gov/13345585/

Olofsson, J. (2013). "The Profession of Firefighting Is About Teamwork, It Is About Trusting Each Other": Masculine enactments and generational discrepancies within the Swedish Fire Service. *Culture, Society and Masculinities, 5*(1), 75–88. https://www.researchgate.net/publication/274674023_The_Profession_of_Firefighting_Is_About_Teamwork_It_Is_About_Trusting_Each_Other_Masculine_Enactments_and_Generational_Discrepancies_Within_the_Swedish_Fire_Service

Olthuis, J. V., Kaltenbach, E., Giberson, E., Saryeddine, T., Asmundson, G. J. G., Carleton, R. N., Cramm, H., Crombach, A., Devlin, J., Mack, J., Lingley, P. P., Rao, S., Sullivan, M., Wozney, L., & McGrath, P. J. (2023). Paraprofessional delivery of online narrative exposure therapy for firefighters. *Journal of Traumatic Stress, 36*(4), 772–784. https://psycnet.apa.org/record/2023-81764-001

Omodei, M. M., McLennan, J., & Reynolds, C. (2005a). Decision making under stress in dynamic environments. In B. S. Fiske (Ed.), *Firefighter safety and behavior* (pp. 75–102). Elsevier.

Omodei, M. M., McLennan, J., & Reynolds, C. (2005b, April). Identifying why even well-trained firefighters make unsafe decisions: A human factors interview protocol [conference report]. In *Proceedings of the eighth international wildland firefighter safety summit—Human factors—10 years later*. Bushfire Cooperative Research Centre. https://www.naturalhazards.com.au/crc-collection/downloads/d2_3_report_1_2005_human_factors_interview_protocol_0.pdf

Onyedire, N. G., Ekoh, A. T., Chukwuorji, J. C., & Ifeagwazi, C. M. (2017). Posttraumatic stress disorder (PTSD) symptoms among firefighters: Roles of resilience and locus of control. *Journal of Workplace Behavioral Health, 32*(4), 227–248. https://psycnet.apa.org/record/2018-01661-002

Oreg, S. (2007). Personality, context, and resistance to organizational change. *European Journal of Work and Organizational Psychology, 15*(1), 73–101. Retrieved from https://www.tandfonline.com/doi/abs/10.1080/13594320500451247

Orosa, J. A., Santos, R., & Pérez, J. A. (2011). A practical case study of the relationship between work risk prevention and fatigue at work in Spanish merchant ships. *Human Factors & Ergonomics in Manufacturing & Service Industries, 21*(5), 484–492. https://www.researchgate.net/publication/230212519_A_Practical_Case_Study_of_the_Relationship_between_Work_Risk_Prevention_and_Fatigue_at_Work_in_Spanish_Merchant_Ships

Oster, C., Morello, A., Venning, A., Redpath, P., & Lawn, S. (2017). The health and wellbeing needs of veterans: A rapid review. *BMC Psychiatry, 17*(1), 414. https://doi.org/10.1186/s12888-017-1547-0

Oxford University Press. (2022). *Oxford English dictionary* (12th ed.). Retrieved from https://www.oed.com

Ozer, E. J., Best, S. R., Lipsey, T. L., & Weiss, D. S. (2003). Predictors of posttraumatic stress disorder and symptoms in adults: A meta-analysis. *Psychological Bulletin, 129*(1), 52–73. https://pubmed.ncbi.nlm.nih.gov/12555794/

Packer, I. K., & Grisso, T. (2011). *Specialty competencies in forensic psychology*. Oxford University Press.

Palendeng, R. S., Kairupan, S. B., & Bulo, L. (2024). Implementation of fire incident response time service policy in Manado City Fire Service. *Technium Social Sciences Journal, 66*:84–96. https://techniumscience.com/index.php/socialsciences/article/view/12020

Papazoglou, K., Blumberg, D. M., Chiongbian, V. B., Tuttle, B. M., Kamkar, K., Chopko, B., Milliard, B., Aukhojee, P., & Koskelainen, M. (2020). The role of moral injury in PTSD among law enforcement officers: A brief report. *Frontiers in Psychology, 11*:310. https://pubmed.ncbi.nlm.nih.gov/32194477/

Park, J., & Fletcher, A. (2018). The US firefighter's perception and lived experience with station work uniform: Occupational safety concerns in public appearance. *International Journal of Fashion Design, Technology & Education, 11*(1), 113–122. https://www.tandfonline.com/doi/full/10.1080/17543266.2017.1332244

Park, J., & Langseth-Schmidt, K. (2016). Anthropometric fit evaluation of firefighters' uniform pants: A sex comparison. *International Journal of Industrial Ergonomics, 56*, 1–8. https://www.sciencedirect.com/science/article/abs/pii/S0169814116300841

Paulus, D. J., Vujanovic, A. A., Schuhmann, B. B., Smith, L. J., & Tran, J. (2017). Main and interactive effects of depression and posttraumatic stress on alcohol dependence among urban male firefighters. *Psychiatry Research*, 25169–25175. https://pubmed.ncbi.nlm.nih.gov/28189939/

Payne, N., & Kinman, G. (2019). Job demands, resources and work-related well-being in UK firefighters. *Occupational Medicine, 69*(8/9), 604–609. https://pubmed.ncbi.nlm.nih.gov/31925427/

Pennington, M. L., Carpenter, T. P., Synett, S. J., Torres, V. A., Teague, J., Morissette, S. B., Knight, J., Kamholz, B. W., Keane, T. M., Zimering, R. T., & Gulliver, S. B. (2018). The influence of exposure to natural disasters on depression and PTSD symptoms among firefighters. *Disaster Medicine and Public Health Preparedness, 12*(3), 362–369. https://pubmed.ncbi.nlm.nih.gov/29223176/

Pennington, M. L., Carpenter, T. P., Synett, S. J., Torres, V. A., Teague, J., Morissette, S. B., Knight, J., Kamholz, B. W., Keane, T. M., Zimering, R. T., & Gulliver, S. B. (2018). The influence of exposure to natural disasters on depression and PTSD symptoms among firefighters. *Prehospital and Disaster Medicine, 12*(3), 362–369. https://pubmed.ncbi.nlm.nih.gov/29223176/

Pennsylvania General Assembly. (2024). Act 121 of 2024 (SB 365): Workers' Compensation Act—compensation for post-traumatic stress injury (first responders). https://www.legis.state.pa.us/cfdocs/legis/li/uconsCheck.cfm?act=121&sessInd=0&yr=2024 (law information) and bill text (PN 1944).

Petrie, K., Milligan-Saville, J., Gayed, A., et al. (2018). Prevalence of PTSD and common mental disorders among ambulance personnel: A systematic review and meta-analysis. *Social Psychiatry and Psychiatric Epidemiology, 53*(9), 897–909. https://doi.org/10.1007/s00127-018-1539-5

Petruzzello, S. J., Poh, P. Y. S., Greenlee, T. A., Goldstein, E., Horn, G. P., & Smith, D. L. (2016). Physiological, perceptual and psychological responses of career versus volunteer firefighters to live-fire training drills. *Stress & Health, 32*(4), 328–336. https://pubmed.ncbi.nlm.nih.gov/25393336/

Perez v. Denver Fire Department, No. 17-1128 (10th Cir. Feb. 7, 2018). https://law.justia.com/cases/federal/appellate-courts/ca10/17-1128/17-1128-2018-02-07.html

Pietrzak, R. H., Goldstein, M. B., Malley, J. C., Rivers, A. J., Johnson, D. C., Morgan, C. A., 3rd, & Southwick, S. M. (2010). Posttraumatic growth in Veterans of Operations Enduring Freedom and Iraqi Freedom. Journal of affective disorders, 126(1-2), 230–235. https://doi.org/10.1016/j.jad.2010.03.021

Pines, A., & Maslach, C. (1978). Characteristics of staff burnout in mental health settings. *Hospital & Community Psychiatry, 29*(4), 233–237.

Pinto, R. J., Henriques, S. P., Jongenelen, I., Carvalho, C., & Maia, Â. C. (2015). The strongest correlates of PTSD for firefighters: Number, recency, frequency, or perceived threat of traumatic events. *Journal of Traumatic Stress, 28*(5), 434–440. https://pubmed.ncbi.nlm.nih.gov/26389531/

Platt, M., Barton, J., & Freyd, J. J. (2009). A betrayal trauma perspective on domestic violence. In E. Stark & E. S. Buzawa (Eds.), *Violence against women in families and relationships* (Vol. 1, pp. 185–207). Greenwood Press.

Ployhart, R. E., & Holtz, B. C. (2008). The diversity–validity dilemma: Strategies for reducing racioethnic and sex subgroup differences and adverse impact in selection. *Personnel Psychology, 61*(1), 153–172. https://psycnet.apa.org/record/2008-01770-007

Pompper, D. (2021). On re-considering the first as a news value to avoid stereotyping. *The Howard Journal of Communications, 32*(1), 1–23. https://www.tandfonline.com/doi/full/10.1080/10646175.2020.1823283

Poston, W. S. C., Haddock, C. K., Jahnke, S. A., Jitnarin, N., Day, R. S., & Daniels, I. D. (2014). Health disparities among racial and ethnic minority firefighters. *Journal of Health Disparities Research and Practice*, 7(5), Article 8. https://digitalscholarship.unlv.edu/jhdrp/vol7/iss5/8

Pouliot, L., & De Leo, D. (2006). Critical issues in psychological autopsy studies. *Suicide and Life-threatening Behavior, 36*(5), 491–510. https://pubmed.ncbi.nlm.nih.gov/17087629/

Powers, M. B., Halpern, J. M., Ferenschak, M. P., Gillihan, S. J., & Foa, E. B. (2010). A meta-analytic review of prolonged exposure for posttraumatic stress disorder. *Clinical Psychology Review, 30*(6), 635–641. https://doi.org/10.1016/j.cpr.2010.04.006

Prati, G., & Pietrantoni, L. (2010). The relation of perceived and received social support to mental health among first responders: A meta-analytic review. *Journal of Community Psychology, 38*(3), 403–417. https://psycnet.apa.org/record/2010-05706-009

President's Conference on Fire Prevention. (1947, May 6–8). Fire prevention and control: A report on national fire safety. *U.S. Government Printing Office*. https://www.firehero.org/wp-content/uploads/2019/02/truman-report-1947.pdf

Psarros, C., Theleritis, C., Kokras, N., Lyrakos, D., Koborozos, A., Kakabakou, O., Tzanoulinos, G., Katsiki, P., & Bergiannaki, J. D. (2018). Personality characteristics and individual factors associated with PTSD in firefighters one month after extended wildfires. *Nordic Journal of Psychiatry, 72*(1), 17–23. https://pubmed.ncbi.nlm.nih.gov/28871848/

Public Safety Testing. (n.d.). Written exam requirements—firefighter. Retrieved from https://www.publicsafetytesting.com/information-center/test-requirements-firefighter-written/

Public Safety Officer Support Act of 2022, Pub. L. No. 117-172, 136 Stat. 2098 (Aug. 16, 2022). https://www.congress.gov/117/plaws/publ172/PLAW-117publ172.pdf

Purdum, T. (2023). "The volunteering days are gone": All-hazard incarcerated firefighters and rural disinvestment. *Rural Sociology, 88*(2), 312–336. https://onlinelibrary.wiley.com/doi/abs/10.1111/ruso.12477

Qi, H., Zhou, Z., Irizarry, J., Lin, D., Zhang, H., Li, N., & Cui, J. (2024). Automatic identification of causal factors from fall-related accident investigation reports using machine learning and ensemble learning approaches. *Journal of Management in Engineering, 40*(1), 1–17. https://www.researchgate.net/publication/377036580_Automatic_Identification_of_Causal_Factors_from_Fall-Related_Accident_Investigation_Reports_Using_Machine_Learning_and_Ensemble_Learning_Approaches

Quigley, D. D., Dworsky, M., Qureshi, N., Ashwood, J. S., O'Hollaren, K., & Meredith, L. S. (2021). *Posttraumatic stress in California's workers' compensation system: A study of mental health presumptions for firefighters and peace officers under Senate Bill 542*. (Research Report No. RR-A1391-1). RAND Corporation. https://doi.org/10.7249/RRA1391-1

Quinn, T. D., Marsh, S. M., Oldham, K., Wurzelbacher, S. J., & Naber, S. J. (2023). Workers' compensation injury claims among firefighters in Ohio, 2001–2017. *Journal of Safety Research, 85*, 147–156. https://pubmed.ncbi.nlm.nih.gov/37330864/

Radler, M. (2011). Amending the EEOC's disability discrimination regulations to protect employees with post-traumatic stress disorder. *The George Washington Law Review, 80*, 1546. https://www.gwlr.org/wp-content/uploads/2018/04/80-Geo.-Wash.-L.-Rev.-1546.pdf

Rajaratnam, S. M. W., Barger, L. K., Lockley, S. W., Shea, S. A., Wang, W., Landrigan, C. P., O'Brien, C. S., Qadri, S., Sullivan, J. P., Cade, B. E., Epstein, L. J., White, D. P., & Czeisler, C. A. (2011). Sleep disorders, health, and safety in police officers. *JAMA, 306*(23), 2567–2578. https://pubmed.ncbi.nlm.nih.gov/22187276/

Rank, O. (1978a). Art and artist: Creative urge and personality development (C. F. Atkinson, Trans.). W. W. Norton. (Original work published 1932).

Rank, O. (1978b). The myth of the birth of the hero. Johns Hopkins University Press. (Original work published 1932) https://www.press.jhu.edu/books/title/3380/myth-birth-hero?srsltid=AfmBOooh5hq7xzc4k3bLd8aDtyIUztc7VAZ02y0aWwnBTXvD7tU84oag

Reason, J. (1990). *Human error*. Cambridge University Press.

Reason, J. (1997). *Managing the risks of organizational accidents*. Ashgate. https://www.scirp.org/reference/referencespapers?referenceid=1716897

Regehr, C., Hill, J., & Glancy, G. (2000). Individual predictors of traumatic reactions in firefighters. *The Journal of Nervous and Mental Disease, 188*(6), 333–339. https://pubmed.ncbi.nlm.nih.gov/10890341/

Regehr, C., & Hill, J. (2001). Evaluating the efficacy of crisis debriefing groups. *Social Work With Groups, 23*(3), 69–79. https://doi.org/10.1300/J009v23n03_06

Regehr, C., Hill, J., & Goldberg, G. (2003). Postmortem inquiries and trauma responses in paramedics and firefighters. *Journal of Interpersonal Violence, 18*(6), 607–622. https://psycnet.apa.org/record/2003-00888-004

Regehr, C., Hill, J., Knott, T., & Sault, B. (2002). Social support, self-efficacy and trauma in new recruits and experienced firefighters. *Stress and Health, 18*(4), 189–193. https://www.researchgate.net/publication/227752360_Social_support_self-efficacy_and_trauma_in_new_recruits_and_experienced_firefighters

Regehr, C., & Millar, D. (2007). Situation critical: High demand, low control, and low support in paramedic organizations. *Traumatology, 13*(1), 49–58. https://doi.org/10.1177/1534765607299912

Reid, R. C., Temko, J., Moghaddam, J. F., & Fong, T. W. (2012). Shame, rumination, and self-compassion in men assessed for hypersexual disorder. *Journal of Psychiatric Practice, 18*(4), 233–240. https://pubmed.ncbi.nlm.nih.gov/25036581/

Reimer, R., & Eriksen, C. (2018). The wildfire within: Gender, leadership and wildland fire culture. *International Journal of Wildland Fire, 27*(11), 715–726. https://www.publish.csiro.au/wf/wf17150

Reinach, S., & Viale, A. (2006). Application of a human error framework to conduct train accident/incident investigations. *Accident Analysis & Prevention, 38*(2), 396–406. https://pubmed.ncbi.nlm.nih.gov/16310153/

Matter of Reith v. City of Albany, 2021 N.Y. Slip Op. 07339 (App. Div. 3d Dep't Dec. 23, 2021).

Repper, J., & Carter, T. (2011). A review of the literature on peer support in mental health services. *Journal of Mental Health, 20*(4), 392–411. https://pubmed.ncbi.nlm.nih.gov/21770786/

Ricci v. DeStefano, 557 U.S. 557 (2009).

Riccucci, N. M., & Riccardelli, M. (2015). The use of written exams in police and fire departments: Implications for social diversity. *Review of Public Personnel Administration, 35*(4), 352–366. https://www.researchgate.net/publication/285406632_The_Use_of_Written_Exams_in_Police_and_Fire_Departments_Implications_for_Social_Diversity

Richard, J., Rebinsky, R., Suresh, R., Kubic, S., Carter, A., Cunningham, J. E. A., Ker, A., Williams, K., & Sorin, M. (2022). Scoping review to evaluate the effects of peer support on the mental health of young adults. *BMJ Open, 12*(8), e061336. https://pubmed.ncbi.nlm.nih.gov/35926986/

Roberts, N. A., & Levenson, R. W. (2001). The remains of the workday: Impact of job stress and exhaustion on marital interaction in police couples. *Journal of Marriage and Family, 63*(4), 1052–1067. https://psycnet.apa.org/record/2001-09225-011

Robinson, R. C., & Mitchell, J. T. (1993). Evaluation of psychological debriefings. *Journal of Traumatic Stress, 6*, 367–382. https://psycnet.apa.org/record/1994-02913-001

Robison, M., Rice, T. B., Hom, M. A., Chu, C., Anestis, M. D., Joiner, T. E., & Stanley, I. H. (2025). Suicide plans involving a firearm and levels of suicidal intent among firefighters. *Crisis: The Journal of Crisis Intervention and Suicide Prevention, 46*(2), 78–84. https://psycnet.apa.org/record/2025-86325-001

Rose, S., Bisson, J., & Wessely, S. (2002). Psychological debriefing for preventing posttraumatic stress disorder (PTSD). *Cochrane Database of Systematic Reviews, 2*, CD000560. https://pubmed.ncbi.nlm.nih.gov/12076399/

Rose, S., Bisson, J., & Wessely, S. (2003). A systematic review of single-session psychological interventions ('debriefing') following trauma: Are they effective in preventing PTSD? *Psychiatric Quarterly, 74*(3), 299–314. https://pubmed.ncbi.nlm.nih.gov/12792122/

Rose, S., Brewin, C. R., Andrews, B., & Lirk, M. (1999). A randomized controlled trial of individual psychological debriefing for victims of violent crime. *Psychological Medicine, 29*, 793–799. https://pubmed.ncbi.nlm.nih.gov/10473306/

Rossi, P. H., Lipsey, M. W., & Henry, G. T. (2018). *Evaluation: A systematic approach* (8th ed.). SAGE Publications.

Roth, S. L., Andrews, K., Protopopescu, A., Lloyd, C., O'Connor, C., Losier, B. J., Lanius, R. A., & McKinnon, M. C. (2022). Mental health symptoms in public safety personnel: Examining the effects of adverse childhood experiences and moral injury. *Child Abuse & Neglect, 123*, 105394. https://pubmed.ncbi.nlm.nih.gov/34808481/

Rotter, J. B. (1966). Generalized expectancies for internal versus external control of reinforcement. *Psychological Monographs: General and Applied, 80*(1), 1–28. https://psycnet.apa.org/record/2011-19211-001

Rowan-White, B., & Williams, J. (2024). Research-based community risk reduction at the company level. Fire Engineering. Retrieved from https://www.fireengineering.com/fire-safety/research-based-community-risk-reduction-at-the-company-level/

Rudman, J. S., Farcas, A., Salazar, G. A., Hoff, J., Crowe, R. P., Whitten-Chung, K., Torres, G., Pereira, C., Hill, E., Jafri, S., Page, D. I., von Isenburg, M., Haamid, A., & Joiner, A. P. (2023).

Diversity, equity, and inclusion in the United States emergency medical services workforce: A scoping review. *Prehospital Emergency Care, 27*(4), 385–397. https://pubmed.ncbi.nlm.nih.gov/36190493/

Russo, B. R. (2013). *Women firefighters' strategies for advancement in the fire service: Breaking down barriers in gender-based occupations*. Oklahoma State University.

Ruzek, J. I., Kuhn, E., Jaworski, B. K., Owen, J. E., & Ramsey, K. M. (2017). Mobile mental health interventions following war and disaster. *MHealth, 3*, 13. https://pubmed.ncbi.nlm.nih.gov/28293610/

Ryerson, D., & Whitlock, R. (2005a). *Fire service human factors: A systems approach to safety*. Firehouse Publications.

Ryerson, M., & Whitlock, C. (2005b). Use of human factors analysis for wildland fire accident investigations. Proceedings of the eighth international wildland Fire Safety summit, Missoula, USA (April 26-28, 2005).

Sadownik, A. (2023). Bronfenbrenner: Ecology of human development in ecology of collaboration. https://www.researchgate.net/publication/373383997_Bronfenbrenner_Ecology_of_Human_Development_in_Ecology_of_Collaboration

Saks, A., & Ashforth, B. (2002). Socialization tactics and newcomer information acquisition. *International Journal of Selection and Assessment, 5*:48–61. https://doi.org/10.1111/1468-2389.00044. https://www.researchgate.net/publication/229734517_Socialization_Tactics_and_Newcomer_Information_Acquisition

Salas, E., Sims, D. E., & Burke, C. S. (2005). Is there a "big five" in teamwork? *Small Group Research, 36*(5), 555–599. https://doi.org/10.1177/1046496405277134. (Original work published 2005).

Salas, E., & Maurino, D. (2010). *Human factors in aviation* (2nd ed.). Academic Press.

Salina, S. J. D., & Wallace, W. C. (2025). A qualitative exploration of motivations for entry into the firefighting profession in Trinidad and Tobago. *International Journal of Emergency Services, 14*(1), 87–102. https://doi.org/10.1108/IJES-08-2024-0049

Salters-Pedneault, K., Ruef, A. M., & Orr, S. P. (2010). Personality and psychophysiological profiles of police officer and firefighter recruits. *Personality and Individual Differences, 49*(3), 210–215. https://psycnet.apa.org/record/2010-09948-011

Salzer, M. S. (2002). Consumer-delivered services as a best practice in mental health care delivery and the development of practice guidelines: Mental Health Association of Southeastern Pennsylvania Best Practices Team Philadelphia. *Psychiatric Rehabilitation Skills, 6*(3), 355–382. https://www.tandfonline.com/doi/abs/10.1080/10973430208408443

SAMHSA. (2015). Core competencies for peer workers in behavioral health services. U.S. Department of Health and Human Services, Substance Abuse and Mental Health Services Administration. https://www.samhsa.gov/technical-assistance/brss-tacs/peer-support-workers/core-competencies

Sanford, K., Kruse, M. I., Proctor, A., Torres, V. A., Pennington, M. L., Synett, S. J., & Gulliver, S. B. (2017). Couple resilience and life wellbeing in firefighters. *The Journal of Positive Psychology, 12*(6), 660–666. https://psycnet.apa.org/record/2017-31938-016

Sanko, S., Kashani, S., Ito, T., Guggenheim, A., Fei, S., & Eckstein, M. (2020). Advanced practice providers in the field: Implementation of the Los Angeles Fire Department Advanced Provider Response Unit. *Prehospital Emergency Care, 24*(5), 693–703. https://pubmed.ncbi.nlm.nih.gov/31621447/

Sarabia, J. R., Dellor, E., Freisthler, B., & Kieninger, K. (2024). Exploring the association between post–critical incident intervention preferences and self-reported coping self-efficacy among firefighters. *Journal of Traumatic Stress, 37*(3), 504–515. https://pubmed.ncbi.nlm.nih.gov/38476048/

Sarialioglu, S., Ugurlu, Ö., Aydin, M., Vardar, B., & Wang, J. (2020). A hybrid model for human-factor analysis of engine-room fires on ships: HFACS-PV&FFTA. *Ocean Engineering, 217*, 1–19. https://www.researchgate.net/publication/344210385_A_hybrid_model_for_human-factor_analysis_of_engine-room_fires_on_ships_HFACS-PVFFTA

Sattler, D. N., Boyd, B., & Kirsch, J. (2014). Trauma-exposed firefighters: Relationships among posttraumatic growth, post traumatic stress, resource availability, coping and critical incident stress debriefing experience. *Stress and health: journal of the International Society for the Investigation of Stress, 30*(5), 356–365. https://pubmed.ncbi.nlm.nih.gov/25476961/

Sawhney, G., Jennings, K. S., Britt, T. W., & Sliter, M. T. (2018). Occupational stress and mental health symptoms: Examining the moderating effect of work recovery strategies in firefighters. *Journal of Occupational Health Psychology, 23*(3), 443–456. https://pubmed.ncbi.nlm.nih.gov/28604019/

Scarborough, R. C. (2017). Risk a lot to save a lot: How firefighters decide whose life matters. *Sociological Forum, 32*(S1), 120–143. Risk_a_Lot_to_Save_a_Lot_How_Firefighters_Decide_Whose_Life_Matters

Scarlett, M. P., Rogers, W. T., Adams, E. M., Dreger, R. W., & Petersen, S. R. (2021). Evidence for validity and reliability, and development of performance standards and cut-scores for job-related tests of physical aptitude for structural firefighters. *Journal of Occupational and Environmental Medicine, 63*(11), 992–1002. https://pubmed.ncbi.nlm.nih.gov/34739443/

Schäfer, S. K., Sopp, M. R., Staginnus, M., Lass-Hennemann, J., & Michael, T. (2020). Correlates of mental health in occupations at risk for traumatization: A cross-sectional study. *BMC Psychiatry, 20*(1), 335. https://pubmed.ncbi.nlm.nih.gov/32586338/

Schenk, L., & Johanson, G. (2021). Management of bias and conflict of interest among occupational exposure limit expert groups. *Regulatory Toxicology and Pharmacology, 123*, 104929. https://doi.org/10.1016/j.yrtph.2021.104929

Schim, S. M., Doorenbos, A. Z., Miller, J., & Benkert, R. (2003). Development of a cultural competence assessment instrument. *Journal of Nursing Measurement, 11*(1), 29–40. https://doi.org/10.1891/jnum.11.1.29.52062

Schlichthorst, M., Ozols, I., Reifels, L., & Morgan, A. (2020). Lived experience peer support programs for suicide prevention: A systematic scoping review. *International Journal of Mental Health Systems, 14*, 1–12. https://pubmed.ncbi.nlm.nih.gov/32817757/

Schröder-Hinrichs, J. U., Baldauf, M., & Ghirxi, K. T. (2011). Accident investigation reporting deficiencies related to organizational factors in machinery space fires and explosions. *Accident Analysis & Prevention, 43*(3), 1187–1196. https://pubmed.ncbi.nlm.nih.gov/21376918/

Schuhmann, B. B., Henderson, S. N., Black, R. A., Van Hasselt, V. B., Klimley Margres, K., Masias, E. V., & LeDuc, T. J. (2022). A behavioral-analytic model for assessing stress in firefighters. *Behavior Modification, 46*(2), 267–293. https://pubmed.ncbi.nlm.nih.gov/33435721/

Schumm, J. A., & Chard, K. M. (2012). Alcohol and stress in the military. *Military Behavioral Health, 1*(1), 17–25. https://pubmed.ncbi.nlm.nih.gov/23584106/

Seijts, G., Gandz, J., Crossan, M., & Reno, M. (2015). Character matters: Character dimensions' impact on leader performance and outcomes. *Organizational Dynamics, 44*(1), 65–74. https://psycnet.apa.org/record/2015-11153-011

Selkirk, G. A., McLellan, T. M., & Wong, J. (2004). Active versus passive cooling during work in warm environments while wearing firefighting protective clothing. *Journal of Occupational & Environmental Hygiene, 1*(8), 521–531. https://pubmed.ncbi.nlm.nih.gov/15238305/

Senge, P. M. (1990). The fifth discipline: The art and practice of the learning organization. *Doubleday*. https://www.e-education.psu.edu/geog468/sites/www.e-education.psu.edu.geog468/files/TheFifthDiscipline.pdf

Senger, A. R., McGrew, S. J., Gallagher, M. W., & Vujanovic, A. (2023). Associations of resilience and hope with mental and physical health among firefighters. *Journal of Clinical Psychology, 79*(9), 2124–2136. https://pubmed.ncbi.nlm.nih.gov/37212250/

Serrano, D. M., Rufino, K. A., Tran, J. K., & Vujanovic, A. A. (2020). Association between sleep disturbances and suicide risk among firefighters: The moderating role of mindfulness. *Mindfulness, 11*, 2793–2803. https://psycnet.apa.org/record/2020-64919-001

Shakespeare-Finch, J., & Obst, P. L. (2011). The development of the 2-way social support scale: A measure of giving and receiving emotional and instrumental support. *Journal of Personality Assessment, 93*(5), 483–490. https://pubmed.ncbi.nlm.nih.gov/21859288/

Shalev, A. Y., Ankri, Y., Israeli-Shalev, Y., Peleg, T., Adessky, R., & Freedman, S. (2012). Prevention of posttraumatic stress disorder by early treatment: Results from the Jerusalem Trauma outreach and prevention study. *Archives of General Psychiatry, 69*(2), 166–176. https://pubmed.ncbi.nlm.nih.gov/21969418/

Shalev, A., Cho, D., & Marmar, C. R. (2024). Neurobiology and treatment of posttraumatic stress disorder. *American Journal of Psychiatry, 181*(8), 705–719. https://doi.org/10.1176/appi.ajp.20240536

Shappell, S., & Wiegmann, D. (2003). A human error approach to aviation accident analysis: The human factors analysis and classification system. Ashgate. https://www.researchgate.net/publication/345694423_A_Human_Error_Approach_to_Aviation_Accident_Analysis_The_Human_Factors_Analysis_and_Classification_System

Shaw, R. (Ed.). (2012). *Community based disaster risk reduction*. Emerald Group Publishing.

Shaw v. Kittitas Valley Fire, 539 P.3d 907 (Wash. Ct. App. 2024).

Shreffler, K. M., Meadows, M. P., & Davis, K. D. (2011). Firefighting and fathering: Work-family conflict, parenting stress, and satisfaction with parenting and child behavior. *Fathering: A Journal of Theory, Research, and Practice about Men as Fathers, 9*(2), 169–188. https://psycnet.apa.org/record/2011-13049-003

Shultz, J. M., Forbes, D., & Fikretoglu, D. (2013). Psychological first aid: Rapid proliferation and the search for evidence. *Disaster Health, 1*(2), 110–114. https://doi.org/10.4161/dish.26006

Sidanius, J., & Pratto, F. (1999). *Social dominance: An intergroup theory of social hierarchy and oppression*. Cambridge University Press.

Silverman, M. M. (2006). The language of suicidology. *Suicide and Life-threatening Behavior, 36*(5), 519–532. https://pubmed.ncbi.nlm.nih.gov/17087631/

Sintos v. City of Chicago, No. 1:21-cv-05327, 2025 U.S. Dist. LEXIS 124899 (N.D. Ill. July 1, 2025).

Sippel, L. M., Watkins, L. E., Pietrzak, R. H., Hoff, R., & Harpaz-Rotem, I. (2018). The unique roles of emotional numbing and arousal symptoms in relation to social connectedness among military veterans in residential treatment for PTSD. *Psychiatry, 81*(3), 271–282. doi: https://doi.org/10.1080/00332747.2017.1395313. Epub 2018 Jul 17. https://pubmed.ncbi.nlm.nih.gov/30015602/

Siwinski v. The Retirement Board of the Firemen's Annuity and Benefit Fund of the City of Chicago, 2019 IL App (1st) 180388 (Ill. App. Ct. Feb. 1, 2019).

Skeffington, P. M., Rees, C. S., Mazzucchelli, T. G., & Kane, R. T. (2016). The primary prevention of PTSD in firefighters: Preliminary results of an RCT with 12-month follow-up. *PLoS One, 11*(7), e0155873. https://pubmed.ncbi.nlm.nih.gov/27382968/

Skerrett, D. M., Kõlves, K., & De Leo, D. (2012). *Suicidal behaviours in LGB populations: A literature review of research trends*. Australian Institute for Suicide Research and Prevention. https://www.griffith.edu.au/__data/assets/pdf_file/0034/359755/suicidal-behaviours-in-LGB-populations.pdf

Skerrett, D. M., Kõlves, K., & De Leo, D. (2014). Suicides among lesbian, gay, bisexual, and transgender populations in Australia: An analysis of the Queensland suicide register. *Asia-Pacific Psychiatry, 6*(4), 440–446. https://pubmed.ncbi.nlm.nih.gov/24692051/

Skerrett, D. M., Kõlves, K., & De Leo, D. (2015). Are LGBT populations at a higher risk for suicidal behaviors in Australia? Research findings and implications. *Journal of Homosexuality, 62*(7), 883–901. https://pubmed.ncbi.nlm.nih.gov/25569508/

Skinner, B. F. (1953). *Science and human behavior*. New York: Macmillan. https://archive.org/details/dli.ernet.448915

Skinner, B. F. (1974). *About Behaviorism: By BF Skinner*. Knopf.

Simek, R. (1993). *Dictionary of northern mythology* (Angela Hall, Trans.). Boydell & Brewer. ISBN: 0-85991-369-4. https://archive.org/details/dictionaryofnort0000sime

Smith, R. L., & Lyons, W. (1980). The impact of fire fighter unionization on wages and working hours in American cities. *Public Administration Review, 40*(6), 568–574. https://doi.org/10.2307/3110309

Smith, T. B., Domenech Rodríguez, M., & Bernal, G. (2011). Culture. *Journal of Clinical Psychology, 67*(2), 166–175. https://doi.org/10.1002/jclp.20757

Smith, T. D., Dyal, M. A., & DeJoy, D. M. (2023). Firefighter stress, anxiety, and diminished compliance-oriented safety behaviors: Consequences of passive safety leadership in the fire service? *Fire, 6*. https://pubmed.ncbi.nlm.nih.gov/39703438/

Smith, C. P., & Freyd, J. J. (2013). Dangerous safe havens: Institutional betrayal exacerbates sexual trauma. *Journal of Traumatic Stress, 26*(1), 119–124. https://pubmed.ncbi.nlm.nih.gov/23417879/

Smith, C. P., & Freyd, J. J. (2014). Institutional betrayal. *American Psychologist, 69*(6), 575–587. https://psycnet.apa.org/record/2014-36500-001

Smith, T. D., Balogun, A. O., Hughes, K., Dyal, M.-A., & DeJoy, D. M. (2024). Safety climate and seat belt use in the fire service. *Traffic Injury Prevention, 25*(8), 1055–1061. https://doi.org/10.1080/15389588.2024.2362834

Solomon, P. (2004). Peer support/peer provided services underlying processes, benefits, and critical ingredients. *Psychiatric Rehabilitation Journal, 27*(4), 392–401. https://pubmed.ncbi.nlm.nih.gov/15222150/

Sommerfeld, A., Wagner, S. L., Harder, H. G., & Schmidt, G. (2017). Behavioral health and firefighters: An intervention and interviews with Canadian firefighters. *Journal of Loss & Trauma, 22*(4), 307–324. https://psycnet.apa.org/record/2017-17463-004

Soner, O., Asan, U., & Celik, M. (2015). Use of HFACS–FCM in fire prevention modeling on board ships. *Safety Science, 77*(1), 25–41. https://www.sciencedirect.com/science/article/abs/pii/S092575351500065X?via%3Dihub

Souza, E. M. d. (2022). Can mothers be heroes? Maternity and maternal body work in military firefighters. *Journal of Contemporary Administration, 26*(Suppl 1), e210193. https://www.researchgate.net/publication/362583119_Can_Mothers_Be_Heroes_Maternity_and_Maternal_Body_Work_in_Military_Firefighters

Spector, P. E. (1988). Development of the work locus of control scale. *Journal of Occupational Psychology, 61*(4), 335–340. https://bpspsychub.onlinelibrary.wiley.com/doi/10.1111/j.2044-8325.1988.tb00470.x

Stack, S., & Tsoudis, O. (1997). Suicide risk among correctional officers: A logistic regression analysis. *Archives of Suicide Research, 3*(3), 183–186. https://link.springer.com/article/10.1023/A:1009677102357

Stajkovic, A. D., & Luthans, F. (2003). Behavioral management and task performance in organizations: Conceptual background, meta-analysis, and test of alternative models. *Personnel Psychology, 56*(1), 155–194. https://psycnet.apa.org/record/2003-02432-008

Stamatis, A., Papadakis, Z., & Beitia, P. (2024). Concurrent validity and interrater reliability assessment of two mental toughness instruments in firefighting: A two-wave longitudinal study. *Behavioral Sciences, 14*(7), 523. https://pubmed.ncbi.nlm.nih.gov/39062346/

Stanley, I. H., Hom, M. A., Hagan, C. R., & Joiner, T. E. (2015). Career prevalence and correlates of suicidal thoughts and behaviors among firefighters. *Journal of Affective Disorders, 187*, 163–171. https://doi.org/10.1016/j.jad.2015.08.007

Stanley, I. H., Boffa, J. W., Hom, M. A., Kimbrel, N. A., & Joiner, T. E. (2017). Differences in psychiatric symptoms and barriers to mental health care between volunteer and career firefighters. *Psychiatry Research, 247*, 236–242. https://pubmed.ncbi.nlm.nih.gov/27930964/

Stanley, I. H., Boffa, J. W., Hom, M. A., Stage, D. L., & Joiner, T. E. (2019a). PTSD symptoms and suicidal thoughts and behaviors among firefighters. *Journal of Psychiatric Research, 62*, 79–85. https://pubmed.ncbi.nlm.nih.gov/27810667/

Stanley, I. H., Hom, M. A., Chu, C., Dougherty, S. P., Gallyer, A. J., Spencer-Thomas, S., Shelef, L., Fruchter, E., Comtois, K. A., Gutierrez, P. M., Sachs-Ericsson, N. J., & Joiner, T. E. (2019b). Perceptions of belongingness and social support attenuate PTSD symptom severity among firefighters: A multistudy investigation. *Psychological Services, 16*(4), 543–555. https://pmc.ncbi.nlm.nih.gov/articles/PMC6163099/

Stanley, I. H., Hom, M. A., Gai, A. R., & Joiner, T. E. (2018). Wildland firefighters and suicide risk: Examining the role of social disconnectedness. *Psychiatry Research, 266*:269–274. https://pubmed.ncbi.nlm.nih.gov/29573853/

Stanley, I. H., Hom, M. A., Gallyer, A. J., Gray, J. S., & Joiner, T. E. (2020). Suicidal behaviors among American Indian/Alaska native firefighters: Evidence for the role of painful and provocative events. *Transcultural Psychiatry, 57*(2), 275–287. https://psycnet.apa.org/record/2020-33173-004

Stanley, I. H., Hom, M. A., Hagan, C. R., & Joiner, T. E. (2016a). Career prevalence and correlates of suicidal thoughts and behaviors among firefighters. *Journal of Affective Disorders, 187*, 163–171. https://pubmed.ncbi.nlm.nih.gov/26339926/

Stanley, I. H., Hom, M. A., & Joiner, T. E. (2016b). A systematic review of suicidal thoughts and behaviors among police officers, firefighters, EMTs, and paramedics. *Clinical Psychology Review, 44*, 25–44. https://doi.org/10.1016/j.cpr.2015.12.002

Stanley, I. H., Hom, M. A., Spencer-Thomas, S., & Joiner, T. E. (2017a). Examining anxiety sensitivity as a mediator of the association between PTSD symptoms and suicide risk among women firefighters. *Journal of Anxiety Disorders*, 5094–5102. https://pubmed.ncbi.nlm.nih.gov/28645017/

Stanley, I. H., Hom, M. A., Spencer-Thomas, S., & Joiner, T. E. (2017). Suicidal thoughts and behaviors among women firefighters: An examination of associated features and comparison of pre-career and career prevalence rates. Journal of affective disorders, 221, 107–114. https://pubmed.ncbi.nlm.nih.gov/28641147/

Stanley Abler v. Mayor & City Council of Baltimore, No. 22-1630 (4th Cir. Aug. 28, 2023) (unpublished). https://law.justia.com/cases/federal/appellate-courts/ca4/22-1630/22-1630-2023-08-28.html

Stanley, I. H., Lebeaut, A., Betz, M. E., Wright, A., & Vujanovic, A. A. (2024). Firearm ownership and storage practices among United States firefighters and emergency medical services personnel. *Psychological Services, 21*(2), 206–213. https://doi.org/10.1037/ser0000780

Stanley v. City of Sanford, 606 U.S. (2025). https://www.supremecourt.gov/opinions/24pdf/23-997_6579.pdf

Steinberg, L., & Vujanovic, A. A. (2024). The appearance of multidimensionality: Exploring the case for unidimensionality of the PTSD checklist for DSM-5 using a firefighter sample. *Psychological Assessment, 36*(3), 235–241. https://psycnet.apa.org/doiLanding?doi=10.1037%2Fpas0001300

Sterud, T., Ekeberg, O., & Hem, E. (2006). Health status in the ambulance services: A systematic review. *BMC Health Services Research, 6*, 82. https://doi.org/10.1186/1472-6963-6-82

Stinchcomb, J. B., & Ordaz, F. (2007). The integration of two "brotherhoods" into one organizational culture: A psycho-social perspective on merging police and fire and emergency services. *Public Organization Review, 7*, 143–161.

Stout, J. W., Beidel, D. C., Brush, D., & Bowers, C. (2021). Sleep disturbance and cognitive functioning among firefighters. *Journal of Health Psychology, 26*(12), 2248–2259. https://pubmed.ncbi.nlm.nih.gov/32126834/

Stout, R. A., & Kostamo, S. M. (2021). Burnout, compassion fatigue, and vicarious trauma among wildfire responders. *Journal of Ethnographic & Qualitative Research*, 16(1), 35–50. https://wmpllc.org/ojs/index.php/jem/article/view/3086

Substance Abuse and Mental Health Services Administration. (2014). Trauma-informed care in behavioral health services (TIP Series 57; HHS Publication No. SMA14-4816). U.S. Department of Health and Human Services. https://library.samhsa.gov/sites/default/files/sma14-4816.pdf

Substance Abuse and Mental Health Services Administration. (2022). Incorporating peer support into substance use disorder treatment services (TIP Series 64). https://archive.org/details/tip-64

Sue, S. (2006). Cultural competency: From philosophy to research and practice. *Journal of Community Psychology, 34*(2), 237–245. https://onlinelibrary.wiley.com/doi/abs/10.1002/jcop.20095

Sue, D. W., Arredondo, P., & McDavis, R. J. (1992). Multicultural counseling competencies and standards: A call to the profession. *Journal of Counseling & Development, 70*(4), 477–486. https://psycnet.apa.org/record/1992-25074-001

Sue, S., Zane, N., Nagayama Hall, G. C., & Berger, L. K. (2009). The case for cultural competency in psychotherapeutic interventions. *Annual Review of Psychology, 60*, 525–548. https://doi.org/10.1146/annurev.psych.60.110707.163651

Sue, S., Cheng, J. K. Y., Saad, C. S., & Chu, J. P. (2012). Asian American mental health: A call to action. *American Psychologist, 67*(7), 532–544. https://pubmed.ncbi.nlm.nih.gov/23046304/

Sussman, S., & Sussman, A. N. (2011). Considering the definition of addiction. *International Journal of Environmental Research and Public Health, 8*(10), 4025–4038. https://pubmed.ncbi.nlm.nih.gov/22073026/

Swann, W. B. Jr., Gómez, Á., Huici, C., Morales, J. F., & Hixon, J. (2012). Identity fusion: The interplay of personal and social identities in extreme group behavior. *Journal of Personality and Social Psychology, 96*(5), 995–1011. Retrieved from https://www.researchgate.net/publication/24309947_Identity_Fusion_The_Interplay_of_Personal_and_Social_Identities_in_Extreme_Group_Behavior

Tajfel, H., & Turner, J. C. (1979). An integrative theory of intergroup conflict. In W. G. Austin, & S. Worchel (Eds.), *The social psychology of intergroup relations* (pp. 33–47). Brooks/Cole.

Tamrakar, T., Langtry, J., Shevlin, M., Reid, T., & Murphy, J. (2020). Help-seeking behavior among UK firefighters: A latent class analysis. *European Journal of Psychotraumatology, 11*(1), 1721144. https://pubmed.ncbi.nlm.nih.gov/32158515/

Taylor, N. A., Peoples, G. E., & Petersen, S. R. (2016). Load carriage, human performance, and employment standards. *Applied Physiology, Nutrition, and Metabolism = Physiologie appliquee, nutrition et metabolisme, 41*(6 Suppl 2), S131–S147. https://doi.org/10.1139/apnm-2015-0486

Taylor, J. A., Lee, J., Shepler, L. J., Davis, A. L., Zohar, D., & Resick, C. R. (2019). Development and validation of the fire service safety climate scale. *Safety Science, 118*, 126–136. https://doi.org/10.1016/j.ssci.2019.05.007

Teoh, K. R. H., Lima, E., Vasconcelos, A., Nascimento, E., & Cox, T. (2019). Trauma and work factors as predictors of firefighters' psychiatric distress. *Occupational Medicine, 69*(8/9), 598–603. https://pubmed.ncbi.nlm.nih.gov/31960054/

Thapaliya, S., Sharma, P., & Upadhyaya, K. (2017). Suicide and self harm in Nepal: A scoping review. *Asian Journal of Psychiatry, 32*, 20–26. https://pubmed.ncbi.nlm.nih.gov/29202423/

Thayer, J. F., & Lane, R. D. (2000). A model of neurovisceral integration in emotion regulation and dysregulation. *Journal of Affective Disorders, 61*(3), 201–216. https://pubmed.ncbi.nlm.nih.gov/11163422/

The National WWII Museum. (n.d.). Our War Too: Women in Service. Retrieved from https://www.nationalww2museum.org/visit/exhibits/traveling-exhibits/our-war-too-women-service

The Philadelphia Contributionship. (n.d.). History. Retrieved from https://1752.com/about-us/history/

The White House. (2022, August 16). Bills signed: H.R. 2992, H.R. 5313, H.R. 6943, and S. 3451. https://bidenwhitehouse.archives.gov/briefing-room/legislation/2022/08/16/bills-signed-h-r-2992-h-r-5313-h-r-6943-and-s-3451/

Thoits, P. A. (2013). Self, identity, stress, and mental health. In C. S. Aneshensel, J. C. Phelan, & A. Bierman (Eds.), *Handbook of the sociology of mental health* (2nd ed., pp. 357–377). Springer. https://doi.org/10.1007/978-94-007-4276-5_18

Thurnell-Read, T., & Parker, A. (2008). Men, masculinities and firefighting: Occupational identity, shop-floor culture and organisational change. *Emotion, Space and Society, 1*(2), 127–134. https://doi.org/10.1016/j.emospa.2009.03.001

Tippett, J. B. (2007). Near-miss reporting: Sharing our lessons learned. *Fire Engineering, 160*(6), 105.

Tobia, M., Smith, D. L., Jahnke, S. A., & LeDuc, T. J. (2024). Occupational medical evaluations in the U.S. fire service: State of the art review [Presentation/PDF]. https://c36a7b585371cb8e876b-385db121fa2b55910fed97d2d3aaf4f8.ssl.cf1.rackcdn.com//2768752-950202-001.pdf

Tokar, D. M., Fischer, A. R., & Subich, L. M. (1998). Personality and vocational behavior: A selective review of the literature, 1993–1997. *Journal of Vocational Behavior, 53*(2), 115–153. https://doi.org/10.1006/jvbe.1998.1660

Tomaka, J., Magoc, D., Morales-Monks, S. M., & Reyes, A. C. (2017). Posttraumatic stress symptoms and alcohol-related outcomes among municipal firefighters. *Journal of Traumatic Stress, 30*(4), 416–424. https://pubmed.ncbi.nlm.nih.gov/28699663/

Traffic Safety. (n.d.) Washington, DC: U.S. Department of Defense. Retrieved from https://apps.dtic.mil/sti/pdfs/ADA291196.pdf

Truman, H. S. (1947). Fire prevention and control: A report on national fire safety. U.S. Government Printing Office. https://www.firehero.org/wp-content/uploads/2019/02/truman-report-1947.pdf

Turecki, G., & Brent, D. A. (2016). Suicide and suicidal behavior. *The Lancet, 387*(10024), 1227–1239. https://pubmed.ncbi.nlm.nih.gov/26385066/

Underwood, P., & Waterson, P. (2013). *Accident analysis models and methods: Guidance for safety professionals*. Loughborough University. Report. https://hdl.handle.net/2134/13865

U.S. Attorney's Manual. (n.d.) Washington, DC: U.S. Department of Justice. https://www.justice.gov/archives/usam/united-states-attorneys-manual

U.S. Census Bureau. (2021). The population and housing characteristics of the United States: 2020 Census brief (C2020BR-06). U.S. Department of Commerce. https://www2.census.gov/library/publications/decennial/2020/census-briefs/c2020br-06.pdf

U.S. Congress. (2003). S. 459 — Hometown heroes survivors benefits act of 2003, 108th Congress (2003–2004). Congress.gov. https://www.congress.gov/bill/108th-congress/senatebill/459

U.S. Department of Defense. (2021, August 27). *DoD motor vehicle and traffic safety (DoDI 6055.04)*. Office of the Under Secretary of Defense for Personnel and Readiness. https://www.esd.whs.mil/Portals/54/Documents/DD/issuances/dodi/605504p.pdf

U.S. Department of Justice. (2017, August 1). Department of Justice Policy on Seat Belt Use. https://www.justice.gov/archives/usam/eousa-resource-manual-154-department-justice-policy-seat-belt-use#:~:text=It%20is%20the%20policy%20of,the%20vehicle%20is%20in%20motion

U.S. Department of Justice. (n.d.). About the Department of Justice. U.S. Department of Justice. Retrieved November 21, 2024, from https://www.justice.gov/about

U.S. Department of Health and Human Services. (2001). *Report of a surgeon general's working meeting on the integration of mental health services and primary health care*. U.S. Department of Health and Human Services, Substance Abuse and Mental Health Services Administration. https://www.ncbi.nlm.nih.gov/books/NBK44335/

U.S. Department of Labor Wage & Hour Division. (2022, May). Fact Sheet #28O: Mental health conditions and the FMLA. https://www.dol.gov/agencies/whd/fact-sheets/28o-mental-health

U.S. Equal Employment Opportunity Commission. (2008, September 3). Applying performance and conduct standards to employees with disabilities. https://www.eeoc.gov/laws/guidance/applying-performance-and-conductstandards-employees-disabilities

U.S. Equal Employment Opportunity Commission. (2011). Regulations to implement the Equal Employment Provisions of the Americans with Disabilities Act, as amended (29 C.F.R. part 1630). (Final rule). https://www.ecfr.gov/current/title-29/subtitle-B/chapter-XIV/part-1630

U.S. Fire Administration. (2014). National Safety Culture Change Initiative: Changing the culture of the fire service. United States Fire Administration. https://www.usfa.fema.gov/downloads/pdf/publications/fa_342.pdf

U.S. Fire Administration. (2016). Risk management practices in the fire service. Federal Emergency Management Agency. https://www.usfa.fema.gov/downloads/pdf/publications/risk_management_practices.pdf

U.S. Fire Administration. (n.d.). *Emerging health and safety issues among women in the fire service [report]*. Federal Emergency Management Agency/U.S. Fire Administration. https://

www.usfa.fema.gov/downloads/pdf/publications/emerging_health_safety_issues_women_fire_service.pdf
U.S. Fire Administration. (2018). Vacant residential building fires (Topical Fire Report Series, Volume 18, Issue 9). U.S. Department of Homeland Security. https://www.usfa.fema.gov/downloads/pdf/statistics/v18i9.pdf
U.S. Fire Administration. (2022). Fire department overall run profile, 2020. *Topical Fire Report Series, 22*(2) Federal Emergency Management Agency. https://www.usfa.fema.gov/downloads/pdf/statistics/v22i2.pdf
U.S. Fire Administration. (2023). Firefighter fatalities in the United States in 2022 (2022 annual report). Federal Emergency Management Agency. Retrieved from https://www.usfa.fema.gov/downloads/pdf/publications/firefighter-fatalities-2022.pdf
U.S. Fire Administration. (2024). Behavioral health: 2024 U.S. Fire administrator's summit on fire prevention and control. https://www.usfa.fema.gov/downloads/pdf/summit/2024/2024-summit-workgroup-report.pdf
U.S. Fire Administration. (n.d.). About the U.S. Fire Administration. U.S. Department of Homeland Security. https://www.usfa.fema.gov/about/
U.S. Fire Administration (USFA). (2014). National Safety Culture Change Initiative. U.S. Department of Homeland Security https://www.usfa.fema.gov/downloads/pdf/publications/fa_342.pdf
U.S. Fire Administration (USFA). (2018). Vacant residential building fires (2013–2015). FEMA. https://www.usfa.fema.gov/downloads/pdf/statistics/v18i9.pdf
U.S. Fire Administration (USFA). (2022). Firefighter fatalities in the United States in 2022. Federal Emergency Management Agency (FEMA). Retrieved from https://www.usfa.fema.gov/downloads/pdf/publications/firefighter-fatalities-2022.pdf
United States Code. (1990). Americans with disabilities Act of 1990, 42 U.S.C. § 12113(b). https://uscode.house.gov
United States Fire Administration. (n.d.). About us. Federal Emergency Management Agency. https://www.usfa.fema.gov/
United States Special Operations Command (USSOCOM). (2017). Psychological Autopsy Study of Suicides among United States Special Operations Forces. https://www.socom.mil/FOIA/Documents/Psychological%20Autopsy%20Study%20of%20Suicides%20among%20United%20States%20Special%20Operations%20Forces.pdf
United States v. City of Durham, North Carolina, No. 1:24-cv-00838 (M.D.N.C. Oct. 7, 2024).
United States v. Giles, No. 40482 (A.F. Ct. Crim. App. Jan. 26, 2024).
United States v. City of New York, 637 F. Supp. 2d 77 (E.D.N.Y. 2010).
Ursano, R. J., Heeringa, S. G., Stein, M. B., Jain, S., & The Army STARRS Team. (2017). Risk factors associated with attempted suicide among US Army soldiers without a history of mental health diagnosis. *JAMA Psychiatry, 74*(6), 617–626. https://pubmed.ncbi.nlm.nih.gov/30167650/
Vaillancourt-Morel, M. P., Godbout, N., Labadie, C., Runtz, M., Lussier, Y., & Sabourin, S. (2019). Avoidant and compulsive sexual behaviors in male and female survivors of childhood sexual abuse. *Child Abuse & Neglect, 92*:116–127. https://pubmed.ncbi.nlm.nih.gov/25435106/
Valencia v. Haines City, No. 8:21-cv-1748-TPB-AAS, 2023 U.S. Dist. LEXIS 25026 (M.D. Fla. Feb. 14, 2023).
Van der Kolk, B. A. (2014). The body keeps the score: Brain, mind, and body in the healing of trauma. Viking.
Van Emmerik, A. A., Kamphuis, J. H., Hulsbosch, A. M., & Emmelkamp, P. M. (2002). Single session debriefing after psychological trauma: A meta-analysis. *Lancet, 360*(9335), 766–771. https://pubmed.ncbi.nlm.nih.gov/12241834/
Van Hasselt, V. B., Bourke, M. L., & Schuhmann, B. B. (2022). Firefighter stress and mental health: Introduction to the special issue. *Behavior Modification, 46*(2), 259–266. https://doi.org/10.1177/01454455211064955
van Schie, K., van den Hout, M. A., Engelhard, I. M., & van Oorsouw, K. (2025). Adverse effects of eye movement desensitization and reprocessing: A systematic review of random-

ized controlled trials. *Current Opinion in Psychology, 58*, 102155. https://doi.org/10.1016/j.copsyc.2025.102155
Vargas de Barros, V., Martins, L. F., Saitz, R., Bastos, R. R., & Ronzani, T. M. (2013). Mental health conditions, individual and job characteristics and sleep disturbances among firefighters. *Journal of Health Psychology, 18*(3), 350–358. https://pubmed.ncbi.nlm.nih.gov/22517948/
Varone, C. (2022, June 1). California firefighter files fourth race discrimination lawsuit. Fire Law Blog. https://www.firelawblog.com/2022/06/01/california-firefighter-files-fourth-race-discrimination-lawsuit/
Varone, C. (2022, May 9). California firefighter sues alleging race discrimination. Fire Law Blog. Retrieved from https://www.firelawblog.com/2022/05/09/california-firefighter-sues-alleging-race-discrimination
Varone, C. (2024, August 19). Los Angeles Fire Department (LAFD) Captain's Claims Reverse Discrimination. Fire Law Blog. Retrieved from https://www.firelawblog.com/2024/08/19/lafd-captain-claims-reverse-discrimination/
Varone, C. (2024, July 8). Rochester Settles Firefighter's Racism Suit. Fire Law Blog. Retrieved from https://www.firelawblog.com/2024/07/08/rochester-settles-firefighters-racism-suit/
Varone, C. (2024, November 13). Fired Colorado FireFighter Alleges Race and Gender Discrimination. Fire Law Blog. Retrieved from https://www.firelawblog.com/2024/11/13/fired-colorado-firefighter-alleges-race-and-gender-discrimination/
Varone, C. (2025, July 3). Court rules in favor of Chicago Fire applicant denied employment due to mental health history. Fire Law Blog. Retrieved from https://www.firelawblog.com/2025/07/03/court-rules-in-favor-of-chicago-fire-applicant-denied-employment-due-to-mental-health-history/
Vaughan, D. (1996). *The challenger launch decision: Risky technology, culture, and deviance at NASA*. University of Chicago Press.
Vaulerin, J., Colson, S. S., Emile, M., Scoffier-Mériaux, S., & d'Arripe-Longueville, F. (2016b). The big five personality traits and French Firefighter burnout: The mediating role of achievement goals. *Journal of Occupational and Environmental Medicine, 58*(4), e128–e132. https://pubmed.ncbi.nlm.nih.gov/27058490/
Vaulerin, J., d'Arripe-Longueville, F., Emile, M., Colson, S. S., & d'Arripe-Longueville, F. (2016a). Physical exercise and burnout facets predict injuries in a population-based sample of French career firefighters. *Applied Ergonomics, 54*, 131–135. https://pubmed.ncbi.nlm.nih.gov/26851472/
Vecchi, G. M., Van Hasselt, V. B., & Romano, S. J. (2005). Crisis (hostage) negotiation: Current strategies and issues. *Aggression and Violent Behavior, 10*(5), 533–551. https://doi.org/10.1016/j.avb.2004.10.001
Violanti, J. M., & Paton, D. (1999). *Police trauma: Psychological aftermath of civilian combat*. Charles C Thomas Publisher. https://psycnet.apa.org/record/1999-02836-000
Vissel, L. M., & Wells, R. (2017). *Health program planning and evaluation: A practical, systematic approach for community health* (4th ed.). Jones & Bartlett Learning.
Vivaldi, R. A., & Rose, S. E. (2024). A cross-cultural study of children's graphic representations of men- and women-dominated occupations. *British Journal of Developmental Psychology, 42*(4), 461–477. https://psycnet.apa.org/record/2024-99837-001
Vujanovic, A. A. (2023). Behavioral health in the fire service. International Society for Traumatic Stress Studies. https://istss.org/clinicians-corner-behavioral-health-in-the-fire-service-anka-a-vujanovic-phd/
Vulcan Society v. City of New York. (2012). Settlement agreement. NAACP Legal Defense Fund. https://www.naacpldf.org/case-issue/united-states-america-vulcan-society-inc-v-city-new-york/
Wagner, S. L., & Martin, C. A. (2012). Can firefighters' mental health be predicted by emotional intelligence and proactive coping? *Journal of Loss & Trauma, 17*(1), 56–72. https://psycnet.apa.org/record/2012-00190-005
Wagner, S. L., Martin, C. A., & McFee, J. A. (2009). Investigating the 'rescue personality'. *Traumatology, 15*(3), 5–12. https://psycnet.apa.org/record/2009-17906-002

Wagner, S. L., McFee, J. A., & Martin, C. A. (2010). Mental health implications of fire service membership. *Traumatology, 16*(2), 26–32. https://psycnet.apa.org/record/2010-13580-004

Wagner, S. L., & Pasca, R. (2022). Firefighters: Hostility and world assumptions. *Journal of Community Safety & Well-Being, 7*(4), 164–167. https://www.journalcswb.ca/index.php/cswb/article/view/205

Wagner, S. L., Pasca, R., & Regehr, C. (2019). Firefighters and empathy: Does it hurt to care too much? *Journal of Loss & Trauma, 24*(3), 238–250. https://psycnet.apa.org/record/2019-19882-001

Wagstaff, A. S., & Sigstad Lie, J. A. (2011). Shift and night work and long working hours—a systematic review of safety implications. *Scandinavian Journal of Work, Environment & Health, 37*(3), 173–185. https://pubmed.ncbi.nlm.nih.gov/21290083/

Walker, B. (2022). *Community risk reduction principles and practices*. Jones & Bartlett Learning.

Washington State Legislature. (2018). *Senate Bill 6214: Industrial insurance coverage for post-traumatic stress disorders of law enforcement and firefighters*. Washington State. Retrieved from https://app.leg.wa.gov/billsummary?BillNumber=6214&Year=2017

Watson v. City of Miami Beach, 177 F.3d 932 (11th Cir. 1999).

Weaver, M. D., Wang, H. E., Fairbanks, R. J., & Patterson, D. (2012). The association between EMS workplace safety culture and safety outcomes. *Prehospital Emergency Care, 16*(1), 43–52. https://pmc.ncbi.nlm.nih.gov/articles/PMC3533489/

Webb, R. A., & Chertok, J. (Producers). (1972–1977). Emergency! [TV series]. Universal Television.

Weger, H., Jr., Castle, G. R., & Emmett, M. C. (2010). Active listening in peer interviews: The influence of message paraphrasing on perceptions of listening skill. *International Journal of Listening, 24*(1), 34–49. https://doi.org/10.1080/10904010903466311

Wessel v. Wilmette Firefighters' Pension Fund, 2024 IL App (1st) 230565 (Ill. App. Ct. Feb. 9, 2024).

Wheldon, K., & Wolf, G. (2022). Psychological employment screening in the fire service: Reducing workplace risk through collaboration. *Fire Service Psychology Association Journal, 1*(1), 15–22. https://firepsychology.org/wp-content/uploads/2023/07/FIRE_PreemploymentScreening.pdf

White, M., & Epston, D. (1990). *Narrative means to therapeutic ends*. W. W. Norton & Company.

Whitman, M. R., Corey, D. M., & Ben-Porath, Y. S. (2023). Associations between MMPI-3 and psychosocial history findings obtained in pre employment evaluations of public safety candidates. *Assessment, 30*(7), 2128–2145. https://pubmed.ncbi.nlm.nih.gov/36510659/

Wickens, C. D., Hollands, J. G., Banbury, S., & Parasuraman, R. (2013). *Engineering psychology and human performance* (4th ed.). Pearson. https://isulibrary.isunet.edu/index.php?lvl=notice_display&id=8949

Wiegmann, D. A., & Shappell, S. A. (2003). *A human error approach to aviation accident analysis: The human factors analysis and classification system*. Ashgate. https://www.researchgate.net/publication/345694423_A_Human_Error_Approach_to_Aviation_Accident_Analysis_The_Human_Factors_Analysis_and_Classification_System

Wild, J., El-Salahi, S., Degli Esposti, M., & Thew, G. R. (2020). The effectiveness of interventions aimed at improving wellbeing and resilience to stress in first responders: A systematic review. *European Psychologist, 25*(4), 252–271. https://ora.ox.ac.uk/objects/uuid:9c49d3e0-97ce-4002-9e0b-ed1e2cdef3ae/download_file?safe_filename=WildetalAAM2020.pdf&type_of_work=Journal+article

Wilkie, T., Tajirian, T., & Stergiopoulos, V. (2022). Advancing physician wellness, engagement and excellence in a mental health setting: A Canadian perspective. *Health Promotion International, 37*(1), 1–8. https://pubmed.ncbi.nlm.nih.gov/33942064/

Williams, D. R., & Mohammed, S. A. (2009). Discrimination and racial disparities in health: Evidence and needed research. *Journal of Behavioral Medicine, 32*(1), 20–47. https://pubmed.ncbi.nlm.nih.gov/19030981/

Williamson, V., Murphy, D., & Greenberg, N. (2020). COVID-19 and experiences of moral injury in front-line key workers. *Occupational Medicine, 70*(5), 317–319. https://pmc.ncbi.nlm.nih.gov/articles/PMC7184422/

Wisco, B. E., Marx, B. P., Holowka, D. W., Vasterling, J. J., Han, S. C., Chen, M. S., Gradus, J. L., Nock, M. K., Rosen, R. C., & Keane, T. M. (2014). Traumatic brain injury, PTSD, and current suicidal ideation among Iraq and Afghanistan U.S. veterans. *Journal of Traumatic Stress, 27*(2), 244–248. https://pmc.ncbi.nlm.nih.gov/articles/PMC9040387/

Whybrow, D., Jones, N., & Greenberg, N. (2015). Promoting organizational well-being: A comprehensive review of trauma risk management. *Occupational medicine (Oxford, England), 65*(4), 331–336. https://doi.org/10.1093/occmed/kqv024

Whybrow, D., Jones, N., & Greenberg, N. (2015). A comprehensive review of trauma risk management (TRiM). *Occupational Medicine, 65*(4), 331–335. https://doi.org/10.1093/occmed/kqv074

Wójcik, M., & Siatkowski, I. (2023). The effect of cranial techniques on the heart rate variability response to psychological stress test in firefighter cadets. *Scientific Reports, 13*(1), 7780. https://pubmed.ncbi.nlm.nih.gov/37179419/

Wolffe, T. A. M., Clinton, A., Robinson, A., Turrell, L., & Stec, A. A. (2023a). Contamination of UK firefighters personal protective equipment and workplaces. *Scientific Reports, 13*(1), 65. https://pubmed.ncbi.nlm.nih.gov/36627304/

Wolffe, T. A. M., Turrell, L., Robinson, A., Dickens, K., Clinton, A., Maritan-Thomson, D., & Stec, A. A. (2023b). Culture and awareness of occupational health risks among UK firefighters. *Scientific Reports, 13*(1), 1–12. https://pubmed.ncbi.nlm.nih.gov/36627294/

Wolkow, A. P., Barger, L. K., O'Brien, C. S., Sullivan, J. P., Qadri, S., Lockley, S. W., Czeisler, C. A., & Rajaratnam, S. M. W. (2019). Associations between sleep disturbances, mental health outcomes and burnout in firefighters, and the mediating role of sleep during overnight work: A cross-sectional study. *Journal of Sleep Research, 28*(6), e12869. https://doi.org/10.1111/jsr.12869

Won, G. H., Lee, J. H., Choi, T. Y., Yoon, S., Kim, S. Y., & Park, J. H. (2020). The effect of a mental health promotion program on Korean firefighters. *International Journal of Social Psychiatry, 66*(7), 675–681. https://pubmed.ncbi.nlm.nih.gov/32500791/

Wong, Y. J., Ho, M. R., Wang, S. Y., & Miller, I. S. K. (2017). Meta-analyses of the relationship between conformity to masculine norms and mental health-related outcomes. *Journal of Counseling Psychology, 64*(1), 80–93. https://pubmed.ncbi.nlm.nih.gov/27869454/

Woodman, S., Bearman, C., & Hayes, P. (2021). Understanding skill decay and skill maintenance in first responders. *Australian Journal of Emergency Management*. Central Queensland University, Appleton Institute. https://knowledge.aidr.org.au/resources/ajem-October-2021-understanding-skill-decay-and-skill-maintenance-in-first-responders/

World Health Organization. (2023, October 13). *Burns: Fact Sheet*. https://www.who.int/news-room/fact-sheets/detail/burns

World Health Organization. (2019). International classification of diseases for mortality and morbidity statistics (11th revision). https://icd.who.int/en/

Wright, T. (2008). Lesbian firefighters: Shifting the boundaries between masculinity and femininity. *Journal of Lesbian Studies, 12*(1), 103–114. https://pubmed.ncbi.nlm.nih.gov/19042297/

Wu, B., Wang, J., Cai, H., Shen, Y., Qu, B., & Fu, Y. (2024). Research on the analysis method of production safety accidents based on accident event causal association diagram. *Mining, Metallurgy & Exploration, 1*(1), 1–14. https://www.researchgate.net/publication/384307882_Research_on_the_Analysis_Method_of_Production_Safety_Accidents_Based_on_Accident_Event_Causal_Association_Diagram

Yang, T., Jiang, X., & Cheng, H. (2022). Employee recognition, task performance, and OCB: Mediated and moderated by pride. *Sustainability, 14*(3), 1631. https://doi.org/10.3390/su14031631

Yellin, E. (2004). *Our Mothers' War: American women at home and at the front during World War II*. Free Press.

Yerkes, R. M. (Ed.). (1921). *Psychological examining in the U.S. Army: Memoirs of the National Academy of Sciences (Vol. 15)*. U.S. Government Printing Office.
Yoder, J. D., & Aniakudo, P. (1997). "Outsider within" the firehouse: Subordination and difference in the social interactions of African American women firefighters. *Gender & Society, 11*(3), 324–341. https://psycnet.apa.org/record/1997-06625-003
Yoder, J. D., & McDonald, T. W. (1998). Measuring sexist discrimination in the workplace: Support for the validity of the schedule of sexist events. *Psychology of Women Quarterly, 22*(3), 487–491. https://journals.sagepub.com/doi/10.1111/j.1471-6402.1998.tb00170.x
Young, P. M., Partington, S., Wetherell, M. A., Gibson, S. C., & A., & Partington, E. (2014). Stressors and coping strategies of UK firefighters during on-duty incidents. *Stress And Health: Journal Of The International Society For The Investigation Of Stress, 30*(5), 366–376. https://pubmed.ncbi.nlm.nih.gov/25312623/
Yu, Y., Fu, M., Yang, F., & Guo, J. (2023, April). The Relationship Between Effort-Reward Imbalance and Depressive Symptoms Among Chinese Firefighters: Moderating by Coping Styles. *Journal of Occupational and Environmental Medicine, 65*(4), 300–306. https://doi.org/10.1097/JOM.0000000000002739
Zarei, E. (2023). Advanced system engineering approaches to dynamic modeling of human factors and system safety in sociotechnical systems (Doctoral dissertation, Memorial University of Newfoundland). https://memorial.scholaris.ca/items/0c54b53d-d851-457a-8e94-6555f2861eac
Zegel, M., Leonard, S. J., McGrew, S. J., & Vujanovic, A. A. (2024). Firefighter relationship satisfaction: Associations with mental health outcomes. *American Journal of Family Therapy, 52*(4), 404–417. https://pubmed.ncbi.nlm.nih.gov/39184064/
Zhang, S., Jiang, J., Hao, L., Yu, Y., Zhang, Q., & Meng, H. (2023). What matters most? Network analysis of mental health, recovery experiences, sleep, and fatigue among career firefighters. *Stress & Health: Journal of the International Society for the Investigation of Stress, 39*(3), 663–672. https://pubmed.ncbi.nlm.nih.gov/36538510/
Zhang, Y., Jing, L., & Sun, C. (2018). Systems-based analysis of China-Tianjin port fire and explosion: A comparison of HFACS, AcciMap, and STAMP. *Journal of Failure Analysis and Prevention, 18(6),*1386–1400. https://www.researchgate.net/publication/327490983_Systems-Based_Analysis_of_China-Tianjin_Port_Fire_and_Explosion_A_Comparison_of_HFACS_AcciMap_and_STAMP
Zhang, J., Wieczorek, W., Conwell, Y., Tu, X. M., Wu, B. Y., Xiao, S., & Jia, C. (2010). Characteristics of young rural Chinese suicides: a psychological autopsy study. Psychological medicine, 40(4), 581–589. https://pubmed.ncbi.nlm.nih.gov/19656428/

Yerkes, R. M. (Ed.) (1921). *Psychological examining in the U.S. Army. Memoirs of the National Academy of Sciences* (vol. 15). U.S. Government Printing Office.

Yoder, J. D., & Aniakudo, P. (1997). "Outsider within" the firehouse: Subordination and difference in the social interactions of African American women firefighters. *Gender & Society, 11*(3), 324–341. [illegible]

[illegible]

Index

K. Wheldon, *Fire Service Psychology*,
https://doi.org/10.1007/978-3-032-02126-7

If you have any concerns about our products,
you can contact us on
ProductSafety@springernature.com

In case Publisher is established outside the EU,
the EU authorized representative is:
Springer Nature Customer Service Center GmbH
Europaplatz 3, 69115 Heidelberg, Germany

Printed by Libri Plureos GmbH
in Hamburg, Germany